Editorial Advisory Board

The Diabetes Carbohydrate and Fat Gram Guide

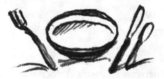

Quick, Easy Meal Planning Using Carbohydrate and Fat Gram Counts

Lea Ann Holzmeister, RD, CDE

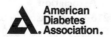

American Diabetes Association.

THE AMERICAN DIETETIC ASSOCIATION

Book Acquisitions: Susan Reynolds
Book Editor: Karen Lombardi Ingle
Production Coordinator: Peggy M. Rote
Production Manager: Carolyn R. Segree
Text design and typography: Harlowe Typography, Inc.
Cover design: Renée Boudreau

Library of Congress Cataloging-in-Publication Data

Holzmeister, Lea Ann.
    The diabetes carbohydrate and fat gram guide / by Lea
Ann Holzmeister.
        p.   cm.
    ISBN 0-945448-75-9 (pb)
    1. Diabetes—Diet therapy.   2. Food exchange lists.
    3. Food—Carbohydrate content—Tables.   4. Food—Fat
    content—Tables.
    I. Title.
    RC662.H66   1997
    616.4'620654—dc21   97-19169
                                                    CIP

Printed in the United States of America

American Diabetes   **The American Dietetic**
  Association   **Association**
1660 Duke Street   216 West Jackson Boulevard
Alexandria, Virginia 22314   Chicago, Illinois 60606

Dedication

To Jeff, Erin, Adam, and Emily

Acknowledgments

Thanks to Richard Ziriax for his expert technical support and collaboration.

Thanks to Madelyn L. Wheeler, MS, RD, FADA, CDE and Patti Bazel Geil, MS, RD, CDE for their valuable review comments.

Contents

Introduction

Since its discovery hundreds of years ago, diabetes has been linked with what people eat. What people with diabetes are advised to eat and how they plan their meals has changed over the years. The latest American Diabetes Association (ADA) *Nutrition Recommendations and Principles for People With Diabetes Mellitus* (published each year in January as Supplement 1 of the journal *Diabetes Care*) emphasizes individuality and flexibility, which are essential for helping people with diabetes follow a healthy eating plan.

Many people with diabetes use some type of meal planning system to help them meet their individual nutrition goals. Just as there is no one diet that is right for everyone with diabetes, there is also no one meal planning approach that meets everyone's needs.

It is important to know your own nutrition goals. A registered dietitian (RD) can help you determine your individual nutrition goals and develop a meal plan based on your food preferences, lifestyle, blood glucose and blood lipid (fat) levels, overall health, and abilities. Your doctor may be able to recommend a dietitian. Or call The American Dietetic Association at 1-800-366-1655 for a referral to a local dietitian.

Types of Meal Planning Approaches

Four types of meal planning approaches are described in this book: carbohydrate counting, fat gram counting, food exchange system, and calorie counting. The advantages and disadvantages of each are discussed, and information about where to learn more is provided.

It is important to select a meal planning approach that you are comfortable using and that will work toward achieving your goals. You do not have to use the same approach your entire life. As your individual nutrition goals change, so may your meal planning approach. Before switching though, it is a good idea to consult with your dietitian.

Carbohydrate Counting

Carbohydrate counting has been used for many years in Europe and is becoming increasingly popular in the United States. The three main nutrients in the foods we eat are carbohydrate, protein, and fat. The carbohydrate in foods affects your blood glucose level more than protein or fat. In carbohydrate counting, you count only carbohydrate.

To use carbohydrate counting, you must know your total carbohydrate allotment for the day. Your dietitian can help you determine this. Together, you and your dietitian will make a carbohydrate counting meal plan based on your usual food intake, lifestyle, diabetes medications, and physical activity. Once you have your carbohydrate counting meal plan, you'll need to become familiar with the carbohydrate content in foods. Carbohydrate is found in many foods, such as grains, vegetables, fruits, milk, and table sugar. It is important to count all carbohydrate regardless of its source.

The two main types of carbohydrate are sugars and starches. According to ADA's nutrition recommendations, it is more important to eat the same amount of carbohydrate at meals and snacks each day than to focus on the type of carbohydrate eaten. Research has shown that sugars do not raise blood glucose any more than starches. This means that you can eat foods that contain sugar as long as you count them as part of your total carbohydrate allotment for the day. Keep in mind that foods high in sugar are often high in fat and calories and low in vitamins and minerals, so they contribute little to the overall healthfulness of your diet.

Carbohydrate counting can provide some advantages over other meal planning approaches. Some people feel that focusing on only one nutrient makes this system easier. With the focus on carbohydrate, food and insulin can be matched more precisely. Matching food and insulin increases flexibility in meal and snack times. This can be particularly helpful when your appetite varies or your schedule changes. Also, insulin can be matched to carbohydrate eaten at specific times during the day. For example, some people need more insulin at breakfast for each gram of carbohydrate eaten. Thus, carbohydrate counting may be most appropriate for people with type 1 diabetes who take insulin.

One disadvantage of carbohydrate counting is that when you focus only on carbohydrate, it is easy to lose sight of the overall nutritional quality of foods. For example, counting the carbohydrate in ice cream but ignoring its fat content may lead you to eat it more often. Too much fat in the diet increases your risk of heart disease, cancer, and weight gain. If you pay no attention to the overall nutritional quality of foods, you may end up eating a diet that is too high in fat or protein.

To learn more about carbohydrate counting, contact your dietitian. The American Diabetes Association and The American Dietetic Association have jointly published three instructional booklets on carbohydrate counting: *Carbohydrate Counting: Getting Started, Carbohydrate Counting: Moving On,* and *Carbohydrate Counting: Using Carbohydrate/Insulin Ratios.* You can obtain these booklets from your dietitian.

Fat Gram Counting

Fat gram counting has been around since the 1980s, when it was introduced as a tool to teach low-fat eating to reduce the risk of cancer. Since that time, it has also been used for teaching heart-healthy eating for heart disease and reduced-calorie eating for weight reduction. Fat gram counting may be particularly useful for people with type 2 diabetes who are overweight. Fat provides two and a half times as many calories per gram as carbohydrate or protein.

The first step in using fat gram counting is to establish a daily calorie requirement based on your height, weight, activity level, and weight goal. Your dietitian can help you determine this. Then, based on your nutrition goals, a daily fat gram goal will be determined. In fat gram counting, you keep a record of the foods you eat and their fat content.

There are some advantages to fat gram counting. It is simple, and it allows a considerable amount of flexibility and control over your food choices. With fat gram counting, you will usually improve the overall quality of your food choices, because you will tend to select lower fat foods, such as fruits, vegetables, grains, and low-fat dairy products. Like carbohydrate counting, you are focusing on only one nutrient. This can be especially appealing when weight loss is the primary goal and other approaches have not worked.

One disadvantage of fat gram counting is that it does not take into consideration foods that may affect your blood glucose. Therefore, your blood glucose values may be inconsistent.

To learn more about fat gram counting, contact your dietitian. Your local American Heart Association may also have additional information on fat gram counting programs.

Food Exchange System

For many years, the food exchange system has been used as a meal planning approach for people with diabetes, regardless of the type of diabetes and how it is treated. This system groups foods with similar nutritional value into lists with the goal of helping people with diabetes eat consistent amounts of nutrients. Each food has approximately the same number of calories, carbohydrate, protein, and fat as the other foods on the same list. Any food on a list can be traded or "exchanged" for any other food on the same list.

To use the exchange system, you need an individualized meal plan that tells you how many exchanges from each list to select for meals and snacks. Your dietitian can help you design your individualized meal plan and teach you how to use this system.

The American Diabetes Association and The American Dietetic Association's *Exchange Lists for Meal Planning* booklet groups food into three broad groups: the carbohydrate group, the meat and meat substitutes group, and the fat group.

The carbohydrate group includes five lists: the starch list, the fruit list, the milk list, the other carbohydrates list, and the vegetable list. The meat and meat substitutes group includes four lists: the very lean list, the lean list, the medium-fat list, and the high-fat list. The fat group includes a monounsaturated fats list, a polyunsaturated fats list, and a saturated fats list. In addition to these lists, there is a free foods list, a combination foods list, and a fast foods list.

One advantage of the food exchange system is its emphasis on more than one nutrient and the importance of the overall nutritional content of foods. This system also encourages consistency in the timing and amount of your meals and snacks.

People desiring to lose weight might find this approach useful for learning the caloric and fat values of foods. Food exchanges can also be used as a reference for those using carbohydrate counting. Each serving of a food in the carbohydrate group counts as 15 grams of carbohydrate.

One disadvantage of this system is the level of understanding needed to grasp the concept of "exchanging" foods. It also requires learning where a food that is not listed fits. To learn more about the food exchange system for meal planning, contact your dietitian.

Calorie Counting

Calorie counting has been used for many years as a way to achieve weight loss, weight gain, or weight maintenance. This approach is most appropriate for people who are overweight and do not take insulin. Even modest weight loss improves blood glucose levels.

To use calorie counting, you and your dietitian establish a calorie goal that will help you achieve your weight goal. Your weight goal will be based on your current weight, height, and activity level. If you desire to lose weight, your calorie goal will be set lower than your usual intake of calories. If you wish to maintain your current weight, your calorie goal will be set at a calorie level similar to your current intake of calories.

You keep records of the foods you eat and their calorie content. A periodic comparison of your food records and weekly weight can give you feedback on how you are progressing toward your weight goal. These records can also help you identify problem areas. For example, you might realize after reviewing your records that you tend to overeat when away from home. Knowing this information will help you and your dietitian develop strategies for changing this behavior.

The main advantage of calorie counting is the expanded choice of foods, which gives you more flexibility in what you eat. You decide whether and how a food might fit into your meal plan. For example, say your daily calorie goal is 1,500 calories, and a food you want to eat contains 600 calories. You can eat that food as long as you plan what other foods you'll eat that day to add up to the remaining 900 calories. Your serving size, too, is based on how you want to "spend" your calories. You might decide you can work in only half a serving of pasta salad, or you might choose to have a double serving of pasta salad.

One disadvantage of calorie counting might be the amount of time involved in keeping records and calculating the calorie content of foods. Also, because this approach does not guide you toward making nutritionally balanced choices, you may end up with a high-fat diet or one low in essential vitamins and minerals. Your dietitian can provide you with basic nutrition guidelines by which to select your foods to ensure that you meet your nutrition goals as well.

Estimating Serving Sizes

The success of any meal planning approach depends on how accurately you estimate your serving sizes. Therefore, it is essential to train your eyes to do this. Equip your kitchen with measuring spoons, measuring cups, and a food scale. Use these tools to measure and weigh foods consistently for 2 weeks or until you have trained your eyes to recognize what a cup of pasta looks like on your plate or where a cup of milk fills your favorite glass.

Without some practice, it is surprisingly easy to mistakenly pour yourself one cup instead of a half cup of juice. A cup of juice has twice the carbohydrate and calories as a half cup of juice. This might tip you over your calorie or carbohydrate goal. If you did this with two to three foods each day, it could spoil your efforts at weight loss and blood glucose control.

Of course, it is not practical to measure servings when you eat out in a restaurant, but training your eyes will help. Fortunately, the serving sizes of fast foods are fairly standardized among restaurants, i.e., a taco at any Taco Bell restaurant is likely to be the same size.

How Food Counts Can Work For You

The meal planning approach you select will determine what you will "count" in your diet. But using a meal planning approach to guide your food choices is only a starting point. To reach your individual goals (e.g., blood glucose, blood lipids, weight, general health), you need to respond every day to blood glucose changes and periodically to other indicators of your progress (e.g., blood lipid levels, weight gain or loss).

Food Counts and Blood Glucose

Making the connection between what you eat and how it affects your blood glucose level can be a very powerful step toward achieving your blood glucose goals. Once you have recorded your food intake and blood glucose values, you can learn to analyze the data to see how individual foods and meals affect your blood glucose. You can then try adjusting food intake, physical activity, and diabetes medications.

Food Counts and Blood Lipids

Counting total fat and saturated fat in your diet while keeping tabs on your blood lipid levels (total cholesterol, HDL [high-density lipoprotein] cholesterol, LDL [low-density lipoprotein] cholesterol, and triglycerides) allows you to determine whether your meal plan is helping you to achieve your blood lipid goals. Suppose you have been advised to follow a diet with less than 70 grams of fat and less than 25 grams of saturated fat per day in an attempt to reduce your total cholesterol from 250 to 200 mg/dl. By comparing your food records of fat and saturated fat intake to your blood lipid levels over time, you can determine how close you are coming to your blood lipid goals.

Using This Book of Food Counts

This book is intended to be a comprehensive listing of both generic and brand name foods that are available nationally. The nutrition information comes from several sources, including the Food Processor, a nutrient analysis software program from ESHA Research in Salem, Oregon; the American Diabetes Association and The American Dietetic Association's *Exchange Lists for Meal Planning* nutrient database; a variety of food-processing companies, fast-food franchises, and Nutrition Facts from food labels.

Foods are listed alphabetically by food category. Nutrient information for foods from mixes (e.g., puddings and cakes) reflect values after the food has been prepared according to package directions.

This book lists the calories, carbohydrate, fat, saturated fat, and sodium of many foods. These particular nutrients were selected because they are the most commonly monitored by people with diabetes (see Table 1).

The nutrient values you use will depend on your meal planning approach. You may need one, two, or even more of the values to figure out how a food fits in your plan.

Values have been rounded to the nearest calorie, gram (g), or milligram (mg) per serving (a gram is a unit of mass and weight in the metric system; an ounce is about 30 grams). The serving sizes listed in this book are those most commonly used. Similar foods will have the same serving

TABLE 1. American Diabetes Association Nutrient Recommendations

Calories: Most adults require 1,800 to 2,500 calories per day. However, your calorie needs are best determined by your dietitian.

Carbohydrate: Carbohydrates raise your blood glucose level. You might get 50% or more of your daily calories from carbohydrates. Your dietitian can help you determine how much carbohydrate you need in a day.

Fat: Fat contributes to weight gain. Most people need no more than 30% of their daily calories from fat. People who are over-weight are advised to get no more than 20 to 25% of their daily calories from fat.

Saturated Fat: Saturated fat can raise your blood cholesterol level. Most people should get no more than 10% of their daily calories from saturated fat. People with high LDL cholesterol levels are advised to get less than 7% of their daily calories from saturated fat.

Sodium: Sodium has been linked to high blood pressure (hypertension). People with normal blood pressure should get no more than 2,400 to 3,000 milligrams of sodium per day. People with moderately high blood pressure are advised to get 2,400 milligrams or less of sodium per day, and people with high blood pressure and kidney disease are advised to get 2,000 milligrams or less of sodium per day.

sizes. The serving size may be very different from the amount you serve yourself or eat. If your serving size is different, ask your dietitian to help you recalculate the numbers.

The exchange values of foods have been calculated using the "rounding off method" (Wheeler ML, Franz M, Barrier PH, Holler H, Cronmiller N, Delahanty LM: Macronutrient and energy database for the 1995 Exchange Lists for Meal Planning: A rationale for clinical practice decisions. *J Am Diet Assoc* 96:1167–1170, 1996). Table 2 shows the amount of nutrients in one serving from each list.

Some of the foods in this book have a nutrient claim, such as "reduced-fat" or "low-calorie," as part of their name. These claims have standard meanings set by the Food and Drug Administration (FDA). Some of these terms and their meanings are listed in Table 3.

TABLE 2. Nutrient Content of Exchange Lists

Groups/Lists	Carb. (g)	Prot. (g)	Fat (g)	Cal.
Carbohydrate Group				
Starch List	15	3	1 or less	80
Fruit List	15	0	0	60
Milk List				
Skim/Low-Fat	12	8	0–3	90
Reduced-Fat	12	8	5	120
Whole	12	8	8	150
Other Carbohydrates List	15	varies	varies	varies
Vegetable List	5	2	0	25
Meat and Meat Substitutes Group				
Very Lean List	0	7	0–1	35
Lean List	0	7	3	55
Medium-Fat List	0	7	5	75
High-Fat List	0	7	8	100
Fat Group				
Monounsaturated Fats List	0	0	5	45
Polyunsaturated Fats List	0	0	5	45
Saturated Fats List	0	0	5	45
Free Foods List	5 or less	varies	varies	less than 20
Combination Foods List	varies	varies	varies	varies
Fast Foods List	varies	varies	varies	varies

Adapted from the American Diabetes Association and The American Dietetic Association: *Exchange Lists for Meal Planning*. Alexandria, VA, 1995, p. 3.

TABLE 3. Nutrient Claims on Food Labels

Term	Meaning
Calorie-Free	Less than 5 calories per serving
Cholesterol-Free	Less than 2 mg of cholesterol per serving and 2 g or less of saturated fat per serving
Extra Lean	Less than 5 g of fat, 2 g of saturated fat, and 95 mg of cholesterol per serving
Fat-Free	Less than 0.5 g of fat per serving
Lean	Less than 10 g of fat, 4.5 g of saturated fat, and 95 mg of cholesterol per serving
Light or Lite	33.3% fewer calories or 50% less fat per serving than comparison food
Low-Calorie	40 calories or less per serving
Low-Cholesterol	20 mg or less of cholesterol per serving and 2 g or less of saturated fat per serving
Low-Fat	3 g or less of fat per serving
Low-Saturated Fat	1 g or less of saturated fat per serving and 15% or less of calories from saturated fat
Low-Sodium	140 mg or less of sodium per serving
Reduced	25% less per serving than comparison food
Saturated Fat-free	Less than 0.5 g of saturated fat per serving
Sodium-Free	Less than 5 mg of sodium per serving
Sugar-Free	Less than 0.5 g of sugar per serving

APPETIZERS AND DIPS

Products	Cal.	Carb. (g)	Fat (g)	Sat. Fat (g)	Sodium (mg)	Exchanges
Dip, Jalapeño Pepper Bean (2 Tbsp)	46	6	2	<1	382	1/2 strch
Mushrooms, Stuffed w/Meat (2)	113	8	7	2	279	1/2 carb., 1 fat
BREAKSTONE						
Dip, Bacon & Onion Sour Cream (2 Tbsp)	60	2	5	3	170	1 fat
Dip, French Onion Sour Cream (2 Tbsp)	50	2	4	3	160	1 fat
Dip, Jalapeño Cheddar Sour Cream (2 Tbsp)	60	2	4	3	170	1 fat
Dip, Toasted Onion Sour Cream (2 Tbsp)	50	2	4	3	180	1 fat
CHUN KING						
Egg Rolls, Chicken (1)	170	25	5	3	450	1-1/2 carb., 1 fat
Egg Rolls, Pork (1)	170	23	6	2	390	1-1/2 carb., 1 fat
Egg Rolls, Shrimp (1)	150	24	4	<1	420	1-1/2 carb., 1 fat
Mini Egg Rolls, Chicken (6)	200	29	7	2	255	2 carb., 1 fat

APPETIZERS AND DIPS

Products	Cal.	Carb. (g)	Fat (g)	Sat. Fat (g)	Sodium (mg)	Exchanges
Mini Egg Rolls, Pork & Shrimp (6)	210	28	8	2	250	2 carb., 1 fat
Mini Egg Rolls, Shrimp (6)	185	29	6	1	350	2 carb., 1 fat
FRITO-LAY						
Dip, French Onion (2 Tbsp)	60	4	5	3	230	1 fat
Dip, Hot Bean (2 Tbsp)	35	5	1	0	220	1/2 strch
Dip, Jalapeño & Cheddar Cheese (2 Tbsp)	50	3	3	1	280	1 fat
Dip, Jalapeño Bean (2 Tbsp)	40	6	1	<1	140	1/2 strch
Dip, Mild Cheddar Cheese (2 Tbsp)	50	4	3	1	240	1 fat
FRITOS						
Dip, Chili Cheese (2 Tbsp)	45	3	3	1	310	1 fat
KNUDSEN						
Dip, Premium Bacon & Onion Sour Cream (2 Tbsp)	60	2	5	3	170	1 fat
Dip, Premium French Onion Sour Cream (2 Tbsp)	50	2	4	3	160	1 fat
Dip, Premium Nacho Cheese Sour Cream (2 Tbsp)	60	3	4	3	200	1 fat

KRAFT

Dip, Avocado (2 Tbsp)	60	4	4	3	240	1 fat
Dip, Bacon & Horseradish (2 Tbsp)	60	3	5	3	220	1 fat
Dip, Clam (2 Tbsp)	60	3	4	3	250	1 fat
Dip, French Onion (2 Tbsp)	60	4	4	3	230	1 fat
Dip, Green Onion (2 Tbsp)	60	4	4	3	190	1 fat
Dip, Jalapeño (2 Tbsp)	60	3	4	3	260	1 fat
Dip, Premium Bacon & Horseradish (2 Tbsp)	50	2	5	3	200	1 fat
Dip, Premium Bacon & Onion (2 Tbsp)	60	2	5	3	160	1 fat
Dip, Premium Blue Cheese (2 Tbsp)	45	2	4	3	200	1 fat
Dip, Premium Clam (2 Tbsp)	45	2	4	3	210	1 fat
Dip, Premium Creamy Cucumber (2 Tbsp)	50	2	4	3	140	1 fat
Dip, Premium Creamy Onion (2 Tbsp)	45	2	4	3	160	1 fat
Dip, Premium French Onion (2 Tbsp)	50	2	4	3	160	1 fat
Dip, Premium Jalapeño Cheese (2 Tbsp)	60	1	5	3	250	1 fat
Dip, Ranch (2 Tbsp)	60	3	4	3	210	1 fat

APPETIZERS AND DIPS

Products	Cal.	Carb. (g)	Fat (g)	Sat. Fat (g)	Sodium (mg)	Exchanges
LA CHOY						
Egg Rolls, Chicken (1)	170	25	5	3	450	1-1/2 carb., 1 fat
Egg Rolls, Moo Shu (1)	190	25	7	2	330	1-1/2 carb., 1 fat
Egg Rolls, Pork (1)	170	23	6	2	390	1-1/2 carb., 1 fat
Egg Rolls, Shrimp (1)	150	24	4	<1	420	1-1/2 carb., 1 fat
Egg Rolls, Sweet & Sour Chicken (1)	180	29	4	1	300	2 carb., 1 fat
Mini Egg Rolls, Chicken (7)	215	34	6	2	450	2 carb., 1 fat
Mini Egg Rolls, Chinese-Style Vegetables w/Lobster (7)	205	33	6	2	345	2 carb., 1 fat
Mini Egg Rolls, Pork & Shrimp (7)	215	33	6	2	445	2 carb., 1 fat
Mini Egg Rolls, Shrimp (7)	205	34	5	1	495	2 carb., 1 fat
LAY'S						
Dip, Low-Fat Sour Cream & Onion (2 Tbsp)	40	6	1	0	230	1/2 carb.

MARIE'S

Dip, Bacon Ranch (2 Tbsp)	150	3	16	2	200	3 fat
Dip, Fiesta Bean (2 Tbsp)	140	2	14	2	160	3 fat
Dip, Homestyle Ranch (2 Tbsp)	150	3	15	2	140	3 fat
Dip, Parmesan Garlic (2 Tbsp)	140	2	14	2	140	3 fat
Dip, Premium Nacho Cheese (2 Tbsp)	60	2	5	3	270	1 fat
Dip, Spinach (2 Tbsp)	140	3	14	2	200	3 fat
Dip, Sun-Dried Tomato (2 Tbsp)	140	2	14	2	135	3 fat

OLD EL PASO

Dip, Black Bean (2 Tbsp)	20	4	0	0	150	free
Dip, Cheese 'n Salsa, Mild/Medium (2 Tbsp)	40	3	3	1	300	1 fat
Dip, Chunky Salsa, Mild/Medium (2 Tbsp)	15	3	0	0	230	free
Dip, Jalapeño (2 Tbsp)	30	4	1	0	125	free

PROGRESSO

Artichoke Hearts (2)	35	6	0	0	240	1 vegetable
Cherry Peppers, Drained (2 Tbsp)	30	2	2	0	30	1 vegetable

APPETIZERS AND DIPS

Products	Cal.	Carb. (g)	Fat (g)	Sat. Fat (g)	Sodium (mg)	Exchanges
Eggplant Appetizer (2 Tbsp)	30	2	2	0	130	1 vegetable
Fried Peppers, Drained (2 Tbsp)	60	3	5	<1	60	1 fat
Hot Cherry Peppers (1)	15	3	0	0	250	free
Olive Salad, Drained (2 Tbsp)	25	1	3	0	360	1 fat
Olives, Oil-Cured (6)	80	3	6	<1	330	1 fat
Pepper Salad, Drained (2 Tbsp)	25	1	2	0	80	1/2 fat
Peppers, Roasted (1/2)	10	1	0	0	60	free
Tuscan Peppers, Drained (3)	10	1	0	0	330	free
TOSTITOS						
Con Queso, Low-Fat (2 Tbsp)	40	5	2	1	280	carb.
Con Queso, Salsa (2 Tbsp)	40	5	2	<1	650	1/2 carb.
Dip, Black Bean (2 Tbsp)	0	5	0	0	190	free
Salsa, Mild/Medium/Hot (2 Tbsp)	15	3	0	0	230	free

BEVERAGES

Products	Cal.	Carb. (g)	Fat (g)	Sat. Fat (g)	Sodium (mg)	Exchanges
Beer, Alcoholic Beverage (12 oz)	146	13	0	0	18	3 fat
Beer, Light (12 oz)	99	5	0	0	11	2 fat
Club Soda (12 oz)	0	0	0	0	75	free
Coffee, Brewed (8 oz)	5	<1	<1	<1	5	free
Coffee, Cappuccino Mix & Water (6 oz)	61	11	2	2	104	1 carb.
Coffee, Demitasse (8 oz)	5	<1	0	<1	5	free
Coffee, Espresso (8 oz)	5	<1	0	<1	5	free
Coffee, Instant, Prepared (8 oz)	5	<1	<1	<1	7	free
Cola-Type Soda (12 oz)	152	39	<1	<1	15	2-1/2 carb.
Cream Soda (12 oz)	189	49	0	0	45	3 carb.
Diet Cola/Coke w/Aspartame (12 oz)	4	<1	0	0	21	free
Fruit Drink Powder & Water, Low-Calorie (8 oz)	43	11	0	0	50	1/2 carb.

BEVERAGES

Products	Cal.	Carb. (g)	Fat (g)	Sat. Fat (g)	Sodium (mg)	Exchanges
Fruit Punch Drink, Canned (8 oz)	119	30	<1	<1	56	2 carb.
Ginger Ale (12 oz)	124	32	0	0	26	2 carb.
Grape Soda (12 oz)	160	42	0	0	56	3 carb.
Lemon-Lime Soda (12 oz)	147	38	0	0	41	2-1/2 carb.
Lemonade, Frozen Concentrate & Water (8 oz)	99	26	<1	<1	7	2 carb.
Orange Soda (12 oz)	179	46	0	0	45	3 carb.
Root Beer (12 oz)	152	39	0	0	48	2-1/2 carb.
Tea, Brewed (8 oz)	2	<1	<1	<1	7	free
Tonic Water, Sugar-Free (12 oz)	0	<1	0	0	57	free
Tonic Water/Quinine Water (12 oz)	124	32	0	0	15	2 carb.
Wine, Dry Dessert (4 oz)	149	5	0	0	11	1 fat
Wine, Medium White (4 oz)	80	<1	0	0	6	2 fat
Wine, Nonalcoholic, Light or Regular (8 oz)	15	3	0	0	18	free
Wine, Red (4 oz)	85	2	0	0	6	2 fat

ALL SPORT

Lemon-Lime (8 oz)	70	20	0	0	55	1 carb.
Lemon-Lime, Lite (8 oz)	0	0	0	0	55	free
Orange (8 oz)	70	20	0	0	55	1 carb.
Orange, Lite (8 oz)	0	1	0	0	55	free

CAPRI SUN

Natural Juice Drink, Naui Punch (9.6 oz)	109	28	0	0	20	2 carb.
Natural Juice Drink, Orange (9.6 oz)	100	26	0	0	25	2 carb.
Natural Juice Drink, Pacific Cooler (9.6 oz)	110	29	0	0	20	2 carb.
Natural Juice Drink, Red Berry (9.6 oz)	100	28	0	0	20	2 carb.
Natural Juice Drink, Safari Punch (9.6 oz)	100	25	0	0	20	2 carb.
Natural Juice Drink, Strawberry Cool (9.6 oz)	100	26	0	0	20	2 carb.
Natural Juice Drink, Wild Cherry (9.6 oz)	110	30	0	0	20	2 carb.
Natural Juice Drink, YoYogi Berry (9.6 oz)	100	27	0	0	20	2 carb.

COCA-COLA

Cherry Coke (8 oz)	104	28	0	0	4	2 carb.

BEVERAGES

Products	Cal.	Carb. (g)	Fat (g)	Sat. Fat (g)	Sodium (mg)	Exchanges
Coca-Cola Classic (8 oz)	97	27	0	0	9	2 carb.
Diet Coke (8 oz)	1	<1	0	0	4	free
Fresca (8 oz)	3	<1	0	0	1	free
Minute-Maid Orange (8 oz)	118	32	0	0	0	2 carb.
Sprite (8 oz)	96	26	0	0	23	2 carb.
TAB (8 oz)	<1	<1	0	0	4	free
COUNTRY TIME						
Iced Tea Drink w/Sugar (8 oz)	70	17	0	0	0	1 carb.
Lemonade, Powder & Water (8 oz)	103	27	<1	0	13	2 carb.
Lemonade Drink w/Sugar (8 oz)	70	17	0	0	15	1 carb.
Lemonade Drink, Sugar-Free, Low-Calorie (8 oz)	5	0	0	0	0	free
CRYSTAL LIGHT						
Cranberry Breeze Drink (8 oz)	5	0	0	0	0	free
Iced Tea Drink (8 oz)	5	0	0	0	0	free

Lemonade Drink, Low-Calorie (8 oz)	5	0	0	0	0	free
FRUITOPIA						
Apple Raspberry Embrace (8 oz)	75	19	0	0	24	1 carb.
Born Raspberry Iced Tea (8 oz)	81	22	0	0	<1	1-1/2 carb.
Fruit Integration (8 oz)	125	31	0	0	26	2 carb.
Lemonade Love & Hope (8 oz)	113	28	0	0	26	2 carb.
Strawberry Passion Awareness (8 oz)	124	31	0	0	30	2 carb.
GATORADE						
Sports Drink (8 oz)	60	15	0	0	96	1 carb.
GENERAL FOODS						
Coffee, International Café Amaretto (8 oz)	60	8	3	<1	105	1/2 carb., 1/2 fat
Coffee, International Café Francais (8 oz)	60	7	4	1	25	1/2 carb., 1 fat
Coffee, International Café French Vanilla (8 oz)	60	10	3	<1	55	1/2 carb., 1/2 fat
Coffee, International Café Hazelnut Belgian (8 oz)	70	12	2	<1	65	1 carb.
Coffee, International Café Kahlua (8 oz)	60	10	2	<1	55	1/2 carb.
Coffee, International Café Vienna (8 oz)	70	11	3	<1	110	1 carb.

BEVERAGES

Products	Cal.	Carb. (g)	Fat (g)	Sat. Fat (g)	Sodium (mg)	Exchanges
Coffee, International French Vanilla, Sugar-Free (8 oz)	35	4	2	<1	55	1/2 fat
Coffee, International Italian Cappuccino (8 oz)	50	10	2	<1	50	1/2 carb.
Coffee, International Orange Cappuccino (8 oz)	70	11	2	<1	100	1 carb.
Coffee, International Orange Cappuccino, Sugar-Free (8 oz)	30	3	2	<1	75	1/2 fat
Coffee, International Suisse Mocha (8 oz)	60	8	3	<1	50	1/2 carb., 1/2 fat
Coffee, International Suisse Mocha, Decaf (8 oz)	60	8	3	<1	40	1/2 carb., 1/2 fat
Coffee, International Suisse Mocha, Sugar-Free (8 oz)	30	4	2	<1	30	1/2 fat
HI-C						
LoCal Fruit Punch (8 oz)	43	11	0	0	5	1 carb.
KOOL-AID						
Bursts Soft Drink, Cherry (9.6 oz)	100	25	0	0	35	2 carb.

Cherry Drink, Sugar-Free, Low-Calorie (8 oz)	5	0	0	0	5	free
Cherry Drink w/Sugar (8 oz)	60	16	0	0	0	1 carb.
Fruit Drink Powder & Water (8 oz)	89	23	<1	<1	34	1-1/2 carb.
KRAFT						
Coffee, Suisse Mocha, Decaf, Sugar-Free (8 oz)	30	4	2	<1	75	1/2 fat
MAXWELL HOUSE						
Coffee, Cappuccino (8 oz)	90	18	1	0	65	1 carb.
Coffee, Cinnamon Cappuccino (8 oz)	90	16	2	0	70	1 carb.
Coffee, Cappio Iced Cappuccino (8 oz)	130	24	3	2	120	1-1/2 carb.
Coffee, Mocha Cappuccino (8 oz)	100	17	3	1	70	1 carb., 1/2 fat
Coffee, Vanilla Cappuccino (8 oz)	90	19	1	0	65	1 carb.
NESTEA						
Cool From Nestea (8 oz)	82	22	0	0	33	1-1/2 carb.
Diet Cool From Nestea (8 oz)	1	<1	0	0	27	free
Iced Tea, Earl Grey (8 oz)	68	18	0	0	2	1 carb.
Iced Tea, Lemon-Sweetened (8 oz)	80	22	0	0	<1	1-1/2 carb.

BEVERAGES

Products	Cal.	Carb. (g)	Fat (g)	Sat. Fat (g)	Sodium (mg)	Exchanges
NEW YORK SELTZER						
Black Cherry (8 oz)	90	22	0	0	15	1-1/2 carb.
Black Cherry, Diet (8 oz)	2	0	0	0	15	free
Iced Tea, Lemon Sparkling (8 oz)	90	21	0	0	50	1-1/2 carb.
Iced Tea, Raspberry Sparkling (8 oz)	100	21	0	0	50	1-1/2 carb.
Peach (8 oz)	90	22	0	0	15	1-1/2 carb.
Raspberry (8 oz)	90	22	0	0	15	1-1/2 carb.
Raspberry, Diet (8 oz)	2	0	0	0	15	free
OCEAN SPRAY						
Cran-Raspberry Drink (8 oz)	140	36	0	0	35	2 1/2 carb.
Cranberry Juice Cocktail (8 oz)	140	34	0	0	35	2 carb.
Cranberry Juice Cocktail From Concentrate, Reduced-Calorie (8 oz)	50	13	0	0	35	1 carb.
Fruit Punch (8 oz)	130	32	0	0	35	2 carb.

Lightstyle Cranberry Juice Cocktail, Low-Calorie (8 oz)	40	10	0	0	35	1/2 carb.
Lightstyle Pink Grapefruit Juice Cocktail, Low-Calorie (8 oz)	40	9	0	0	35	1/2 carb.
ReFreshers Citrus Cranberry Juice Drink (8 oz)	120	30	0	0	35	2 carb.
ReFreshers Orange Cranberry Juice Drink (8 oz)	130	33	0	0	35	2 carb.
Ruby Red Grapefruit Juice Drink (8 oz)	130	33	0	0	35	2 carb.
Summer Cooler (8 oz)	120	32	0	0	35	2 carb.
PEPSI COLA						
Mountain Dew (12 oz)	170	46	0	0	70	3 carb.
Diet Pepsi (12 oz)	0	0	0	0	35	free
Regular Pepsi (12 oz)	150	41	0	0	35	3 carb.
POWERADE						
Fruit Punch (8 oz)	72	19	0	0	28	1 carb.
Lemon-Lime (8 oz)	72	19	0	0	28	1 carb.
Orange (8 oz)	72	19	0	0	28	1 carb.

BEVERAGES

Products	Cal.	Carb. (g)	Fat (g)	Sat. Fat (g)	Sodium (mg)	Exchanges
SEVEN UP						
7-Up (12 oz)	151	37	0	0	10	2-1/2 carb.
SLICE						
Cola (12 oz)	160	39	0	0	35	2-1/2 carb.
Lemon–Lime Soda (12 oz)	150	40	0	0	55	2-1/2 carb.
Lemon–Lime Soda, Diet (12 oz)	0	1	0	0	35	free
SNAPPLE						
Apple Crisp Juice (10 oz)	140	36	0	0	30	2-1/2 carb.
Bali Blast Drink (8 oz)	120	30	0	0	10	2 carb.
Cherry Lemonade (8 oz)	130	31	0	0	10	2 carb.
Cherry Lime Rickey Soda (8 oz)	110	27	0	0	0	2 carb.
Creme D'Vanilla Soda (8 oz)	130	33	0	0	0	2 carb.
Kiwi Strawberry Drink, Diet (8 oz)	20	5	0	0	10	free
Mango Madness Drink (8 oz)	110	29	0	0	10	2 carb.

Passion Supreme Juice (10 oz)	160	39	0	0	20	2-1/2 carb.
Tea, Just Plain, Sweetened (8 oz)	70	18	0	0	10	1 carb.
Tea, Just Plain, Unsweetened (8 oz)	0	0	0	0	10	free
Tea, Lemon (8 oz)	100	25	0	0	10	1-1/2 carb.
Tea, Lemon, Diet (8 oz)	0	1	0	0	10	free
Tea, Passion Fruit (8 oz)	110	27	0	0	10	2 carb.
Tea, Raspberry (8 oz)	100	26	0	0	10	2 carb.
Vitamin Supreme (10 oz)	150	38	0	0	20	2-1/2 carb.
SUNNY DELIGHT						
Orange Drink/Ade (8 oz)	127	32	<1	<1	40	2 carb.
TANG						
Orange Drink Mix (2 Tbsp powder)	100	24	0	0	0	1-1/2 carb.
Orange Drink Mix, Sugar-Free (2 Tbsp powder)	30	6	0	0	0	1/2 carb.
TROPICANA						
Apple Raspberry Blackberry (10 oz)	150	37	0	0	20	2-1/2 carb.
Orange Cranberry (10 oz)	160	40	0	0	20	2-1/2 carb.

BEVERAGES

Products	Cal.	Carb. (g)	Fat (g)	Sat. Fat (g)	Sodium (mg)	Exchanges
Orange Cranberry, Light (10 oz)	35	9	0	0	25	1/2 carb.
Orange Raspberry, Light (10 oz)	45	11	0	0	20	1 carb.
Orange Strawberry Banana (10 oz)	140	34	0	0	20	2 carb.
Pink Grapefruit (10 oz)	140	34	0	0	20	2 carb.

BREAD PRODUCTS AND BAKED GOODS

Products	Cal.	Carb. (g)	Fat (g)	Sat. Fat (g)	Sodium (mg)	Exchanges
Bagel (1/2)	98	19	<1	<1	190	1 strch
Bagel, Cinnamon Raisin (1)	195	39	1	<1	229	2-1/2 strch
Baklava (2 x 2-inch piece)	333	29	23	9	291	2 carb., 4 fat
Biscuit (1, 2-1/2-inch)	127	17	6	<1	368	1 strch, 1 fat
Bread, Banana, Homemade (1 slice)	163	27	5	1	151	2 carb., 1 fat
Bread, Buckwheat (1 slice)	71	13	1	<1	100	1 strch
Bread, Butter Croissant (1)	231	26	12	7	424	2 strch, 2 fat
Bread, Cheese (1 slice)	71	12	1	<1	144	1 strch
Bread, Corn (2-oz piece)	152	25	4	<1	375	1 strch, 1 fat
Bread, Cracked Wheat (1 slice)	65	12	1	<1	135	1 strch
Bread, Date Nut (1 slice)	217	30	10	2	140	2 carb., 2 fat
Bread, French (1 slice)	96	18	1	<1	213	1 strch

BREAD PRODUCTS & BAKED GOODS

Products	Cal.	Carb. (g)	Fat (g)	Sat. Fat (g)	Sodium (mg)	Exchanges
Bread, Fruit, No Nuts (1 slice)	150	23	6	2	109	1-1/2 carb, 1 fat
Bread, Indian Fry (5-inch)	296	48	9	2	626	3 strch, 2 fat
Bread, Italian (1 slice)	81	15	1	<1	175	1 strch
Bread, Mixed-Grain (1 slice)	63	12	<1	<1	122	1 strch
Bread, Oat Bran (1 slice)	71	12	1	<1	122	1 strch
Bread, Oatmeal (1 slice)	67	12	1	<1	150	1 strch
Bread, Pita (1/2, 6-inch)	83	17	<1	<1	161	1 strch
Bread, Pita, Whole-Wheat (1)	120	25	1	<1	239	1-1/2 strch
Bread, Potato (1 slice)	69	13	<1	<1	143	1 strch
Bread, Pumpernickel (1 slice)	80	15	1	<1	215	1 strch
Bread, Raisin (1 slice)	69	13	1	<1	98	1 strch
Bread, Rye (1 slice)	83	16	1	<1	211	1 strch
Bread, Sourdough (1 slice)	69	13	<1	<1	152	1 strch
Bread, Sweet Potato (1 slice)	72	13	2	<1	228	1 strch

Bread, Triticale (1 slice)	63	12	<1	<1	136	1 strch
Bread, Vienna (1 slice)	69	13	<1	<1	152	1 strch
Bread, Wheat Bran (1 slice)	89	17	1	<1	175	1 strch
Bread, White (1 slice)	67	12	<1	<1	134	1 strch
Bread, White, Reduced-Calorie (2 slices)	96	20	1	<1	208	1 strch
Bread, Whole-Wheat (1 slice)	70	13	1	<1	149	1 strch
Bread Sticks, Crisp (2, 4-inch)	82	14	2	<1	131	1 strch
Bread Stuffing (1/3 cup)	117	14	6	1	359	1 strch, 1 fat
Bread Stuffing, Homemade (1/2 cup)	171	23	8	2	468	1-1/2 strch, 2 fat
Bun, Hamburger (1/2)	61	11	1	<1	120	1 strch
Bun, Hot Dog (1/2)	61	11	1	<1	120	1 strch
Cream Puff w/Custard Filling (1)	284	25	17	4	375	1-1/2 carb., 3 fat
Crepe/French Pancake (1)	239	22	13	4	274	1-1/2 strch, 3 fat
Croissant, Cheese (1)	236	27	12	6	316	2 strch, 2 fat
Croutons (1 cup)	122	22	2	<1	209	1 strch, 1 fat
Danish Pastry, Cinnamon (1)	349	47	17	4	326	3 carb., 3 fat

BREAD PRODUCTS & BAKED GOODS

Products	Cal.	Carb. (g)	Fat (g)	Sat. Fat (g)	Sodium (mg)	Exchanges
Danish Pastry, Fruit-Filled (1)	335	45	16	3	333	3 carb., 3 fat
Dinner Roll/Bun, French (1)	105	19	2	<1	231	1 strch
Dinner Roll/Bun, Wheat (1)	77	13	2	<1	96	1 strch
Doughnut, Cake (1)	211	25	12	3	273	1-1/2 carb., 2 fat
Doughnut, Cake, w/Chocolate Icing (1)	204	21	13	4	184	1-1/2 carb., 3 fat
Doughnut, Cake, Sugared/Glazed (1)	192	23	10	2	181	1-1/2 carb., 2 fat
Doughnut, Custard-Filled w/Icing (1)	261	34	13	6	125	2 carb., 3 fat
Doughnut, Yeast, Creme-Filled (1)	307	26	21	6	263	2 carb., 4 fat
Doughnut, Yeast, Glazed (1)	242	27	13	4	205	2 carb., 2 fat
Doughnut, Yeast, Jelly-Filled (1)	221	25	12	3	190	1-1/2 carb., 2 fat
Dumpling, Plain (medium)	42	7	1	<1	105	1/2 strch
Egg Bread/Challah (1 slice)	66	11	1	<1	113	1 strch
Eclair, Chocolate w/Custard Filling (1)	246	23	15	4	317	1-1/2 carb., 3 fat
English Muffin (1/2)	67	13	<1	<1	132	1 strch

Item	Cal	Carb	Fat		Sodium	Exchange
French Toast, Frozen (1 slice)	126	19	4	1	292	1 strch, 1 fat
French Toast, Homemade w/2% Milk (1 slice)	149	16	7	2	311	1 strch, 1 fat
Muffin (1)	133	19	5	1	210	1 strch, 1 fat
Muffin, Cheese (1)	184	23	8	3	274	1-1/2 strch, 2 fat
Muffin, Chocolate Chip (1)	190	27	9	3	186	2 strch, 2 fat
Muffin, Cranberry Nut (1)	164	25	5	2	326	1-1/2 strch, 1 fat
Muffin, Oat Bran (1)	154	28	4	<1	224	2 strch, 1 fat
Muffin, Pumpkin w/Raisins & Nuts (1)	181	34	4	<1	154	2 strch, 1 fat
Muffin, Wheat Bran (1)	161	24	7	2	335	1-1/2 strch, 1 fat
Muffin, Whole-Wheat (1)	142	20	6	2	283	1 strch, 1 fat
Muffin, Zucchini w/Nuts (1)	210	26	11	2	169	2 strch, 2 fat
Pancakes, From Mix (2)	166	22	6	2	384	1 strch, 1 fat
Pannetone or Italian Sweetbread (1 slice)	86	15	2	1	96	1 strch
Popover, Homemade w/Whole Milk (1)	122	15	5	1	110	1 strch, 1 fat
Pretzel, Soft (2 oz)	190	38	2	<1	772	2-1/2 strch
Roll, Plain (1)	85	14	2	2	148	1 strch

BREAD PRODUCTS & BAKED GOODS

Products	Cal.	Carb. (g)	Fat (g)	Sat. Fat (g)	Sodium (mg)	Exchanges
Roll, Submarine/Hoagie (1, 5 oz)	392	75	4	<1	783	5 strch
Roll, Whole-Wheat (1)	93	18	2	<1	167	1 strch
Scone (1, 1-1/2 oz)	150	19	7	2	246	1 strch, 1 fat
Scone, Whole-Wheat (1)	145	18	7	2	174	1 strch, 1 fat
Sweet Roll, Cheese (1)	238	29	12	4	236	2 strch, 2 fat
Sweet Roll, Cinnamon Raisin (1)	145	20	7	2	149	1 carb., 1 fat
Sweet Roll, Cinnamon w/Raisins & Nuts, Homemade (1)	196	30	7	2	185	2 carb., 1 fat
Taco Shells (2)	122	16	6	<1	95	1 strch, 1 fat
Tortilla, Corn (1, 6-inch)	56	12	<1	<1	40	1 strch
Tortilla, Flour (1, 7-inch)	114	20	3	<1	167	1 strch
Tortilla, Flour (1, 10-1/2-inch)	185	32	4	1	272	2 strch, 1 fat
Tortilla, Whole-Wheat (1)	73	20	<1	<1	171	1 strch
Waffles, Blueberry (1, 4-inch)	97	16	3	<1	272	1 strch, 1 fat

Waffles, From Mix (1, 4-1/2-inch)	145	17	7	1	256	1 strch, 1 fat
Waffles, Homemade (1)	218	25	11	2	383	1-1/2 strch, 2 fat
Waffles, Low-Fat (1, 4-1/2-inch)	80	17	<1	<1	270	1 strch
AUNT FANNY'S						
Honey Bun, Applesauce (1)	330	43	17	4	300	3 carb., 3 fat
Honey Bun, Banana Cream (1)	350	32	18	4	290	2 carb., 3 fat
Honey Bun, Iced Honey (1)	350	32	18	4	290	2 carb., 3 fat
Honey Bun, Raspberry-Filled (1)	350	45	17	5	290	3 carb., 3 fat
Honey Bun, Regular (1)	360	41	20	5	300	3 carb., 3 fat
Honey Bun, Vanilla Creme (1)	350	32	18	4	290	2 carb., 3 fat
AUNT JEMIMA						
Microwave Pancakes, Blueberry (3)	204	39	4	<1	826	2-1/2 strch
Microwave Pancakes, Buttermilk (3)	180	36	2	<1	860	2-1/2 strch
Microwave Pancakes, Original (3)	183	37	2	<1	801	2-1/2 strch
Pancakes, Blueberry (3)	249	46	4	1	789	3 strch, 1 fat
Pancakes, Buttermilk (3)	240	45	4	<1	778	3 strch

BREAD PRODUCTS & BAKED GOODS

Products	Cal.	Carb. (g)	Fat (g)	Sat. Fat (g)	Sodium (mg)	Exchanges
Pancakes, Original Flavor (3)	246	47	4	1	777	3 strch
Waffles, Apple/Cinnamon (2)	176	29	6	1	503	2 strch, 1 fat
Waffles, Blueberry (2)	175	29	5	1	684	2 strch, 1 fat
Waffles, Buttermilk (2)	179	29	6	1	615	2 strch, 1 fat
Waffles, Original (2)	173	28	6	1	591	2 strch, 1 fat
Waffles, Raisin (2)	200	36	4	NA	526	2-1/2 strch, 1 fat
Waffles, Whole-Grain (2)	154	29	3	<1	676	2 strch
BALLARD						
Extra Light Oven-Ready Biscuit Dough (1)	50	10	<1	<1	165	1/2 strch
Extra Light Oven-Ready Biscuit Dough, Buttermilk (1)	50	10	<1	<1	165	1/2 strch
EGGO						
Mini Waffles (4)	90	14	3	1	190	1 strch
Waffles, Apple Cinnamon (1)	130	18	5	1	250	1 strch, 1 fat

Waffles, Blueberry (1)	130	18	5	1	250	1 strch, 1 fat
Waffles, Buttermilk (1)	120	16	5	1	250	1 strch, 1 fat
Waffles, Common Sense Oat Bran (1)	116	17	4	1	231	1 strch, 1 fat
Waffles, Common Sense Oat Bran, Fruit Nut (1)	120	17	5	1	220	1 strch, 1 fat
Waffles, Homestyle (1)	120	16	5	1	250	1 strch, 1 fat
Waffles, Nutri-Grain (1)	126	19	5	1	263	1 strch, 1 fat
Waffles, Special K (1)	80	16	0	0	120	1 strch
Waffles, Strawberry (1)	130	18	5	1	250	1 strch, 1 fat
ENTENMANN'S						
Buns, Cinnamon (1)	220	31	10	6	190	2 carb., 2 fat
Buns, Fat-Free Cholesterol-Free Apple (1)	150	33	0	0	140	2 carb.
Buns, Fat-Free Cholesterol-Free Blueberry Cheez (1)	140	31	0	0	150	2 carb.
Buns, Fat-Free Cholesterol-Free Cinnamon Raisin (1)	160	36	0	0	125	2-1/2 carb.

BREAD PRODUCTS & BAKED GOODS

Products	Cal.	Carb. (g)	Fat (g)	Sat. Fat (g)	Sodium (mg)	Exchanges
Buns, Fat-Free Cholesterol-Free Pineapple Cheez (1)	140	30	0	0	150	2 carb.
Buns, Fat-Free Cholesterol-Free Raspberry Cheez (1)	160	36	0	0	135	2-1/2 carb.
Danish Pastry Ring, Pecan (1 slice)	230	23	15	3	160	1-1/2 carb., 3 fat
Danish Pastry Ring, Walnut (1 slice)	230	23	14	3	160	1-1/2 carb., 3 fat
Danish Pastry Twist, Raspberry (1 slice)	220	28	11	3	170	2 carb., 2 fat
Donuts, Cinnamon Sugar Variety (1)	310	32	19	4	300	2 carb., 4 fat
Donuts, Crumb-Topped (1)	260	34	13	3	230	2 carb., 3 fat
Donuts, Devil's Food Crumb (1)	250	33	12	4	240	2 carb., 2 fat
Donuts, Glazed Buttermilk (1)	270	36	13	3	280	2-1/2 carb., 3 fat
Donuts, Mini Frosted (2)	270	23	20	6	180	1-1/2 carb., 4 fat
Donuts, Rich Frosted (1)	280	27	19	6	220	2 carb., 4 fat
Donuts, Rich Frosted Variety (1)	400	37	27	8	310	2-1/2 carb., 5 fat

Food						Exchanges
Eclairs, Chocolate (1)	250	44	9	2	220	3 carb., 1 fat
Muffins, Blueberry (1)	160	24	7	2	210	1-1/2 carb., 1 fat
Muffins, Fat-Free Cholesterol-Free Blueberry (1)	120	26	0	0	220	2 carb.
Pastry, Apple Puffs (1)	260	36	12	3	220	2-1/2 carb., 2 fat
Pastry, Cinnamon Filbert Ring (1 slice)	270	27	17	3	190	2 carb., 3 fat
Pastry, Fat-Free Cholesterol-Free Apricot (1 slice)	150	34	0	0	110	2 carb.
Pastry, Fat-Free Cholesterol-Free Black Forest (1 slice)	130	32	0	0	115	2 carb.
Pastry, Fat-Free Cholesterol-Free Cinnamon Apple Twist (1 slice)	150	35	0	0	110	2 carb.
Pastry, Fat-Free Cholesterol-Free LemonTwist (1 slice)	130	31	0	0	140	2 carb.
Pastry, Fat-Free Cholesterol-Free Raspberry Cheez (1 slice)	140	32	0	0	110	2 carb.
Pastry, Fat-Free Cholesterol-Free RaspberryTwist (1 slice)	140	33	0	0	125	2 carb.

BREAD PRODUCTS & BAKED GOODS

Products	Cal.	Carb. (g)	Fat (g)	Sat. Fat (g)	Sodium (mg)	Exchanges
POPEMS, Glazed (6)	240	33	11	3	210	2 carb., 2 fat
POPEMS, Glazed Chocolate (4)	200	29	10	3	190	2 carb., 2 fat
GENERAL MILLS						
Muffin Mix, Apple Cinnamon, Prepared (1)	159	26	5	1	217	2 strch, 1 fat
Muffin Mix, Banana Nut, Prepared (1)	196	33	5	<1	250	2 strch, 1 fat
Muffin Mix, Chocolate Chocolate Chip w/Glaze, Prepared (1)	215	34	8	3	222	2 carb., 2 fat
Muffin Mix, Lemon Poppyseed, Prepared (1)	198	32	7	2	262	2 strch, 1 fat
Muffin Mix, Orange Cranberry, Prepared (1)	242	44	7	2	277	3 strch, 1 fat
Pancake Mix, Complete, Prepared (1)	100	19	2	<1	320	1 strch
Sweet Roll, Quick Rise, Prepared (1)	150	26	4	1	230	2 carb., 1 fat
Waffle Mix, Belgian, Prepared (1)	370	47	17	9	1020	3 strch, 3 fat
Waffle Mix, Complete, Prepared (1)	220	36	7	1	710	2-1/2 strch, 1 fat

GOLD MEDAL

Biscuit Mix, Baking Powder, Prepared (1)	160	25	5	1	460	1-1/2 strch, 1 fat
Biscuit Mix, Buttermilk, Prepared (1)	170	24	8	3	420	1-1/2 strch, 2 fat
Biscuit Mix, Cinnamon Raisin, Prepared (1)	260	41	9	3	560	3 strch, 1 fat
Biscuit Mix, Prepared (1)	160	22	7	2	420	1-1/2 strch, 1 fat
Honey Corn Bread Mix, Prepared (1 slice)	140	26	3	1	290	2 strch, 1 fat
Muffin Mix, Blueberry, Prepared (1)	260	44	7	2	320	3 strch, 1 fat
Muffin Mix, Corn Bread, Prepared (1)	140	25	4	1	290	1-1/2 strch, 1 fat
Muffin Mix, Raisin Bran, Prepared (1)	270	46	8	2	450	3 strch, 2 fat
Pancake Mix, Buttermilk, Prepared (1)	100	18	3	0	300	1 strch, 1 fat

GRANDS

Refrigerated Biscuits, Buttermilk (1)	201	23	10	3	573	1-1/2 strch, 2 fat
Refrigerated Biscuits, Homestyle (1)	192	24	9	2	595	1-1/2 strch, 2 fat
Refrigerated Biscuits, Southern (1)	198	23	10	3	573	1-1/2 strch, 2 fat

HEALTH VALLEY

Fat-Free Healthy Scones, Apple Kiwi (1)	80	15	0	0	160	1 strch

BREAD PRODUCTS & BAKED GOODS

Products	Cal.	Carb. (g)	Fat (g)	Sat. Fat (g)	Sodium (mg)	Exchanges
Fat-Free Healthy Scones, Cinnamon Raisin (1)	80	15	0	0	160	1 strch
Fat-Free Healthy Scones, Cranberry Orange (1)	80	15	0	0	160	1 strch
Fat-Free Healthy Scones, Mountain Blueberry (1)	80	15	0	0	160	1 strch
Fat-Free Healthy Scones, Pineapple Raisin (1)	80	15	0	0	160	1 strch
HUNGRY JACK						
Biscuit Dough, Fluffy (1)	88	11	4	1	285	1 strch, 1 fat
Biscuit Dough, Southern Flaky (1)	89	12	4	<1	298	1 strch, 1 fat
Microwave Pancakes, Blueberry (3)	233	45	4	<1	553	3 strch
Microwave Pancakes, Buttermilk (3)	242	46	4	<1	587	3 strch
Microwave Pancakes, Mini Buttermilk (11)	233	45	4	<1	556	3 strch
Microwave Pancakes, Original (3)	243	47	4	<1	551	3 strch
Refrigerated Biscuits, Fluffy (2)	178	23	8	2	573	1-1/2 strch, 2 fat
KELLOGG'S						
Corn Flake Crumbs (1/4 cup)	100	24	0	0	290	1-1/2 strch

Croutons, Croutettes (1/2 cup)	50	10	0	0	185	1/2 strch
Pop-Tarts Pastry, Apple Cinnamon (1)	210	38	5	1	170	2-1/2 carb., 1 fat
Pop-Tarts Pastry, Blueberry (1)	200	37	5	1	210	2-1/2 carb., 1 fat
Pop-Tarts Pastry, Brown Sugar Cinnamon (1)	210	34	7	1	180	2 carb., 1 fat
Pop-Tarts Pastry, Cherry (1)	200	37	5	1	220	2-1/2 carb., 1 fat
Pop-Tarts Pastry, Cherry, Frosted (1)	200	38	5	1	170	2-1/2 carb., 1 fat
Pop-Tarts Pastry, Chocolate Graham (1)	210	36	6	1	220	2-1/2 carb., 1 fat
Pop-Tarts Pastry, Chocolate Vanilla, Frosted (1)	200	37	5	1	230	2-1/2 carb., 1 fat
Pop-Tarts Pastry, Fudge, Frosted (1)	200	37	5	1	220	2-1/2 carb., 1 fat
Pop-Tarts Pastry, Grape, Frosted (1)	200	38	5	1	200	2-1/2 carb., 1 fat
Pop-Tarts Pastry, Raspberry, Frosted (1)	210	37	6	1	210	2-1/2 carb., 1 fat
Pop-Tarts Pastry, Strawberry (1)	200	37	5	1	190	2-1/2 carb., 1 fat
Pop-Tarts Pastry, Strawberry, Frosted (1)	200	37	5	1	180	2-1/2 carb., 1 fat
Pop-Tarts Pastry, Sugar Cinnamon (1)	220	32	9	1	210	2 carb., 2 fat
Waffles, Common Sense Oat Bran (1)	110	16	4	1	220	1 strch, 1 fat
Waffles, Nutri-Grain Multi-Bran (1)	110	17	5	1	220	1 strch, 1 fat

BREAD PRODUCTS & BAKED GOODS

Products	Cal.	Carb. (g)	Fat (g)	Sat. Fat (g)	Sodium (mg)	Exchanges
Waffles, Nutri-Grain Plain (1)	120	18	5	1	250	1 strch, 1 fat
Waffles, Nutri-Grain Raisin Bran (1)	120	18	5	1	250	1 strch, 1 fat
MARIE CALLENDER'S						
Bread, Original Garlic (1 slice)	190	25	8	2	290	1-1/2 strch, 2 fat
Bread, Parmesan Romano Garlic (1 slice)	200	23	10	3	430	1-1/2 strch, 2 fat
MORTON						
Honey Buns (1)	250	35	10	3	160	2 carb., 2 fat
Mini Honey Buns (1)	160	19	8	2	100	1 carb., 2 fat
NABISCO						
Cake Crumbs, Oreo Base (1/4 cup)	140	23	5	1	260	1-1/2 strch, 1 fat
OLD EL PASO						
Taco Shells, Mini (7)	160	18	10	2	130	1 strch, 2 fat
Taco Shells, Super (2)	190	21	12	2	150	1-1/2 strch, 2 fat
Taco Shells, White Corn (3)	170	18	10	2	30	1 strch, 2 fat

Tortilla, Flour (1)	150	27	3	<1	340	2 strch, 1 fat
Tortillas, Soft Taco (2)	180	33	4	<1	410	2 strch, 1 fat
Tostaco Shells (1)	130	14	7	1	10	1 strch, 1 fat
ORTEGA						
Taco Shells (2)	140	20	7	1	200	1 strch, 1 fat
Tostada Shells (2)	150	18	8	2	190	1 strch, 2 fat
PANCHO VILLA						
Taco Shells (3)	190	19	11	3	0	1 strch, 2 fat
PEPPERIDGE FARM						
Biscuits, Garlic & Cheese (1)	170	24	6	3	510	1-1/2 strch, 1 fat
Biscuits, Original Water (15)	60	11	1	<1	100	1 strch
Bread, 1-1/2-lb Natural Wheat (1 slice)	90	16	2	0	170	1 strch
Bread, 1-1/2-lb Wheat (1 slice)	90	16	2	0	190	1 strch
Bread, 2-lb Family Wheat (1 slice)	70	13	1	0	135	1 strch
Bread, Apple Walnut Swirl (1 slice)	81	14	2	<1	122	1 strch
Bread, Cinnamon (1 slice)	80	14	3	<1	115	1 carb., 1 fat

BREAD PRODUCTS & BAKED GOODS

Products	Cal.	Carb. (g)	Fat (g)	Sat. Fat (g)	Sodium (mg)	Exchanges
Bread, Cinnamon Swirl (1 slice)	81	14	3	<1	117	1 strch, 1 fat
Bread, Classic Dark Pumpernickel (1 slice)	80	15	1	<1	230	1 strch
Bread, Cracked Wheat, Thin-Sliced (1 slice)	70	12	1	0	140	1 strch
Bread, European Bake Shop, French-Style (1 slice)	130	25	2	1	280	1-1/2 strch
Bread, European Bake Shop, Twin French (1 slice)	130	26	2	<1	270	2 strch
Bread, European Bake Shop, Twin Sourdough (1 slice)	130	26	2	<1	270	2 strch
Bread, Garlic (1 slice)	161	14	10	3	251	1 strch, 2 fat
Bread, Garlic Parmesan (1)	161	19	7	2	261	1 strch, 1 fat
Bread, Golden Swirl Vermont Maple (1 slice)	90	15	3	1	100	1 strch, 1 fat
Bread, Hearty Country White (1 slice)	90	19	1	0	190	1 strch
Bread, Hearty Crunchy Oat (1 slice)	100	17	2	0	180	1 strch
Bread, Hearty Honey Wheatberry (1 slice)	100	18	2	0	200	1 strch
Bread, Hearty Russet Potato (1 slice)	90	18	2	<1	260	1 strch

Bread, Hearty Sesame Wheat (1 slice)	100	17	2	0	180	1 strch
Bread, Hearty Slice 7-Grain (1 slice)	100	18	2	0	180	1 strch
Bread, Hearty White (1 slice)	90	19	1	0	190	1 strch
Bread, Jewish Seeded Rye (1)	80	15	1	<1	210	1 strch
Bread, Jewish Seedless Family Rye (1 slice)	80	15	1	<1	210	1 strch
Bread, Large Family White, Thin-Sliced (1 slice)	27	14	2	0	160	1 strch
Bread, Light-Style Oatmeal (1 slice)	48	9	<1	0	107	1/2 strch
Bread, Light-Style Seven-Grain (1 slice)	55	11	<1	0	126	1 strch
Bread, Light-Style Sourdough (3 slices)	130	27	1	0	320	2 strch
Bread, Light-Style Wheat (1 slice)	43	9	<1	<1	97	1/2 strch
Bread, Light Vienna (1 slice)	43	9	<1	<1	100	1/2 strch
Bread, Monterey Jack w/Jalapeño Cheese (1 slice)	200	22	10	4	280	1-1/2 strch, 2 fat
Bread, Mozzarella Garlic (1 slice)	200	21	10	5	280	1-1/2 strch, 2 fat
Bread, Oatmeal, Thin-Sliced (1 slice)	60	11	1	1	160	1 strch
Bread, Old-Fashioned Honey Bran (1 slice)	90	17	1	0	160	1 strch
Bread, Old-Fashioned Oatmeal (1 slice)	80	15	1	0	200	1 strch

BREAD PRODUCTS & BAKED GOODS

Products	Cal.	Carb. (g)	Fat (g)	Sat. Fat (g)	Sodium (mg)	Exchanges
Bread, Onion Rye (1 slice)	80	15	1	<1	210	1 strch
Bread, Party Pumpernickel Slices (8 slices)	110	22	2	0	320	1-1/2 strch
Bread, Party Rye Slices (3 slices)	110	22	2	0	410	1-1/2 strch
Bread, Raisin Cinnamon Swirl (1 slice)	80	14	2	0	105	1 strch
Bread, Raisin w/Cinnamon (1 slice)	80	14	2	0	105	1 strch
Bread, Soft 100% Whole-Wheat (1 slice)	60	11	<1	0	95	1 strch
Bread, Soft Oatmeal (1 slice)	60	12	<1	0	2	1 strch
Bread, Sourdough Garlic (1 slice)	180	20	9	3	220	1 strch, 2 fat
Bread, Thin-Sliced Dijon Rye (2 slices)	100	18	2	<1	340	1 strch
Bread, Two Cheddar Cheese (1 slice)	210	21	11	5	280	1-1/2 strch, 2 fat
Bread, Very Thin-Sliced White (3 slices)	110	23	2	0	270	1-1/2 strch
Bread, Vienna, Thick-Sliced (1)	70	12	1	0	150	1 strch
Bread, White Sandwich (2 slices)	130	23	2	<1	260	1-1/2 strch
Bread, White, Thin-Sliced (1 slice)	80	13	2	0	135	1 strch

Bread, Whole-Wheat, Thin-Sliced (1 slice)	60	11	1	0	120	1 strch
Breadsticks, Brown & Serve (1)	150	28	2	<1	290	2 strch
Bun, Multi-Grain Sandwich (1)	150	24	3	<1	230	1-1/2 strch, 1 fat
Bun, Sourdough Sandwich (1)	170	28	4	2	290	2 strch, 1 fat
Buns/Rolls, 5-inch Sandwich Hearty (1)	209	36	5	2	346	2-1/2 strch, 1 fat
Buns/Rolls, Potato Sandwich (1)	160	28	4	<1	260	2 strch, 1 fat
Croissants, Petite (1)	130	13	8	4	180	1 strch, 2 fat
Croutons, Caesar Homestyle (1/2 oz)	71	8	3	0	183	1/2 strch, 1 fat
Croutons, Cheddar & Romano Cheese (1/2 oz)	61	8	2	0	193	1/2 strch
Croutons, Cheese & Garlic (1/2 oz)	71	8	3	0	162	1/2 strch, 1 fat
Croutons, Italian Homestyle (1/2 oz)	71	8	3	1	132	1/2 strch, 1 fat
Croutons, Olive Oil & Garlic Homestyle (1/2 oz)	61	10	2	0	162	1/2 strch
Croutons, Onion & Garlic (1/2 oz)	61	10	2	0	162	1/2 strch
Croutons, Seasoned (1/2 oz)	71	8	3	0	172	1/2 strch, 1 fat
Croutons, Sourdough Cheese Homestyle (1/2 oz)	61	8	2	0	162	1/2 strch
Danish, Apple (1)	209	29	9	3	189	2 carb., 2 fat

BREAD PRODUCTS & BAKED GOODS

Products	Cal.	Carb. (g)	Fat (g)	Sat. Fat (g)	Sodium (mg)	Exchanges
Danish, Cheese (1)	226	25	11	3	226	1-1/2 strch, 2 fat
Danish, Raspberry (1)	209	29	9	3	189	2 strch, 2 fat
Dinner Rolls, Country-Style Classic (1)	50	7	<1	<1	76	1/2 strch
Dinner Rolls, Hearty Potato Classic (1)	88	13	3	<1	121	1 strch, 1 fat
Dinner Rolls, Parker House (1)	50	7	2	<1	77	1/2 strch
English Muffins (1)	129	26	<1	0	249	2 strch
English Muffins, Cinnamon Raisin (1)	139	28	<1	0	229	2 strch
English Muffins, 7-Grain (1)	129	26	<1	0	229	2 strch
English Muffins, Sourdough (1)	130	26	1	0	250	2 strch
Finger Dinner Rolls w/Poppy Seed (1)	50	7	2	<1	77	1/2 strch
Finger Dinner Rolls w/Sesame Seed (1)	50	7	2	<1	8	1/2 strch
Mini Turnovers, Cherry (1)	140	16	8	2	70	1 carb., 2 fat
Muffins, Apple Oatmeal (1)	159	28	4	<1	189	2 strch, 1 fat
Muffins, Blueberry (1)	141	27	3	0	191	2 strch, 1 fat

Item						Exchanges
Muffins, Bran w/Raisins (1)	149	30	3	<1	259	2 strch, 1 fat
Muffins, Corn (1)	151	27	3	0	191	2 strch, 1 fat
Puff Pastry, Apple Dumplings (1)	290	44	11	3	160	3 carb, 2 fat
Puff Pastry, Apple Mini Turnovers (1)	140	15	8	2	80	1 carb., 2 fat
Puff Pastry, Apple Turnovers, Vanilla Icing (1)	380	53	14	3	190	3-1/2 carb., 2 fat
Puff Pastry, Cherry Turnovers, Vanilla Icing (1)	340	51	13	3	200	3-1/2 carb., 2 fat
Puff Pastry, Raspberry Turnovers, Vanilla Icing (1)	360	53	14	3	190	3-1/2 strch, 2 fat
Puff Pastry, Strawberry Mini Turnover (1)	140	18	7	2	100	1 strch, 1 fat
Rolls, Baked French-Style (1)	130	25	2	1	280	1-1/2 strch
Rolls, Baked French-Style, Sliced (1)	120	24	2	<1	260	1-1/2 strch
Rolls, Cinnamon (1)	249	33	12	3	219	2 carb., 2 fat
Rolls, Deli Classic Soft Hoagie (1)	199	32	5	3	338	2 strch, 1 fat
Rolls, Dijon Frankfurter (1)	140	23	3	2	240	1-1/2 strch, 1 fat
Rolls, European Bake Shop, 3 French, Brown & Serve (1)	240	45	3	<1	490	3 strch
Rolls, European Bake Shop, 6 Club (1)	120	22	2	0	240	1-1/2 strch

BREAD PRODUCTS & BAKED GOODS

Products	Cal.	Carb. (g)	Fat (g)	Sat. Fat (g)	Sodium (mg)	Exchanges
Rolls, European Bake Shop, 9 Sourdough French (1)	100	18	1	0	240	1 strch
Rolls, European Bake Shop, 9 French (1)	100	19	1	0	230	1 strch
Rolls, European Bake Shop, 12 Hearth, Brown & Serve (3)	150	28	2	0	300	2 strch
Rolls, European Bake Shop, Italian, Brown & Serve (1)	130	24	2	1	260	1-1/2 strch
Rolls, Frankfurter, Top- or Side-Sliced (1)	140	24	3	1	270	1-1/2 strch, 1 fat
Rolls, French, Brown & Serve (1/2)	180	34	2	<1	400	2 strch
Rolls, Garlic & Cheese (1)	131	16	5	2	281	1 strch, 1 fat
Rolls, Heat & Serve Butter Crescent (1)	110	13	5	3	160	1 strch, 1 fat
Rolls, Heat & Serve Golden Twist (1)	110	13	4	2	160	1 strch, 1 fat
Rolls, Onion Sliced Sandwich (1)	150	26	3	2	270	2 strch, 1 fat
Rolls, Party Enriched (5)	170	26	5	2	240	2 strch, 1 fat

Food						Exchanges
Rolls, Sandwich Sliced w/Sesame Seeds (1)	140	23	3	2	240	1-1/2 strch, 1 fat
Rolls, 7-Grain, 9 French (1)	80	19	2	0	270	1 strch
Rolls, Sliced Hamburger (1)	130	22	3	1	230	1-1/2 strch, 1 fat
Stuffing, Corn Bread (1/2 cup)	170	33	2	0	480	2 strch
Stuffing, Country-Style (1/2 cup)	140	27	2	0	380	2 strch
Stuffing, Cube (1/2 cup)	140	28	2	0	530	2 strch
Stuffing, Distinctive, Apple Raisin (1/2 cup)	140	27	2	0	520	2 strch
Stuffing, Distinctive, Classic Chicken (1/2 cup)	130	24	2	0	490	1-1/2 strch
Stuffing, Distinctive, Garden Herb (1/2 cup)	150	22	5	1	360	1-1/2 strch, 1 fat
Stuffing, Distinctive, Harvest Vegetable Almond (1/2 cup)	140	23	3	<1	300	1-1/2 strch, 1 fat
Stuffing, Distinctive, Honey Pecan Corn Bread (1/2 cup)	140	23	5	<1	400	1-1/2 strch, 1 fat
Stuffing, Distinctive, Wild Rice Mushroom (2/3 cup)	170	22	6	2	410	1-1/2 strch, 1 fat
Stuffing, Herb-Seasoned (3/4 cup)	170	33	2	0	600	2 strch
Stuffing, Sage & Onion, for Turkeys (1/2 cup)	150	28	2	0	520	2 strch

BREAD PRODUCTS & BAKED GOODS

Products	Cal.	Carb. (g)	Fat (g)	Sat. Fat (g)	Sodium (mg)	Exchanges
Turnovers, Apple (1)	331	48	14	3	181	3 carb., 2 fat
Turnovers, Blueberry (1)	341	45	16	3	201	3 carb., 3 fat
Turnovers, Cherry (1)	321	46	13	3	191	3 carb., 2 fat
Turnovers, Peach (1)	341	47	15	3	181	3 carb., 2 fat
Turnovers, Raspberry (1)	331	47	14	3	191	3 carb., 2 fat
PILLSBURY						
Biscuit Dough, Big Country, Buttermilk (1)	100	14	4	1	298	1 strch, 1 fat
Biscuit Dough, Big Country, Butter-Tastin' (1)	98	13	4	1	298	1 strch, 1 fat
Biscuit Dough, Big Country, Southern (1)	100	14	4	1	298	1 strch, 1 fat
Biscuit Dough, Butter-Tastin' Flaky (1)	87	12	4	<1	288	1 strch, 1 fat
Biscuit Dough, Butter-Type (1)	51	10	<1	<1	165	1/2 strch
Biscuit Dough, Flaky (1)	87	12	4	<1	299	1 strch, 1 fat
Biscuit Dough, Flaky Buttermilk (1)	86	11	4	<1	298	1 strch, 1 fat
Biscuit Dough, Grands, Butter-Tastin' (1)	185	21	10	3	533	1-1/2 strch, 2 fat

Biscuit Dough, Grands, Cinnamon Raisin (1)	185	26	7	2	539	2 strch, 1 fat
Biscuit Dough, Tender Layer Buttermilk (1)	55	9	1	<1	159	1/2 strch
Bread, Ballard Corn (1 piece)	130	23	3	1	520	1-1/2 strch, 1 fat
Bread Machine Mix, Cracked Wheat (1 slice)	130	25	2	0	260	1-1/2 strch
Bread Machine Mix, Crusty White (1 slice)	130	25	2	0	250	1-1/2 strch
Danish Roll Dough & Icing, Cinnamon Raisin (1)	134	20	5	1	246	1 carb., 1 fat
Danish Roll & Icing, Orange (1)	134	20	5	1	265	1 carb, 1 fat
Gingerbread Mix (1 slice)	220	40	5	2	340	2-1/2 carb., 1 fat
Quick Bread Mix, Apple Cinnamon (1 slice)	180	30	6	1	170	2 strch, 1 fat
Quick Bread Mix, Banana (1 slice)	170	26	6	1	200	2 strch, 1 fat
Quick Bread Mix, Blueberry (1 slice)	180	29	6	1	160	2 strch, 1 fat
Quick Bread Mix, Carrot (1 slice)	140	22	5	1	150	1-1/2 strch, 1 fat
Quick Bread Mix, Cranberry (1 slice)	160	30	4	1	150	2 strch, 1 fat
Quick Bread Mix, Date (1 slice)	180	32	4	1	160	2 strch, 1 fat
Quick Bread Mix, Nut (1 slice)	170	27	6	1	190	2 strch, 1 fat
Quick Bread Mix, Pumpkin (1 slice)	170	27	6	1	200	2 strch, 1 fat

BREAD PRODUCTS & BAKED GOODS

Products	Cal.	Carb. (g)	Fat (g)	Sat. Fat (g)	Sodium (mg)	Exchanges
Refrigerated Crescent Rolls, Cheese (2)	212	21	12	3	604	1-1/2 strch, 2 fat
Refrigerated Pipin' Hot Bread Loaf (1 slice)	112	22	<1	<1	345	1-1/2 strch
Refrigerated Rolls w/Icing, Apple Cinnamon (1)	139	21	5	1	309	1-1/2 strch, 1 fat
Roll/Bread Dough, Butterflake (1)	135	20	5	1	527	1 strch, 1 fat
Roll/Bread Dough, Corn Bread Twist (1)	68	9	3	<1	158	1/2 strch, 1 fat
Roll/Bread Dough, Crescent (1)	102	11	6	1	216	1 strch, 1 fat
Roll/Bread Dough, Pizza Crust (1 slice)	89	16	1	<1	174	1 strch
Roll/Bread Dough, Soft Bread Sticks (1)	103	17	2	<1	270	1 strch
Roll/Bun Dough & Icing, Cinnamon (1)	114	17	4	1	268	1 carb., 1 fat
Toaster Strudel Pastries, Apple (1)	180	27	7	2	190	2 carb., 1 fat
Toaster Strudel Pastries, Blueberry (1)	180	26	7	2	200	2 carb., 1 fat
Toaster Strudel Pastries, Cherry (1)	180	27	7	2	200	2 carb., 1 fat
Toaster Strudel Pastries, Cinnamon (1)	190	26	8	2	200	2 carb., 2 fat
Toaster Strudel Pastries, Cream Cheese (1)	190	23	10	4	230	1-1/2 carb., 2 fat

	Cal.	Carb. (g)	Fat (g)	Sat. Fat (g)	Sod. (mg)	Exchanges/Choices
Toaster Strudel Pastries, Cream Cheese & Blueberry (1)	190	24	9	3	220	1-1/2 carb., 2 fat
Toaster Strudel Pastries, Cream Cheese & Strawberry (1)	190	24	9	3	220	1-1/2 carb., 2 fat
Toaster Strudel Pastries, French Toast-Style (1)	190	28	7	2	200	2 carb., 1 fat
Toaster Strudel Pastries, Raspberry (1)	180	26	7	2	200	2 carb., 1 fat
Toaster Strudel Pastries, Strawberry (1)	180	26	7	2	200	2 carb., 1 fat
Turnovers, Flaky Apple (1)	170	22	8	2	331	1-1/2 carb., 2 fat
Turnovers, Flaky Cherry (1)	177	24	8	2	325	1-1/2 carb., 2 fat
PROGRESSO						
Bread Crumbs, Italian-Style (1/4 cup)	110	20	2	0	430	1 strch
Bread Crumbs, Plain (1/4 cup)	100	19	2	0	210	1 strch
SHAKE 'N BAKE						
Coating Mix, BBQ Chicken (1 pkt)	360	72	8	0	3280	5 strch, 1 fat
Coating Mix, BBQ Pork (1 pkt)	280	64	0	0	2000	4 strch
Coating Mix, Honey Mustard (1 pkt)	360	72	8	0	2320	5 strch, 1 fat
Coating Mix, Hot Spicy Chicken (1 pkt)	320	56	8	0	1520	4 strch, 1 fat

BREAD PRODUCTS & BAKED GOODS

Products	Cal.	Carb. (g)	Fat (g)	Sat. Fat (g)	Sodium (mg)	Exchanges
Coating Mix, Hot Spicy Pork (1 pkt)	262	47	3	0	1280	3 strch
Coating Mix, Italian Herb (1 pkt)	320	56	4	0	2400	4 strch
Coating Mix, Mild Country (1 pkt)	280	40	16	8	1920	2-1/2 strch, 3 fat
Coating Mix, Original Chicken (1 pkt)	320	56	8	0	1840	4 strch, 1 fat
Coating Mix, Original Fish (1 pkt)	280	56	6	0	1680	4 strch, 1 fat
Coating Mix, Original Pork (1 pkt)	320	72	0	0	2560	5 strch
Coating Mix, Tangy Honey (1 pkt)	360	80	8	0	2240	5 strch, 1 fat
Potato Mix, Crispy Cheddar (1 pkt)	180	12	12	9	2280	1 strch, 2 fat
Potato Mix, Herb & Garlic (1 pkt)	120	30	0	0	2220	2 strch
STOVE TOP						
Microwave Stuffing, Chicken (1/2 cup)	130	20	4	<1	450	1 strch, 1 fat
Microwave Stuffing, Corn Bread (1/2 cup)	116	19	2	<1	434	1 strch
Stuffing Mix for Beef (1/2 cup)	110	22	1	0	520	1-1/2 strch
Stuffing Mix for Pork (1/2 cup)	110	20	1	0	500	1 strch

Stuffing Mix for Turkey (1/2 cup)	110	20	1	0	490	1 strch
Stuffing Mix, Chicken Flavor (1/2 cup)	110	20	1	0	440	1 strch
Stuffing Mix, Corn Bread (1/2 cup)	110	21	1	0	510	1-1/2 strch
Stuffing Mix, Low-Sodium Chicken (1/2 cup)	110	21	1	0	270	1-1/2 strch
Stuffing Mix, San Francisco (1/2 cup)	110	20	1	0	510	1 strch
Stuffing Mix, Savory Herbs (1/2 cup)	110	20	1	0	510	1 strch
WEIGHT WATCHERS						
Coffee Cake, Cinnamon Streusel (1)	190	35	4	1	190	2 carb., 1 fat
Muffins, Banana Nut (1)	190	32	5	2	280	2 strch, 1 fat
Muffins, Blueberry (1)	250	46	5	1	384	3 strch, 1 fat
Muffins, Chocolate Chocolate Chip (1)	200	39	4	2	250	2-1/2 strch, 1 fat
Muffins, Honey Bran (1)	220	43	4	1	150	3 strch
Rolls, Glazed Cinnamon (1)	200	33	5	2	200	2 carb., 1 fat
WHOLESOME CHOICE						
Bread, Mini Pita Pocket (1)	71	15	0	0	142	1 strch
Bread, White Pita Pocket (1)	150	30	1	0	290	2 strch

CANDY

CANDY

Products	Cal.	Carb. (g)	Fat (g)	Sat. Fat (g)	Sodium (mg)	Exchanges
Almond Roca (1 oz)	122	19	5	3	50	1 carb., 1 fat
Almonds, Chocolate-Coated (1/4 cup)	234	16	18	3	24	1 carb., 4 fat
Almonds, Sugar-Coated (7)	129	20	5	<1	6	1 carb., 1 fat
Butterscotch (5 pieces)	119	29	1	<1	13	2 carb.
Candy Corn (1/4 cup)	179	47	<1	<1	20	3 carb.
Caramel Apple (1 medium)	255	56	4	3	111	1 fruit, 4 carb., 1 fat
Caramels (9 = 1 oz)	271	55	7	5	174	3-1/2 carb., 1 fat
Chewing Gum (1 piece)	14	4	<1	0	<1	free
Chewing Gum, Sugar-Free (1 piece)	11	4	<1	0	<1	free
Cherries, Chocolate-Covered (2)	102	23	3	2	7	1-1/2 carb., 1 fat
Divinity Candy, Homemade (1 oz)	98	25	3	<1	13	1-1/2 carb., 1 fat
Fruit Leather (0.5 oz)	41	11	<1	<1	2	1 carb.
Fudge, Chocolate, Homemade (1 oz)	108	23	3	1	18	1-1/2 carb., 1 fat

Fudge, Chocolate Marshmallow, Homemade (1 oz)	118	20	5	3	29	1 carb., 1 fat
Fudge, Chocolate w/Nuts, Homemade (1 oz)	121	21	5	2	16	1-1/2 carb., 1 fat
Fudge, Vanilla, Homemade (1 oz)	98	22	1	1	18	1-1/2 carb.
Fudge, Vanilla w/Nuts, Homemade (1 oz)	103	18	3	1	15	1 carb., 1 fat
Gumdrops (10 small)	135	35	<1	0	15	2 carb.
Gummy Bears (10 small)	135	35	<1	0	15	2 carb.
Hard Candy, All Flavors (1 oz)	106	28	0	0	11	2 carb.
Jellybeans (10)	40	10	<1	0	3	1/2 carb.
Lollipops (1)	22	6	0	0	2	1/2 carb.
Milk Chocolate Bar w/Almonds (1.5 oz)	216	22	14	7	30	1-1/2 carb., 3 fat
Milk Chocolate Bar w/Peanuts (1.5 oz)	238	17	18	5.2	17	1 carb., 4 fat
Mint Patty, Chocolate-Covered (1 small)	40	9	1	<1	3	1/2 carb.
Peanut Brittle, Homemade (1 oz)	127	19	5	1	127	1 carb., 1 fat
Peanuts, Milk Chocolate-Coated (1/4 cup)	220	21	14	6	18	1-1/2 carb., 3 fat
Peanuts, Yogurt-Covered (1/4 cup)	194	16	13	3	15	1 carb., 3 fat

CANDY

Products	Cal.	Carb. (g)	Fat (g)	Sat. Fat (g)	Sodium (mg)	Exchanges
Penuche Brown Sugar Fudge w/Nuts, Homemade (1 oz)	110	22	2	1	28	1-1/2 carb.
Praline, Homemade (1 oz)	127	17	7	<1	17	1 carb., 1 fat
Raisins, Milk Chocolate-Covered (1/4 cup)	185	33	7	4	17	2 carb., 1 fat
Raisins, Yogurt-Covered (1/4 cup)	190	34	6	4	21	2 carb., 1 fat
Taffy, Homemade (0.5 oz)	56	14	<1	<1	13	1 carb.
Toffee, Homemade (1 oz)	151	19	9	7	51	1 carb., 2 fat
Truffles, Homemade (1 oz)	138	12	9	7	21	1 carb., 2 fat
BREATHSAVERS						
Breath Mints (1)	10	0	0	0	0	free
CADBURY'S						
Caramello Bar (1.6 oz)	220	30	11	NA	55	2 carb., 2 fat
CONCORDE						
Bit-O-Honey Chews (6 = 1.7 oz)	186	39	4	NA	124	2-1/2 carb., 1 fat

DEMET'S						
Turtles (1)	83	10	5	2	16	1/2 carb., 1 fat
ESTEE						
Carmels, Vanilla/Chocolate (5)	150	26	5	1	65	2 carb., 1 fat
Gumdrops (23)	140	36	0	0	0	2-1/2 carb.
Gummy Bears (16)	140	31	0	0	0	2 carb.
Hard Candy, Butterscotch (2)	50	12	0	0	50	1 carb.
Hard Candy, Peppermint (3)	60	14	0	0	0	1 carb.
Lollipops (2)	60	16	0	0	0	1 carb.
Peanut Brittle (1-1/2 oz)	210	28	9	2	115	2 carb., 2 fat
Peanut Butter Cups (5)	200	19	12	5	70	1 carb., 2 fat
Peanuts, Candy-Coated (1/4 cup)	200	23	9	4	45	1-1/2 carb., 2 fat
Raisins, Chocolate-Coated (1/4 cup)	210	19	12	7	45	1 carb., 2 fat
HERSHEY'S						
5th Avenue Bar (2 oz)	261	38	12	NA	104	2-1/2 carb., 2 fat
Chocolate Kisses (6 = 1 oz)	145	17	9	5	23	1 carb., 2 fat

CANDY

Products	Cal.	Carb. (g)	Fat (g)	Sat. Fat (g)	Sodium (mg)	Exchanges
Cookies & Cream Bar (1.6 oz)	270	27	12	6	100	2 carb., 2 fat
Golden Almond Solitaires (3-oz pkg)	455	40	32	NA	46	2-1/2 carb., 6 fat
Golden III Chocolate Bar (3.25 oz)	471	51	30	NA	79	3-1/2 carb., 6 fat
Kit Kat Bar (1.5 oz)	214	26	12	7	42	2 carb., 2 fat
Krackel Bar (1.5 oz)	206	25	11	5	56	1-1/2 carb., 2 fat
Milk Chocolate Bar (1.6 oz)	226	26	14	8	36	2 carb., 3 fat
Milk Chocolate Bar, Symphony (1.5 oz)	219	24	14	NA	36	1-1/2 carb., 3 fat
Mr. Goodbar (1.75 oz)	252	25	16	9	17	1-1/2 carb., 3 fat
Reese's Pieces (1.95-oz pkg)	258	34	11	NA	82	2 carb., 2 fat
Rolos Caramel (10)	260	38	12	NA	93	2-1/2 carb., 2 fat
Skor Bar (1.4 oz)	206	22	13	9	90	1-1/2 carb., 3 fat
Special Dark Sweet Chocolate Bar (1.46 oz)	195	25	12	9	4	1-1/2 carb., 2 fat
Sweet Escapes, Carmel & Peanut Butter (1.4 oz)	150	25	5	2	125	1-1/2 carb., 1 fat
Sweet Escapes, Chocolate Toffee Crisp (1.4 oz)	190	27	8	5	90	2 carb., 2 fat

Sweet Escapes, Triple Chocolate Wafer (1.4 oz)	160	27	5	3	55	2 carb., 1 fat
Whatchamacallit Bar (1.7 oz)	241	28	12	NA	109	2 carb., 2 fat
KRAFT						
Butter Mints (7 = 0.5 oz)	60	14	0	0	25	1 carb.
Caramels (5 = 1.5 oz)	170	32	3	1	110	2 carb., 1 fat
Fudgies (5 = 1.5 oz)	180	32	5	3	90	2 carb., 1 fat
LEAF						
Good & Plenty Licorice (1 oz)	104	26	<1	<1	7	2 carb.
Whoppers Chocolate Malted Milk Balls (10)	144	18	8	5	42	1 carb., 2 fat
M & M MARS						
3 Musketeers Bar (2.16 oz)	251	46	8	4	117	3 carb., 2 fat
Almond Bar (1.8 oz)	234	31	12	5	85	2 carb., 2 fat
Kudos Nutty Fudge Snack Bar (1.3 oz)	200	20	12	NA	55	1 carb., 2 fat
M&M's, Chocolate (1.7-oz pkg)	228	33	11	5	49	2 carb., 2 fat
M&M's, Peanut (1.76-oz pkg)	244	29	13	5	46	2 carb., 3 fat
Milky Way Bar (2.2 oz)	256	44	9	5	146	3 carb., 2 fat

CANDY

Products	Cal.	Carb. (g)	Fat (g)	Sat. Fat (g)	Sodium (mg)	Exchanges
Milky Way Bar (snack size)	75	13	3	1	43	1 carb., 1 fat
Skittles Bite Size (2.3 oz)	260	60	2	NA	30	4 carb.
Snickers Bar (2.1 oz)	267	35	13	7	157	3 carb., 3 fat
Snickers Bar (snack size)	68	9	3	2	40	1/2 carb., 1 fat
Starburst Fruit Chews (6)	232	50	5	NA	33	3 carb., 1 fat
Twix Carmel Cookie Bar (2 oz)	271	37	13	NA	114	2-1/2 carb., 3 fat
Twix Peanut Butter Cookie Bar (1.7 oz, 2 pieces)	245	28	14	NA	143	2 carb., 3 fat
NESTLE						
100 Grand Bar (1.5 oz)	200	30	8	5	75	2 carb., 2 fat
After Eight Mints (1 oz)	119	21	4	2	2	1-1/2 carb., 1 fat
Baby Ruth Bar (2 oz)	281	38	13	6	136	2-1/2 carb., 3 fat
Buncha Crunch Bar (1.4 oz)	200	26	10	5	95	2 carb., 2 fat
Butterfinger BB's (1.7-oz bag)	230	34	10	7	90	2 carb., 2 fat
Butterfinger Bar (2.18 oz)	286	43	11	6	121	3 carb., 2 fat

Item	Cal					Exchanges
Chunky Bar (1.4 oz)	200	22	11	6	20	1-1/2 carb., 2 fat
Crunch Bar (1.4 oz)	198	26	10	6	59	2 carb., 2 fat
Goobers Chocolate-Covered Peanuts (1.4-oz bag)	120	19	13	5	20	1 carb., 3 fat
Milk Chocolate Bar (1 oz)	150	16	9	5	20	1 carb., 2 fat
Nestle Crunch Bar (1.55 oz)	230	28	12	7	60	2 carb., 2 fat
Oh Henry! Bar (2 oz)	246	37	10	4	135	2-1/2 carb., 2 fat
Perugina After Eight Chocolate Mints (5)	190	32	6	4	10	2 carb., 1 fat
Raisinets (1.6 oz)	200	31	8	4	15	2 carb., 2 fat
Turtles Caramel Chocolate (2 = 1.2 oz)	160	20	9	3	30	1 carb., 2 fat
PEARSON						
Nips, Caramel (4 = 1 oz)	122	24	3	3	81	1-1/2 carb., 1 fat
Nips, Chocolate Parfait (4 = 1 oz)	122	22	4	4	71	1-1/2 carb., 1 fat
Nips, Coffee (6 = 1 oz)	130	26	3	2	97	2 carb., 1 fat
Nips, Licorice (1 oz)	120	24	3	3	80	1-1/2 carb., 1 fat
Nips, Peanut Butter Parfait (1 oz)	120	22	4	4	80	1-1/2 carb., 1 fat

CANDY

Products	Cal.	Carb. (g)	Fat (g)	Sat. Fat (g)	Sodium (mg)	Exchanges
PETER PAUL						
Almond Joy Bar (1.75 oz)	227	29	14	8	66	2 carb., 3 fat
Mounds Bar (1.9 oz)	191	31	11	6	66	2 carb., 2 fat
PLANTER'S						
Peanut Bar (3.6 oz)	522	47	34	4	241	3 carb., 7 fat
REESE'S						
Peanut Butter Cups (2 = 1.6 oz)	218	22	14	10	131	1-1/2 carb., 3 fat
TOOTSIE ROLL						
Tootsie Rolls (7 bite-size)	126	31	<1	<1	9	2 carb.
Y & S						
Nibs Cherry (2 oz)	212	52	1	NA	134	3-1/2 carb.
Twizzlers Strawberry (2.5-oz pkg)	263	66	1	NA	197	4-1/2 carb.
YORK						
Peppermint Patty (large, 1.5 oz)	145	33	4	NA	16	2 carb., 1 fat

CEREALS

Products	Cal.	Carb. (g)	Fat (g)	Sat. Fat (g)	Sodium (mg)	Exchanges
Bulgur (1/2 cup)	76	17	<1	0	5	1 strch
Corn Grits, White or Yellow, Cooked (1/2 cup)	73	16	<1	<1	0	1 strch
Corn Grits, White, Cooked (1 pkt)	82	18	<1	<1	343	1 strch
Cream of Rice, Cooked (1/2 cup)	64	14	<1	<1	1	1 strch
Cream of Rye, Cooked (1/2 cup)	54	12	<1	<1	175	1 strch
Cream of Wheat, Cooked (1/2 cup)	66	14	<1	<1	71	1 strch
Farina Cereal, Cooked (1/2 cup)	59	25	<1	<1	0	1-1/2 strch
Farina, Cooked (1/2 cup)	59	13	<1	<1	0	1 strch
Granola, Homemade (1 cup)	594	67	33	6	12	4-1/2 strch, 6 fat
Honey Bran Cereal (1 cup)	119	29	<1	<1	202	2 strch
Kasha or Buckwheat Groats, Cooked (1/2 cup)	91	20	<1	<1	4	1 strch
Millet, Cooked (1/4 cup)	72	14	<1	<1	1	1 strch

CEREALS

Products	Cal.	Carb. (g)	Fat (g)	Sat. Fat (g)	Sodium (mg)	Exchanges
Multi-Grain Cereal, Cooked (1/2 cup)	100	20	1	<1	380	1 strch
Oatmeal Cereal, Cooked (1/2 cup)	73	13	1	<1	1	1 strch
Wheatena, Cooked (1/2 cup)	68	15	<1	<1	3	1 strch
GENERAL MILLS						
Basic 4 (1 cup)	210	42	3	0	330	3 strch
Cheerios (1-1/4 cup)	111	20	2	<1	307	1 strch
Cheerios, Apple Cinnamon (3/4 cup)	120	25	2	0	160	1-1/2 strch
Cheerios, Honey Nut (1 cup)	125	27	<1	<1	299	2 strch
Cheerios, Multi-Grain (1 cup)	110	24	1	0	240	1-1/2 strch
Cinnamon Toast Crunch (3/4 cup)	130	24	4	<1	210	1-1/2 strch
Crispy Wheat 'N Raisins (1 cup)	150	35	<1	<1	204	2 strch
Fiber One (1/2 cup)	91	23	1	<1	133	1-1/2 strch
French Toast Crunch (3/4 cup)	120	26	2	0	170	2 strch
Golden Grahams (1 cup)	150	33	2	1	385	2 strch

Honey Nut Clusters (1 cup)	210	46	3	0	270	3 strch
Hot Oats Cereal (1/2 cup)	148	27	3	<1	1	2 strch
Kix (1 1/3 cup)	120	26	<1	0	270	1-1/2 strch
Kix, Berry Berry (3/4 cup)	120	26	1	0	170	2 strch
Lucky Charms (1 cup)	120	25	1	0	210	1-1/2 strch
Oatmeal Crisp w/Raisins (1 cup)	210	44	3	0	210	3 strch
Raisin Bran (1 cup)	180	43	1	0	240	3 strch
Raisin Nut Bran (1 cup)	221	42	6	1	302	3 strch
Total Corn Flakes (1 cup)	126	28	<1	<1	217	2 strch
Total Whole-Grain (1 cup)	116	26	<1	<1	326	2 strch
Trix (1 cup)	120	26	2	0	200	2 strch
Wheaties (1 cup)	110	24	1	0	220	1-1/2 strch
Wheaties, Honey-Frosted (3/4 cup)	110	24	1	0	200	1-1/2 strch
HEALTH VALLEY						
Fat-Free Crisp Brown Rice, Honey (1 cup)	110	30	0	0	0	2 strch
Fat-Free Puffed Corn, Honey (1 cup)	80	20	0	0	0	1 strch

CEREALS

Products	Cal.	Carb. (g)	Fat (g)	Sat. Fat (g)	Sodium (mg)	Exchanges
Fat-Free Granola O's, Almond (3/4 cup)	120	26	0	0	10	2 strch
Fat-Free Granola O's, Apple Cinnamon (3/4 cup)	120	26	0	0	10	2 strch
Fat-Free Granola O's, Honey Crunch (3/4 cup)	120	26	0	0	10	2 strch
KASHI						
Kashi (1/2 cup)	170	30	3	0	15	2 strch
Kashi Medley (1/2 cup)	100	20	1	0	50	1 strch
Puffed Kashi (1 cup)	70	13	<1	0	0	1 strch
KELLOGG'S						
All-Bran (1/2 cup)	80	22	1	0	280	1-1/2 strch
All-Bran w/Extra Fiber (1/2 cup)	50	22	1	0	150	1-1/2 strch
Apple Cinnamon Squares (3/4 cup)	180	44	1	0	15	3 strch
Apple Jacks (1 cup)	110	27	0	0	135	2 strch
Apple Raisin Crisp (1 cup)	180	46	0	0	340	3 strch
Blueberry Squares (3/4 cup)	180	44	1	0	15	3 strch

Bran Buds (1/3 cup)	70	24	1	0	210	1-1/2 strch
Cinnamon Mini Buns (3/4 cup)	120	27	<1	0	210	2 strch
Cocoa Krispies (3/4 cup)	120	27	<1	0	190	2 strch
Common Sense Oat Bran (3/4 cup)	110	23	1	0	270	1-1/2 strch
Complete Bran Flakes (3/4 cup)	100	25	<1	0	230	1-1/2 strch
Corn Flakes (1 cup)	110	26	0	0	330	2 strch
Corn Pops (1 cup)	110	27	0	0	95	2 strch
Cracklin' Oat Bran (3/4 cup)	230	40	8	3	180	2-1/2 strch, 2 fat
Crispix (1 cup)	110	26	0	0	230	2 strch
Double Dip Crunch (3/4 cup)	110	27	0	0	160	2 strch
Froot Loops (1 cup)	120	26	1	<1	150	2 strch
Frosted Bran (3/4 cup)	100	26	0	0	200	2 strch
Frosted Flakes (3/4 cup)	120	28	0	0	200	2 strch
Frosted Krispies (3/4 cup)	110	27	0	0	230	2 strch
Frosted Mini-Wheats (1 cup)	190	45	1	0	0	3 strch
Frosted Mini-Wheats, Bite Size (1 cup)	190	45	1	0	0	3 strch

CEREALS

Products	Cal.	Carb. (g)	Fat (g)	Sat. Fat (g)	Sodium (mg)	Exchanges
Fruitful Bran (1-1/4 cup)	170	44	1	0	330	3 strch
Fruity Marshmallow Krispies (3/4 cup)	110	27	0	0	180	2 strch
Healthy Choice Multi-Grain Flakes (1 cup)	100	25	0	0	210	1-1/2 strch
Healthy Choice Multi-Grain Squares (1-1/4 cup)	190	45	1	0	0	3 strch
Healthy Choice Multi-Grain Raisins, Crunchy Oat	200	45	2	0	240	3 strch
Clusters & Almonds						
Just Right w/Crunchy Nuggets (1 cup)	200	46	2	0	340	3 strch
Just Right w/Fruit & Nut (1 cup)	210	46	2	0	288	3 strch
Low-Fat Granola (1/2 cup)	210	43	3	<1	120	3 strch
Low-Fat Granola w/Raisins (2/3 cup)	210	43	3	3	135	3 strch
Mueslix Crispy Blend (2/3 cup)	200	42	3	0	190	3 strch
Mueslix Golden Crunch (3/4 cup)	210	40	5	1	280	2-1/2 strch, 1 fat
Nut & Honey Crunch (1-1/4 cup)	220	45	4	1	370	3 strch
Nut & Honey Crunch O's (3/4 cup)	120	23	3	0	200	1-1/2 strch, 1 fat

Nutri-Grain Almond Raisin (1-1/4 cup)	200	44	3	0	330	3 strch
Nutri-Grain Golden Wheat (3/4 cup)	100	24	<1	0	240	1-1/2 strch
Nutri-Grain Golden Wheat & Raisin (1-1/4 cup)	180	45	1	0	310	3 strch
Pop-Tarts Crunch Frosted Brown Sugar Cinnamon (3/4 cup)	120	26	1	0	160	2 strch
Pop-Tarts Crunch Frosted Strawberry (3/4 cup)	120	27	1	0	125	2 strch
Product 19 (1 cup)	110	25	0	0	280	1-1/2 strch
Raisin Bran (1 cup)	170	43	1	0	310	3 strch
Raisin Squares (3/4 cup)	180	44	1	0	0	3 strch
Rice Krispies (1-1/4 cup)	110	26	0	0	320	2 strch
Rice Krispies, Apple Cinnamon (3/4 cup)	110	27	0	0	220	2 strch
Rice Krispies Treats (3/4 cup)	120	25	2	0	170	1-1/2 strch
Smacks (3/4 cup)	110	26	<1	0	75	2 strch
Special K (1 cup)	110	21	0	0	250	1-1/2 strch
Strawberry Squares (3/4 cup)	180	44	1	0	10	3 strch
Temptations French Vanilla Almond (3/4 cup)	120	24	2	1	210	1-1/2 strch

CEREALS

Products	Cal.	Carb. (g)	Fat (g)	Sat. Fat (g)	Sodium (mg)	Exchanges
Temptations Honey-Roasted Pecan (1 cup)	120	24	3	0	240	1-1/2 strch, 1 fat
MALT-O-MEAL						
Bran Flakes (3/4 cup)	100	24	<1	0	210	1-1/2 strch
Cocoa Comets (3/4 cup)	120	27	1	0	190	2 strch
Corn Bursts (1 cup)	110	27	0	0	95	2 strch
Corn Flakes (1 cup)	110	26	0	0	310	2 strch
Crispy Rice (1 cup)	110	26	0	0	250	2 strch
Frosted Flakes (3/4 cup)	110	27	0	0	200	2 strch
Golden Puffs (3/4 cup)	120	26	0	0	40	2 strch
Hot Wheat Cereal, Chocolate (3 Tbsp dry)	120	28	0	0	0	2 strch
Hot Wheat Cereal, Maple & Brown Sugar (3 Tbsp dry)	120	28	0	0	0	2 strch
Hot Wheat Cereal, Quick (3 Tbsp dry)	120	26	0	0	0	2 strch
Puffed Rice (1 cup)	60	13	0	0	0	1 strch
Puffed Wheat (1 cup)	44	11	0	0	0	1 strch

	Calories	Carbohydrate (g)	Fat (g)	Saturated Fat (g)	Sodium (mg)	Exchanges
Raisin Bran (1 cup)	180	43	1	0	260	3 strch
Toasty O's (1 cup)	110	22	2	0	280	1-1/2 strch
Toasty O's, Apple & Cinnamon (3/4 cup)	120	24	2	0	190	1-1/2 strch
Toasty O's, Honey & Nut (1 cup)	110	24	1	0	270	1-1/2 strch
Tootie Fruities (1 cup)	110	26	1	0	150	2 strch
NABISCO						
100% Bran Cereal (1/3 cup)	80	23	<1	0	120	1-1/2 strch
Frosted Wheat Bites (1 cup)	190	44	1	0	10	3 strch
Fruit Wheat Raspberry Cereal (3/4 cup)	160	40	<1	0	15	2-1/2 strch
Shredded Wheat (2 biscuits)	160	38	<1	0	0	2-1/2 strch
Shredded Wheat, Spoon-Size (1 cup)	170	41	<1	0	0	3 strch
Shredded Wheat & Bran (1-1/4 cup)	200	47	1	0	0	3 strch
Team Flakes (1-1/4 cup)	220	49	0	0	360	3 strch
NATURE VALLEY						
Granola (1 cup)	503	76	20	13	233	5 strch, 3 fat
Granola, Fruit & Nut (1 oz)	130	18	6	1	40	1 strch, 1 fat

CEREALS

Products	Cal.	Carb. (g)	Fat (g)	Sat. Fat (g)	Sodium (mg)	Exchanges
Granola, Cinnamon Raisin (1 oz)	121	20	4	<1	45	1 strch, 1 fat
Granola, LoFat w/Fruit (1 oz)	109	23	1	<1	105	1-1/2 strch
Granola, Toasted Oat (1 oz)	128	19	5	<1	46	1 strch, 1 fat
POST						
100% Bran Cereal (1/2 cup)	89	24	2	<1	229	1-1/2 strch
Alpha-Bits (1 cup)	130	27	1	0	210	2 strch
Banana Nut Crunch (1 cup)	250	43	6	1	200	3 strch, 1 fat
Blueberry Morning (1-1/4 cup)	230	45	4	<1	250	3 strch
Bran Flakes (1 cup)	152	37	<1	<1	431	2-1/2 strch
Bran'ola, Original (1/2 cup)	200	43	3	<1	240	3 strch
Bran'ola, Raisin (1/2 cup)	200	44	3	<1	220	3 strch
Cocoa Pebbles (3/4 cup)	120	25	1	1	160	1-1/2 strch
Corn Toasties (1 cup)	100	24	0	0	270	1-1/2 strch
Cranberry Almond Crunch (1 cup)	220	43	4	0	200	3 strch

Fruit & Fiber, Peach/Raisin/Almond (1 cup)	210	46	3	<1	270	3 strch
Fruit & Fiber, Raisin/Walnut (1 cup)	210	46	3	<1	260	3 strch
Fruity Pebbles (3/4 cup)	110	24	1	<1	150	1-1/2 strch
Grape Nuts (1/2 cup)	200	47	1	0	350	3 strch
Grape Nuts Flakes (3/4 cup)	105	24	1	0	140	1-1/2 strch
Great Grains Crunchy Cereal (2/3 cup)	220	38	6	1	150	2-1/2 strch, 1 fat
Great Grains, Raisin/Date/Pecan (2/3 cup)	210	39	5	<1	150	2-1/2 strch, 1 fat
Hearty Granola (2/3 cup)	280	45	9	1	150	3 strch, 1 fat
Honey Bunches of Oats (3/4 cup)	130	24	3	<1	180	1-1/2 strch, 1 fat
Honey Bunches of Oats & Almonds (3/4 cup)	130	24	3	<1	180	1-1/2 strch, 1 fat
Honeycombs (1 cup)	86	20	<1	<1	124	1 strch
Marshmallow Alpha-Bits (1 cup)	120	25	1	0	160	1-1/2 strch
Raisin Bran (1 cup)	190	46	1	0	300	3 strch
Super Golden Crisp (3/4 cup)	110	25	0	0	40	1-1/2 strch
Toasties Corn Flakes (1 cup)	93	21	<1	<1	252	1-1/2 strch
Waffle Crisp (1 cup)	130	24	3	0	120	1-1/2 strch

CEREALS

Products	Cal.	Carb. (g)	Fat (g)	Sat. Fat (g)	Sodium (mg)	Exchanges
QUAKER						
100% Natural Crispy Whole-Grain w/Raisins, Low-Fat (1/2 cup)	190	40	3	1	95	2-1/2 strch, 1 fat
100% Natural Honey & Raisins (1/2 cup)	220	35	8	4	20	2 strch, 2 fat
100% Natural Oats & Honey (1/2 cup)	220	32	8	4	25	2 strch, 2 fat
100% Natural w/Apple & Cinnamon (1/2 cup)	239	35	10	8	26	2 strch, 2 fat
100% Natural w/Raisins & Dates (1/2 cup)	248	36	10	7	24	2 strch, 2 fat
Cap'n Crunch (3/4 cup)	110	23	2	0	210	1-1/2 strch
Cap'n Crunch w/Crunchberries (3/4 cup)	100	22	2	0	190	1-1/2 strch
Cap'n Crunch's Peanut Butter (3/4 cup)	110	21	3	<1	210	1-1/2 strch, 1 fat
Cinnamon Oat Squares (1 cup)	230	48	3	<1	260	3 strch
Corn Bran (1 cup)	125	30	1	<1	310	2 strch
Crunchy Bran (3/4 cup)	90	23	1	0	250	1-1/2 strch
Honey Graham O's (3/4 cup)	110	23	2	<1	180	1-1/2 strch

Item	Cal				Sod	Exchanges
Instant Hot Oatmeal (1 pkt)	130	22	3	<1	95	1-1/2 strch, 1 fat
Instant Hot Oatmeal, Apple & Cinnamon (1 pkt)	130	26	2	<1	105	2 strch
Instant Hot Oatmeal, Apple, Raisin, & Walnut (1 pkt)	140	27	3	<1	160	2 strch, 1 fat
Instant Hot Oatmeal, Blueberry & Cream (1 pkt)	130	27	3	<1	140	2 strch, 1 fat
Instant Hot Oatmeal, Cinnamon Graham Cookie (1 pkt)	150	30	3	<1	170	2 strch, 1 fat
Instant Hot Oatmeal, Cinnamon Spice (1 pkt)	170	36	2	0	290	2-1/2 strch
Instant Hot Oatmeal, Cinnamon Toast (1 pkt)	130	27	2	0	160	2 strch
Instant Hot Oatmeal, Honey Nut (1 pkt)	130	25	3	<1	210	1-1/2 strch, 1 fat
Instant Hot Oatmeal, Maple/Brown Sugar (1 pkt)	160	33	2	<1	240	2 strch
Instant Hot Oatmeal, Peaches & Cream (1 pkt)	130	27	2	<1	150	2 strch
Instant Hot Oatmeal, Radical Raspberry (1 pkt)	150	29	3	<1	170	2 strch, 1 fat
Instant Hot Oatmeal, Raisin/Date/Walnut (1 pkt)	130	27	3	<1	240	2 strch, 1 fat
Instant Hot Oatmeal, Raisin Spice (1 pkt)	160	32	2	<1	250	2 strch
Instant Hot Oatmeal, Strawberries & Cream (1 pkt)	130	27	2	<1	160	2 strch
Instant Hot Oatmeal, Strawberries 'N Stuff (1 pkt)	150	30	2	<1	170	2 strch

CEREALS

Products	Cal.	Carb. (g)	Fat (g)	Sat. Fat (g)	Sodium (mg)	Exchanges
King Vitamin (1-1/2 cup)	120	26	1	0	260	2 strch
Kretschmer Honey Crunch Wheat Germ (1-2/3 Tbsp)	50	8	1	0	0	1/2 strch
Kretschmer Toasted Wheat Bran (1/4 cup)	30	10	1	0	0	1/2 strch
Kretschmer Wheat Germ (2 Tbsp)	50	6	1	0	0	1/2 strch
Life (3/4 cup)	120	25	2	0	170	1-1/2 strch
Life, Cinnamon (1 cup)	190	39	2	0	220	2-1/2 strch
Life, Cinnamon (3/4 cup)	120	26	1	0	140	2 strch
Mother's Hot Oat Bran (1/2 cup)	150	24	3	1	0	1-1/2 strch, 1 fat
Mother's Instant Hot Oatmeal (1/2 cup)	150	27	3	<1	0	2 strch, 1 fat
Mother's Multi-Grain Hot Cereal (1/2 cup)	130	29	2	0	10	2 strch
Mother's Whole-Wheat Natural Hot Cereal (1/2 cup)	130	30	1	0	0	2 strch
Oat Bran (1-1/4 cup)	210	41	3	<1	210	3 strch
Oat Squares (1 cup)	220	44	3	<1	260	3 strch
Old-Fashioned Hot Oats (1/2 cup)	150	27	3	<1	0	2 strch, 1 fat

Food	Calories	Carbs	Fat		Sodium	Exchanges
Popeye Cocoa Blasts (1 cup)	130	29	2	<1	125	2 strch
Popeye Fruit Curls (1 cup)	120	27	1	0	170	2 strch
Popeye Jeepers (1-1/3 cup)	110	24	1	0	140	1-1/2 strch
Popeye Oat'mmms (1 cup)	120	25	2	<1	300	1-1/2 strch
Popeye Sweet Crunch (1 cup)	110	23	2	<1	190	1-1/2 strch
Puffed Rice (1 cup)	50	12	0	0	0	1 strch
Puffed Wheat (1-1/4 cup)	50	11	0	0	0	1 strch
Quick Hot Oats (1/2 cup)	150	27	3	<1	0	2 strch, 1 fat
Quisp (1 cup)	124	25	2	2	241	1-1/2 strch
Shredded Wheat (3 biscuits)	220	50	2	<1	0	3 strch
Sun Country Granola, Almond (1/2 cup)	270	38	9	2	20	2-1/2 strch, 2 fat
Sun Country Granola, Raisin & Date (1/2 cup)	260	43	8	1	15	3 strch, 1 fat
Sweet Puffs (1 cup)	130	30	<1	0	80	2 strch
Toasted Oatmeal, Honey Nut (1 cup)	200	37	5	1	180	2-1/2 strch, 1 fat
Toasted Oatmeal, Original (3/4 cup)	120	25	1	0	210	1-1/2 strch
Unprocessed Bran (1/3 cup)	30	11	0	0	0	1 strch

CEREALS

Products	Cal.	Carb. (g)	Fat (g)	Sat. Fat (g)	Sodium (mg)	Exchanges
RALSTON						
Chex, 100% Whole-Wheat (3/4 cup)	190	41	1	0	390	2 strch
Chex, Bran (1 cup)	156	39	1	<1	455	2-1/2 strch
Chex, Corn (1-1/4 cup)	110	26	0	0	270	2 strch
Chex, Double (1-1/4 cup)	120	27	0	0	230	2 strch
Chex, Multi-Bran (1-1/4 cup)	220	48	1	0	300	3 strch
Chex, Rice (1 cup)	120	27	0	0	230	2 strch
Chex, Wheat (1 cup)	169	38	1	<1	308	2-1/2 strch
Cookie Crisp Multi-Grain Chocolate Chip (1 cup)	120	25	2	0	110	1-1/2 strch
Honey Almond Delight (1 cup)	210	41	3	0	410	3 strch
Hot Cereal (1 cup)	134	28	<1	<1	5	2 strch
Muesli, Blueberry Pecan (1 cup)	200	41	3	2	170	2 strch, 1 fat
Muesli, Cranberry Walnut (3/4 cup)	200	40	3		180	2-1/2 strch, 1 fat
Muesli, Peach Pecan (3/4 cup)	200	39	3	0	170	2-1/2 strch, 1 fat

Muesli, Raspberry Almond (3/4 cup)	220	44	3	0	170	3 strch
Muesli, Strawberry Pecan (1 cup)	210	42	3	0	170	3 strch
Sun Flakes (3/4 cup)	110	23	1	0	210	1-1/2 strch
Tasteeos (1 cup)	94	19	<1	<1	183	1 strch

CHEESE AND CHEESE PRODUCTS

CHEESE AND CHEESE PRODUCTS

Products	Cal.	Carb. (g)	Fat (g)	Sat. Fat (g)	Sodium (mg)	Exchanges
American Processed (1 oz)	106	<1	9	6	406	1 high-fat meat
Cheddar (1 oz)	114	<1	9	6	176	1 high-fat meat
Cheddar/Colby, Low-Fat (1 oz)	49	<1	2	2	174	1 lean meat
Cheese, Fat-Free (1 oz)	37	3	0	0	384	1 very lean meat
Colby & Monterey Jack (1 oz)	110	0	9	6	190	1 high-fat meat
Cottage Cheese, 2%, Low-Fat (1/4 cup)	50	2	1	<1	227	1 very lean meat
Cottage Cheese, 4.5% (1/4 cup)	54	1	2	2	213	1 lean meat
Cottage Cheese, Dry (1/4 cup)	31	<1	<1	<1	5	1 very lean meat
Cottage Cheese, Nonfat (1/4 cup)	35	3	0	0	210	1 very lean meat
Feta (1 oz)	74	1	6	4	313	1 med-fat meat
Goat Cheese, Semi-Soft (1 oz)	103	<1	9	6	146	1 high-fat meat
Monterey Jack (1 oz)	106	0	9	5	152	1 high-fat meat
Mozzarella, Light (1 oz)	65	0	3	2	180	1 lean meat

Mozzarella, Part-Skim (1 oz)	72	<1	5	3	132	1 med-fat meat
Parmesan, Grated (2 Tbsp)	46	<1	3	2	186	1 lean meat
Ricotta, Part-Skim (1/4 cup)	86	3	5	3	78	1 med-fat meat
String Cheese Stick (1)	72	<1	5	3	132	1 med-fat meat
Swiss (1 oz)	107	1	8	5	74	1 high-fat meat
Yogurt Cheese (1 oz)	22	3	<1	<1	22	free
ALPINE LACE						
American (1/4 cup)	89	2	7	4	221	1 high-fat meat
Cheddar, Reduced-Fat (1/4 cup)	89	1	5	3	105	1 med-fat meat
Cheese Product, Fat-Free (1/4 cup)	44	2	0	0	310	1 very lean meat
Cheese Product, Fat-Free, Mozzarella (1/4 cup)	44	2	0	0	310	1 very lean meat
Cheese Product, Fat-Free, Parmesan (1/4 cup)	44	2	0	0	388	1 very lean meat
Colby, Reduced-Fat (1/4 cup)	89	1	6	3	127	1 med-fat meat
Cream Cheese, Fat-Free (2 Tbsp)	34	1	0	0	154	1 very lean meat
Provolone, Reduced-Fat (1/4 cup)	78	1	6	3	133	1 med-fat meat
Swiss, Reduced-Fat (1/4 cup)	100	1	7	4	39	1 high-fat meat

CHEESE AND CHEESE PRODUCTS

Products	Cal.	Carb. (g)	Fat (g)	Sat. Fat (g)	Sodium (mg)	Exchanges
Monterey Jack, Reduced-Fat (1/4 cup)	78	1	5	3	188	1 med-fat meat
Muenster, Reduced-Sodium (1/4 cup)	111	1	10	6	94	1 high-fat meat
BREAKSTONE						
Ricotta (1/4 cup)	110	3	8	5	90	1 high-fat meat
Cottage Cheese, 2% Low-Fat, Small Curd (1/2 cup)	90	4	3	2	380	2 lean meat
Cottage Cheese, 4% Cream, Large Curd (1/2 cup)	120	4	5	4	400	2 lean meat
Cottage Cheese, 4% Cream, Small Curd (1/2 cup)	120	4	5	4	400	2 lean meat
DI GIORNO						
100% Romano, Grated (2 Tbsp)	25	0	2	1	90	free
100% Romano, Shredded (2 Tbsp)	20	0	2	1	70	free
100% Parmesan, Shredded (2 Tbsp)	20	0	2	1	90	free
HEALTHY CHOICE						
Cream Cheese, Fat-Free (2 Tbsp)	34	2	0	0	NA	1 very lean meat
Cream Cheese, Fat-Free, Herb & Garlic (2 Tbsp)	34	2	0	0	NA	1 very lean meat

Food	Calories					Exchange
Cream Cheese, Fat-Free, Strawberry (2 Tbsp)	34	2	0	0	NA	1 very lean meat
Natural Cheddar, Fat-Free, Shredded (1/4 cup)	45	1	0	0	220	1 very lean meat
KNUDSEN						
Cottage Cheese, 2% Low-Fat (1/2 cup)	100	3	3	2	400	2 very lean meat
Cottage Cheese, Nonfat (1/2 cup)	80	4	0	0	370	2 very lean meat
Creamed Cottage Cheese, 4%, Large Curd (1/2 cup)	130	3	5	4	340	2 lean meat
Creamed Cottage Cheese, 4%, Small Curd (1/2 cup)	120	2	5	4	400	2 lean meat
KRAFT						
American Cheese, Old English Sharp Pasteurized Processed (1 oz)	100	<1	9	6	440	1 high-fat meat
American Cheese Product, Harvest Moon (1 slice)	50	1	3	2	280	1 lean meat
American Cheese Spread, Harvest Moon (2/3 oz)	60	2	4	3	270	1 med-fat meat
American Pasteurized Processed Cheese (3/4 oz)	70	1	5	3	350	1 med-fat meat
American Pasteurized Processed Cheese, Light 'N' Lively (3/4 oz)	50	2	3	2	280	1 lean meat

CHEESE AND CHEESE PRODUCTS

Products	Cal.	Carb. (g)	Fat (g)	Sat. Fat (g)	Sodium (mg)	Exchanges
American Pasteurized Processed Cheese, Light 'N' Lively, White (3/4 oz)	50	2	3	2	300	1 lean meat
Baby Swiss (1 oz)	110	0	9	6	110	1 high-fat meat
Blue Cheese, Cold Pack (1 oz)	100	<1	8	6	390	1 high-fat meat
Blue Cheese Crumbles (1 oz)	100	<1	8	6	390	1 high-fat meat
Brick (1 oz)	110	0	9	6	190	1 high-fat meat
Cheddar (1 oz)	110	<1	9	6	180	1 high-fat meat
Cheddar, Natural LoFat (1 oz)	80	0	5	4	220	1 med-fat meat
Cheddar, Shredded (1/4 cup)	120	<1	10	6	190	1 high-fat meat
Chedder, Cracker Barrel Low-Fat Sharp (1 oz)	80	<1	5	3	220	1 med-fat meat
Cheddar, Kraft LoFat Mild, Shredded (1/4 cup)	90	<1	6	4	NA	1 med-fat meat
Cheddar, Kraft LoFat Natural Sharp (1 oz)	80	<1	5	4	220	1 med-fat meat
Cheddar Cold Cheese Food, Cracker Barrel Sharp (2 Tbsp)	100	4	8	5	290	1 high-fat meat

Cheddar Cold Cheese Food, Cracker Barrel Xtra Sharp (2 Tbsp)	100	3	8	0	290	1 high-fat meat
Cheese Food w/Garlic, Pasteurized Processed (1 oz)	90	2	7	5	370	1 high-fat meat
Cheese Food w/Jalapeño, Mexican, Pasteurized Processed (1 slice)	70	2	5	4	330	1 med-fat meat
Cheese Food w/Jalapeño, Pasteurized Processed (1 oz)	90	2	7	5	370	1 high-fat meat
Cheese Spread, Pimento (2 Tbsp)	80	3	6	4	170	1 med-fat meat
Cheese Spread, Pineapple (2 Tbsp)	70	4	5	4	120	1 med-fat meat
Cheese Spread w/Bacon, Pasteurized Processed (2 Tbsp)	90	<1	8	5	570	1 high-fat meat
Cheez Whiz Light Pasteurized Processed Cheese (2 Tbsp)	80	6	3	2	540	1/2 carb., 1 lean meat
Cheez Whiz Pasteurized Processed Cheese Spread (2 Tbsp)	90	2	7	5	560	1 med-fat meat

CHEESE AND CHEESE PRODUCTS

Products	Cal.	Carb. (g)	Fat (g)	Sat. Fat (g)	Sodium (mg)	Exchanges
Cheez Whiz Salsa Cheese Spread, Hot (2 Tbsp)	90	2	7	5	540	1 high-fat meat
Cheez Whiz Salsa Cheese Spread, Mild (2 Tbsp)	90	2	7	5	530	1 high-fat meat
Cheez Whiz Squeezable Cheese Sauce (2 Tbsp)	100	4	8	4	470	2 fat
Cheez Whiz Zap-a-Pack Cheese Sauce (2 Tbsp)	90	3	8	5	580	1 high-fat meat
Colby (1 oz)	110	<1	9	6	180	1 high-fat meat
Colby, Natural LoFat (1 oz)	80	0	5	4	220	1 med-fat meat
Colby & Monterey Jack, Shredded (1/4 cup)	120	<1	10	6	200	1 high-fat meat
Cottage Cheese, 1% Low-Fat (1/2 cup)	80	4	2	1	380	2 very lean meat
Cottage Cheese, 2% Low-Fat (1/2 cup)	90	4	3	2	380	2 very lean meat
Cottage Cheese, Free Nonfat (1/2 cup)	80	5	0	0	440	2 very lean meat
Cottage Cheese w/Skim Milk, Dry Curd (1/4 cup)	45	3	0	0	25	1 very lean meat
Cream Cheese, Philadelphia Brick (1 oz)	100	<1	10	6	90	2 fat
Cream Cheese, Philadelphia Free Nonfat (2 Tbsp)	30	2	0	0	180	1 very lean meat
Cream Cheese, Philadelphia Soft (2 Tbsp)	100	1	10	7	100	2 fat

Cream Cheese, Philadelphia Soft, Chive & Onion (2 Tbsp)	110	2	10	7	110	2 fat
Cream Cheese, Philadelphia Soft, Herb & Garlic (2 Tbsp)	110	2	10	7	180	2 fat
Cream Cheese, Philadelphia Soft, Light (2 Tbsp)	70	2	5	4	150	1 fat
Cream Cheese, Philadelphia Soft, Olive & Pimento (2 Tbsp)	100	2	9	6	170	2 fat
Cream Cheese, Philadelphia Soft, Pineapple (2 Tbsp)	100	4	9	6	100	2 fat
Cream Cheese, Philadelphia Soft, Smoked Salmon (2 Tbsp)	100	1	9	6	200	2 fat
Cream Cheese, Philadelphia Soft, Strawberry (2 Tbsp)	100	5	9	6	65	2 fat
Cream Cheese, Philadelphia Whipped (3 Tbsp)	100	1	11	7	95	2 fat
Cream Cheese w/Chives, Philadelphia Brick (1 oz)	90	<1	9	6	150	2 fat
Cream Cheese w/Pimento, Philadelphia Brick (1 oz)	90	<1	9	6	150	2 fat

CHEESE AND CHEESE PRODUCTS

Products	Cal.	Carb. (g)	Fat (g)	Sat. Fat (g)	Sodium (mg)	Exchanges
Farmers Cheese (1 oz)	100	<1	8	6	190	1 high-fat meat
Four-Cheese Pizza-Style, Shredded (1/4 cup)	90	<1	7	5	230	1 high-fat meat
Gouda (1 oz)	110	<1	9	6	160	1 high-fat meat
Havarti (1 oz)	120	0	11	7	240	1 high-fat meat
Italian Blend, Grated (2 tsp)	25	0	2	1	95	free
Jalapeño Pepper Cheese Spread (2 Tbsp)	89	2	7	4	520	1 high-fat meat
Limburger (1 oz)	90	0	8	5	240	1 high-fat meat
Limburger Cheese Spread, Mohawk Valley (2 Tbsp)	80	0	7	5	500	1 high-fat meat
Monterey Jack (1 oz)	110	0	9	6	190	1 high-fat meat
Monterey Jack, Natural LoFat (1 oz)	80	0	5	4	220	1 med-fat meat
Monterey Jack, Shredded (1/4 cup)	110	<1	9	6	200	1 high-fat meat
Monterey Jack & Pepper, Low-Fat Natural (1 oz)	80	<1	5	4	220	1 med-fat meat
Monterey Jack & Jalapeño Pepper (1 oz)	110	<1	9	6	190	1 high-fat meat
Mozzarella, Fat-Free Natural, Shredded (1/4 cup)	50	2	0	0	280	1 very lean meat

Mozzarella, Imitation, Shredded (1/4 cup)	110	1	8	2	430	1 high-fat meat
Mozzarella, Whole-Milk, Shredded (1/4 cup)	90	<1	7	5	210	1 high-fat meat
Mozzarella, Part-Skim (1 oz)	80	<1	5	4	200	1 med-fat meat
Mozzarella, Part-Skim, String Cheese (1 piece)	80	<1	6	4	240	1 med-fat meat
Muenster (1 oz)	110	0	9	6	190	1 high-fat meat
Nacho Blend Cheese w/Peppers (1 oz)	110	0	9	6	250	1 high-fat meat
Neufchatel, Philadelphia (1 oz)	70	<1	6	4	120	1 med-fat meat
Neufchatel, Philadelphia, Light (1 oz)	71	<1	6	4	122	1 med-fat meat
Neufchatel, Spreadery, Classic Ranch (2 Tbsp)	80	1	7	5	210	1 med-fat meat
Neufchatel, Spreadery, Garden Vegetable (2 Tbsp)	70	2	6	4	230	1 med-fat meat
Neufchatel, Spreadery, Garlic Herb (2 Tbsp)	80	1	7	5	180	1 med-fat meat
Parmesan, Grated (2 tsp)	20	0	2	1	85	free
Pizza Cheese, Smoke-Flavored Mozzarella & Provolone (1/4 cup)	90	<1	7	5	210	1 high-fat meat
Pizza Cheese, Swiss, Shredded (1/4 cup)	110	<1	9	6	45	1 high-fat meat

CHEESE AND CHEESE PRODUCTS

Products	Cal.	Carb. (g)	Fat (g)	Sat. Fat (g)	Sodium (mg)	Exchanges
Pizza Cheese, Taco, Cheddar & Monterey Jack (1/4 cup)	100	<1	8	6	180	1 high-fat meat
Provolone Cheese w/Smoke Flavor (1 oz)	100	<1	7	5	240	1 high-fat meat
Romano, Grated (2 tsp)	25	0	2	1	90	free
Singles Nonfat Pasteurized Processed Cheese Slice (3/4 oz)	30	3	0	0	320	1 very lean meat
Singles Nonfat Pasteurized Processed Sharp Cheddar Cheese (3/4 oz)	30	3	0	0	290	1 very lean meat
Singles Nonfat Pasteurized Processed Swiss Cheese (3/4 oz)	30	3	0	0	290	1 very lean meat
Singles Nonfat Pasteurized Processed White Cheese (3/4 oz)	30	3	0	0	320	1 very lean meat
Singles Pasteurized Processed American Cheese (3/4 oz)	50	2	3	2	330	1 lean meat

Singles Pasteurized Processed Cheese Food w/Pimento (1 slice)	70	2	5	4	290	1 med-fat meat
Singles Pasteurized Processed Monterey Jack Cheese Food (1 slice)	70	2	5	4	290	1 med-fat meat
Singles Pasteurized Processed Sharp Cheddar Cheese (3/4 oz)	50	2	3	2	300	1 lean meat
Singles Pasteurized Processed Sharp Cheddar Cheese Food (1 slice)	70	<1	6	4	300	1 med-fat meat
Singles Pasteurized Processed Swiss Cheese (3/4 oz)	50	2	3	2	270	1 lean meat
Singles Pasteurized Processed Swiss Cheese Food (1 slice)	70	1	5	4	320	1 med-fat meat
Singles Pasteurized Processed White American Cheese (3/4 oz)	50	2	3	2	330	1 lean meat
Spreadery Cheese, Cold, Nacho (2 Tbsp)	80	3	5	3	290	1 med-fat meat
Spreadery Cheese, Cold, Port Wine (2 Tbsp)	80	3	5	3	290	1 med-fat meat

CHEESE AND CHEESE PRODUCTS

Products	Cal.	Carb. (g)	Fat (g)	Sat. Fat (g)	Sodium (mg)	Exchanges
Spreadery Cheese, Cold, Sharp Cheddar (2 Tbsp)	80	3	5	3	290	1 med-fat meat
Spreadery Processed Pimento Cheese Spread (2 Tbsp)	100	3	8	5	320	1 high-fat meat
Squeez-A-Snak Sharp Processed Cheese Spread (2 Tbsp)	90	<1	8	5	440	1 high-fat meat
Swiss Cheese (1 oz)	110	0	9	6	50	1 high-fat meat
Velveeta Cheese Spread (1 oz)	80	3	6	4	420	1 med-fat meat
Velveeta Cheese Spread w/Jalapeño, Mild (1 oz)	80	3	6	4	440	1 med-fat meat
Velveeta Italiana Processed Cheese Spread (1 oz)	80	2	6	4	430	1 med-fat meat
Velveeta Light Processed Cheese (1 oz)	60	3	3	2	420	1 lean meat
Velveeta Shredded Pasteurized Processed Cheese Food (1/4 cup)	130	3	9	6	500	1 high-fat meat
Velveeta Slices Processed Cheese Spread (1 slice)	60	2	5	3	300	1 med-fat meat

LIFETIME

Cheddar, Fat-Free (1/4 cup)	44	1	0	0	244	1 very lean meat
Cheddar, Fat-Free, Sharp (1/4 cup)	44	1	0	0	244	1 very lean meat
Cheese Spread, Olive & Pimento (2 Tbsp)	70	3	6	4	220	1 med-fat meat
Mexican Cheese, Fat-Free, Mild (1/4 cup)	44	1	0	0	244	1 very lean meat
Monterey Jack, Fat-Free (1/4 cup)	44	1	0	0	244	1 very lean meat
Mozzarella, Fat-Free (1/4 cup)	44	1	0	0	244	1 very lean meat
Swiss, Fat-Free (1/4 cup)	44	1	0	0	244	1 very lean meat

SARGENTO

3-Cheese Gourmet Cheddar (1/4 cup)	110	6	9	1	160	1 high-fat meat
4-Cheese Mexican (1/4 cup)	110	6	9	<1	200	1 high-fat meat
4-Cheese Mexican, Light (1/4 cup)	70	3	5	<1	200	1 med-fat meat

STELLA FOODS

Aged Provolone (1 oz)	100	<1	8	5	290	1 high-fat meat
Blue Cheese (1 oz)	100	<1	8	5	390	1 high-fat meat
Feta (1 oz)	80	1	6	5	310	1 med-fat meat

CHEESE AND CHEESE PRODUCTS

Products	Cal.	Carb. (g)	Fat (g)	Sat. Fat (g)	Sodium (mg)	Exchanges
Fontinella (1 oz)	100	.5	7	4	330	
Italian Cheese, Sharp (1 oz)	100	<1	7	5	330	1 high-fat meat
Lorraine Cheese (1 oz)	110	<1	9	5	30	1 high-fat meat
Lorraine Cheese w/Chive & Onion (1 oz)	110	<1	9	5	30	1 high-fat meat
Mozzarella (1 oz)	80	<1	6	4	180	1 med-fat meat
Mozzarella, Whole-Milk (1 oz)	90	<1	7	5	180	1 high-fat meat
Parmesan, Dried Grated (1 Tbsp)	35	0	3	2	130	1 fat
Provolone, Lite (1 oz)	70	<1	4	2	120	1 med-fat meat
Provolone, Mello (1 oz)	100	<1	7	4	290	1 high-fat meat
Ricotta, Whole-Milk (1/4 cup)	120	3	8	5	240	1 high-fat meat
Romano, Dried Grated (1 Tbsp)	35	0	3	2	130	1 fat
WEIGHT WATCHERS						
Cheddar, Natural Mild Yellow (1/4 cup)	88	1	6	3	197	1 med-fat meat
Cheddar, Sharp Yellow (1/4 cup)	88	1	6	3	197	1 med-fat meat

Cheddar Cheese Slices, Fat-Free, Sharp (2 slices)	30	2	0	0	310	1 very lean meat
Cottage Cheese, 1% (1/2 cup)	90	4	1	<1	460	2 very lean meat
Cottage Cheese, 2% (1/2 cup)	106	5	2	2	541	2 very lean meat
Cream Cheese, Light (2 Tbsp)	40	1	3	2	105	1 fat
Monterey Jack, Natural (1/4 cup)	88	1	6	3	197	1 med-fat meat
Parmesan Italian Topping, Fat-Free, Grated (1 tsp)	15	2	0	0	45	free
Swiss Cheese Slices, Fat-Free (2 slices)	30	2	0	0	280	1 very lean meat
White Cheese Slices, Fat-Free (2 slices)	30	2	0	0	310	1 very lean meat
Yellow Cheese Slices, Fat-Free (2 slices)	30	2	0	0	310	1 very lean meat

COMBINATION FOODS & FROZEN ENTREES

COMBINATION FOODS AND FROZEN ENTREES

Products	Cal.	Carb. (g)	Fat (g)	Sat. Fat (g)	Sodium (mg)	Exchanges
Beef Burgundy (1 cup)	285	10	11	3	110	1/2 carb., 5 lean meat
Beef Stroganoff & Noodles (1 cup)	342	21	20	8	454	1-1/2 carb., 2 med-fat meat, 2 fat
Beef w/Macaroni & Tomato Sauce, Homemade (1 cup)	284	25	11	4	841	1-1/2 carb., 2 med-fat meat
Burrito, Beef (1)	262	30	11	6	746	2 carb., 1 med-fat meat, 1 fat
Burrito, Ham & Cheese Flavor (3.5 oz)	210	29	6	2	350	2 carb., 1 fat
Cabbage Rolls, Stuffed (8 oz)	234	26	11	3	654	2 carb., 1 med-fat meat, 1 fat
Chicken & Noodles, Homemade (1 cup)	367	26	19	6	600	2 carb., 2 med-fat meat, 2 fat
Chicken a la King, Homemade (1 cup)	468	12	34	13	760	1 carb., 3 med-fat meat, 4 fat
Chicken Tetrazzini (1 cup)	372	28	20	7	813	2 carb., 2 med-fat meat, 2 fat
Chiles Rellenos (1)	425	7	35	17	620	1/2 carb., 3 med-fat meat, 4 fat
Chili Con Carne w/Beans & Rice (1 cup)	297	46	8	4	1162	3 carb., 2 fat
Chili Con Carne, w/o Beans (1 cup)	350	21	19	7	1407	1-1/2 carb., 3 med-fat meat, 1 fat

Chimichanga, Beef & Bean (1)	249	26	12	3	242	2 carb., 1 med-fat meat, 1 fat
Chop Suey, Shrimp, w/Noodles (1 cup)	277	22	12	2	937	1-1/2 carb., 2 med-fat meat
Chop Suey & Noodles, Beef (1 cup)	425	31	25	5	818	2 carb., 2 med-fat meat, 3 fat
Chow Mein, Beef, No Noodles/Rice (2 cups)	160	13	3	1	2373	1 carb., 2 lean meat
Chow Mein, Beef, Shrimp, w/Noodles (1 cup)	277	22	12	2	937	1-1/2 carb., 2 med-fat meat
Corndog (1)	460	56	19	5	973	4 carb., 1 med-fat meat, 3 fat
Corned Beef Hash, Canned (1 cup)	398	24	25	12	1188	1-1/2 carb., 2 med-fat meat, 3 fat
Curry, Beef (1 cup)	437	13	32	7	1323	1 carb., 3 med-fat meat, 3 fat
Eggplant Parmesan (1 cup)	320	17	22	10	683	1 carb., 2 med-fat meat, 2 fat
Enchilada, Beef & Cheese (1)	323	31	18	9	1319	2 carb., 1 med-fat meat, 3 fat
Enchilada, Chicken (1)	197	16	9	4	302	1 carb., 2 med-fat meat
Fajita, Chicken (1)	405	50	13	3	439	3 carb., 2 med-fat meat, 1 fat
Goulash, Beef, w/Noodles (1 cup)	341	23	14	4	457	1-1/2 carb., 3 med-fat meat
Lasagna (8 oz)	302	27	12	NA	885	2 carb., 2 med-fat meat
Macaroni & Cheese (1 cup)	228	26	10	4	730	2 carb., 2 med-fat meat
Manicotti w/Meat & Tomato Sauce (1)	303	21	15	8	526	1-1/2 carb., 2 med-fat meat, 1 fat

COMBINATION FOODS & FROZEN ENTREES

Products	Cal.	Carb. (g)	Fat (g)	Sat. Fat (g)	Sodium (mg)	Exchanges
Meat Loaf, Beef & 1/3 Pork (1 slice)	221	5	15	5	389	2 med-fat meat, 1 fat
Meat Tamale (1)	183	16	10	4	229	1 carb., 1 med-fat meat, 1 fat
Meat Tortellini (1 cup)	372	33	15	5	797	2 carb., 3 med-fat meat
Moo Goo Gai Pan (1 cup)	281	12	20	5	327	2 vegetable, 2 med-fat meat, 2 fat
Pepper, Stuffed Green Bell (1)	236	20	13	5	203	1 carb., 1 vegetable, 2 med-fat meat, 2 fat
Pizza, Cheese, Thin Crust (1/4 of 10-inch)	317	28	17	7	770	2 carb., 2 med-fat meat, 1 fat
Pizza, Meat, Thin Crust (1/4 of 10-inch)	368	29	21	7	1000	2 carb., 2 med-fat meat, 2 fat
Pot Pie (7 oz)	450	35	28	NA	778	2 carb., 2 med-fat meat, 4 fat
Quesadilla (1)	199	21	10	4	255	1-1/2 carb., 2 fat
Quiche Lorraine (1/8 pie)	508	20	39	18	549	1 carb., 3 med-fat meat, 5 fat
Ravioli, Cheese w/Tomato Sauce (1)	336	38	14	6	1541	2-1/2 carb., 1 med-fat meat, 2 fat
Salad, Carrot Raisin (1/2 cup)	202	21	14	2	117	1/2 fruit, 2 vegetable, 3 fat
Salad, Chef-Style (1-1/2 cup)	267	5	16	8	743	1 vegetable, 3 med-fat meat

Salad, Egg (1/2 cup)	293	2	28	6	333	1 med-fat meat, 5 fat
Salad, Potato, No Egg (1/2 cup)	134	16	7	1	345	1 carb., 1 fat
Salad, Seafood (1/2 cup)	166	3	12	2	274	2 med-fat meat
Salad, Shrimp (1/2 cup)	141	3	9	2	196	2 med-fat meat
Salad, Three-Bean (1/2 cup)	70	7	4	<1	257	1/2 carb., 1 fat
Salad, Tuna (1/2 cup)	192	10	10	2	412	1/2 carb., 2 med-fat meat
Salad, Waldorf (1/2 cup)	199	6	20	3	121	1/2 fruit, 4 fat
Salmon Patty/Cake (4.5 oz)	261	14	16	4	657	1 carb., 2 med-fat meat, 1 fat
Shepherd's Pie, Beef (1 cup)	287	31	10	3	702	2 carb., 2 med-fat meat
Sloppy Joe Gravy/Sauce, Beef (1 cup)	380	24	23	9	1246	1-1/2 carb., 2 med-fat meat, 3 fat
Spaghetti w/Meatballs (1 cup)	258	29	10	2	1220	2 carb., 2 med-fat meat
Shrimp, Stuffed (1 cup)	276	9	14	3	694	1/2 carb., 4 lean meat
Shrimp w/Noodles & Cheese Sauce (1 cup)	350	24	15	6	698	1-1/2 carb., 3 med-fat meat
Souffle, Cheese, Homemade (1 cup)	195	5	14	5	291	2 med-fat meat, 1 fat
Souffle, Spinach (1 cup)	219	3	18	7	763	2 med-fat meat, 2 fat
Sukiyaki (1 cup)	175	6	8	3	762	1/2 carb., 3 lean meat

COMBINATION FOODS & FROZEN ENTREES

Products	Cal.	Carb. (g)	Fat (g)	Sat. Fat (g)	Sodium (mg)	Exchanges
Swedish Meatballs w/Cream Sauce (1 cup)	404	17	23	10	1157	1 carb., 4 med-fat meat, 1 fat
Sweet & Sour Pork w/Rice (1 cup)	269	40	6	2	906	2-1/2 carb., 1 med-fat meat
Taco, Chicken (1)	175	10	8	3	107	1/2 carb., 2 med-fat meat
Tostada, Bean & Cheese (1)	223	27	10	5	543	2 carb., 1 med-fat meat, 1 fat
Tostada, Bean & Chicken (1)	253	19	11	5	435	1 carb., 2 med-fat meat
Tuna-Noodle Casserole (9 oz)	259	34	8	NA	1043	2 carb., 2 med-fat meat
Turkey-Noodle Casserole (1 cup)	326	29	13	4	732	2 carb., 2 med-fat meat, 2 fat
ARMOUR CLASSICS						
Chicken & Noodle Dinner (11 oz)	280	30	9	5	550	2 carb., 2 med-fat meat
Chicken Fettuccine Dinner (10 oz)	230	25	8	NA	520	1-1/2 carb., 2 med-fat meat
Chicken Mesquite Dinner (9.6 oz)	280	39	13	NA	630	2-1/2 carb., 2 med-fat meat, 1 fat
Chicken Parmigiana Dinner (10.9 oz)	360	25	18	6	1020	1-1/2 carb., 3 med-fat meat, 1 fat
Chicken, Wine & Mushroom Dinner (10 oz)	260	20	11	5	540	1 carb., 2 med-fat meat
Glazed Chicken Dinner (10.9 oz)	280	20	14	4	740	1 carb., 2 med-fat meat, 1 fat

Meat Loaf Dinner (11.4 oz)	300	33	10	5	600	2 carb., 2 med-fat meat
Salisbury Steak (11.4 oz)	330	20	18	8	1310	1 carb., 3 med-fat meat, 1 fat
Swedish Meatballs Dinner (10 oz)	300	20	17	7	940	1 carb., 3 med-fat meat
Turkey & Dressing Dinner (11.4 oz)	270	34	7	4	1020	2 carb., 2 lean meat
Veal Parmigiana Dinner (11.4 oz)	400	35	22	11	1050	2 carb., 1 med-fat meat, 3 fat
ARMOUR LITE						
Beef Pepper Steak Dinner (11 oz)	210	29	4	2	870	2 carb., 1 med-fat meat
Chicken Burgundy Dinner (10 oz)	210	20	5	2	760	1 carb., 2 lean meat
Shrimp Creole Dinner (10 oz)	220	49	5	0	720	3 carb., 1 fat
Sweet & Sour Chicken (11 oz)	220	38	1	0	520	2-1/2 carb., 1 very lean meat
AUNT JEMIMA						
French Toast (2 pieces)	166	27	4	1	554	2 carb., 1 fat
French Toast, Cinnamon Swirl (2 pieces)	166	27	4	1	516	2 carb., 1 fat
BANQUET						
Beef Enchilada Meal (11 oz)	380	54	12	5	1330	3-1/2 carb., 1 med-fat meat, 1 fat
Breaded Chicken Patty Meal (10.2 oz)	380	31	21	5	1270	2 carb., 2 med-fat meat, 2 fat

COMBINATION FOODS & FROZEN ENTREES

Products	Cal.	Carb. (g)	Fat (g)	Sat. Fat (g)	Sodium (mg)	Exchanges
Cheese Enchilada Meal (11 oz)	340	56	6	3	1500	4 carb., 1 med-fat meat
Chicken & Dumplings w/Gravy Meal (10 oz)	260	35	8	3	780	2 carb., 1 med-fat meat, 1 fat
Chicken Chow Mein Meal (9 oz)	210	28	7	2	850	2 carb., 1 med-fat meat
Chicken Fried Beef Steak Meal (10 oz)	400	39	20	6	1180	2-1/2 carb., 1 med-fat meat, 3 fat
Chicken Parmigiana Meal (9.5 oz)	290	27	15	4	900	2 carb., 2 med-fat meat, 1 fat
Chicken Enchilada Meal (11 oz)	360	54	10	3	1580	3-1/2 carb., 1 med-fat meat, 1 fat
Extra Helping Chicken Fried Beef Steak Dinner (18.65 oz)	800	73	44	14	2050	5 carb., 2 med-fat meat, 6 fat
Extra Helping Chicken Parmigiana Dinner (19 oz)	650	64	33	8	1770	4 carb., 2 med-fat meat, 5 fat
Extra Helping Meat Loaf Dinner (19 oz)	650	49	38	16	2140	3 carb., 3 med-fat meat, 5 fat
Extra Helping Mexican-Style Dinner (22 oz)	820	100	34	14	2060	6-1/2 carb., 2 med-fat meat, 5 fat
Extra Helping Salisbury Steak Dinner (19 oz)	740	52	46	19	1860	3-1/2 carb., 3 med-fat meat, 6 fat

Extra Helping Turkey & Gravy w/Dressing Dinner (18.8 oz)	560	63	20	5	1910	4 carb, 3 med-fat meat, 1 fat
Gravy & Beef Patty Meal (9.5 oz)	300	21	20	8	1060	1-1/2 carb, 1 med-fat meat, 3 fat
Pasta Favorites, Chicken Lo Mein (10.5 oz)	270	43	6	1	1060	3 carb, 1 fat
Pasta Favorites, Chicken Pasta Primavera (10.5 oz)	330	40	13	5	930	3 carb, 1 med-fat meat, 2 fat
Pasta Favorites, Fettuccine Alfredo (10.5 oz)	370	39	18	8	940	2-1/2 carb, 1 med-fat meat, 3 fat
Pasta Favorites, Lasagna w/Meat Sauce (10.5 oz)	290	39	9	2	900	2-1/2 carb, 1 med-fat meat, 1 fat
Pasta Favorites, Macaroni & Cheese (10.5 oz)	350	47	12	4	960	3 carb, 1 med-fat meat, 1 fat
Pasta Favorites, Vegetable Lasagna (10.5 oz)	260	41	6	2	850	3 carb, 1 fat
Pasta Favorites, White Cheddar Broccoli (10.5 oz)	350	48	12	5	900	3 carb, 1 med-fat meat, 1 fat
Mexican-Style Combination Meal (11 oz)	380	55	11	5	1370	3-1/2 carb, 1 med-fat meat, 1 fat
Oriental-Style Chicken Meal (9 oz)	260	34	9	3	610	2 carb, 1 med-fat meat, 1 fat
Pork Cutlet Meal (10.25 oz)	410	37	24	6	940	2-1/2 carb, 1 med-fat meat, 4 fat

COMBINATION FOODS & FROZEN ENTREES

Products	Cal.	Carb. (g)	Fat (g)	Sat. Fat (g)	Sodium (mg)	Exchanges
Pot Pie, Beef (7 oz)	330	38	15	7	1000	2-1/2 carb., 3 fat
Pot Pie, Chicken (7 oz)	350	36	18	7	950	2-1/2 carb., 4 fat
Pot Pie, Vegetable Cheese (7 oz)	390	49	18	8	1000	3 carb., 4 fat
Salisbury Steak Meal (9.5 oz)	310	28	16	7	910	2 carb., 2 med-fat meat, 1 fat
Southern Fried Chicken Meal (8.75 oz)	530	44	30	8	1610	3 carb., 2 med-fat meat, 4 fat
Turkey & Gravy w/Dressing Meal (9.25 oz)	270	31	10	3	1100	2 carb., 2 med-fat meat
Veal Parmigiana Meal (9 oz)	320	35	14	5	960	2 carb., 1 med-fat meat, 2 fat
White Meat Fried Chicken Meal (8.75 oz)	470	33	28	11	1100	2 carb., 2 med-fat meat, 4 fat
BETTY CROCKER						
Hamburger Helper Cheeseburger Macaroni (1 cup)	360	32	16	6	1000	2 carb., 2 med-fat meat, 1 fat
Hamburger Helper Lasagna (1 cup)	280	30	10	4	950	2 carb., 2 med-fat meat
Hamburger Helper Stroganoff (1 cup)	320	30	13	5	830	2 carb., 2 med-fat meat, 1 fat
Tuna Helper Creamy Pasta (1 cup)	300	31	13	4	910	2 carb., 1 med-fat meat, 1 fat

Food	Cal	Carb			Sodium	Exchanges
Tuna Helper Tetrazzini (1 cup)	310	33	12	3	1010	2 carb., 2 med-fat meat
Tuna Helper Tuna Melt (1 cup)	300	33	12	3	870	2 carb., 1 med-fat meat, 1 fat

BIRD'S EYE CLASSIC

Food	Cal	Carb			Sodium	Exchanges
Broccoli w/Cauliflower Carrot Butter (1/2 cup)	53	8	2	1	241	2 vegetable
Broccoli w/Cheese Sauce (1/2 cup)	70	7	3	2	423	1 vegetable, 1 fat
Cauliflower w/Cheese Sauce (1/2 cup)	64	7	3	2	382	1 vegetable, 1 fat
Peas & Potatoes w/Cream Sauce (1/2 cup)	75	12	2	<1	378	1 strch
Small Onions w/Cream Sauce (1/2 cup)	58	10	2	<1	325	2 vegetable
Sweet Corn w/Butter Sauce (1/2 cup)	115	23	3	1	216	1-1/2 strch, 1 fat

BRIGHTON'S

Food	Cal	Carb			Sodium	Exchanges
Potato, Cheese & Bacon (9.6 oz)	352	48	13	NA	855	3 carb., 3 fat
Potato, Cheese Sauce w/Ham (10.3 oz)	347	44	12	NA	878	3 carb., 1 med-fat meat, 1 fat
Potato, Classic Combination (9.7 oz)	326	42	13	NA	1248	3 carb., 3 fat
Potato Entree, Broccoli Cheese (10.3 oz)	337	46	12	NA	775	3 carb., 2 fat

BUDGET GOURMET

Food	Cal	Carb			Sodium	Exchanges
Beef SirloinTips w/Country Gravy (10 oz)	310	21	18	NA	570	1-1/2 carb., 2 med-fat meat, 2 fat

COMBINATION FOODS & FROZEN ENTREES

Products	Cal.	Carb. (g)	Fat (g)	Sat. Fat (g)	Sodium (mg)	Exchanges
Chicken & Fettuccine (10 oz)	400	29	21	NA	740	2 carb., 3 med-fat meat, 1 fat
French Recipe Chicken (10 oz)	260	21	10	NA	790	1-1/2 carb., 2 med-fat meat
Ham & Asparagus Au Gratin (9 oz)	280	33	10	NA	1130	2 carb., 1 med-fat meat, 1 fat
Linguine w/Scallops & Clams (9.6 oz)	280	28	11	NA	630	2 carb., 1 med-fat meat, 1 fat
Pepper Steak & Rice (10 oz)	300	39	9	NA	800	2-1/2 carb., 1 med-fat meat, 1 fat
Seafood Newburg (10 oz)	350	43	12	NA	660	3 carb., 1 med-fat meat, 1 fat
Side Dish, Country-Style Corn (5.8 oz)	140	19	5	NA	290	1 carb., 1 fat
Side Dish, Macaroni & Cheese (5.4 oz)	210	23	8	NA	370	1-1/2 carb., 1 med-fat meat, 1 fat
Side Dish, New England Vegetables (5.6 oz)	210	18	10	NA	290	1 carb., 1 med-fat meat, 1 fat
Side Dish, Oriental Rice w/Vegetables (5.8 oz)	210	27	10	NA	310	2 carb., 2 fat
Side Dish, Pasta Alfredo w/Broccoli (5.6 oz)	200	17	8	NA	390	1 carb., 2 med-fat meat
Side Dish, Rice Pilaf & Green Beans (5.6 oz)	240	35	9	NA	350	2 carb., 2 fat
Side Dish, Spinach Au Gratin (6 oz)	120	14	5	NA	410	1 carb., 1 fat
Side Dish, Spring Vegetables w/Cheese (5 oz)	90	10	3	NA	290	2 vegetables, 1 fat

Food	Calories	Carb. (g)	Fat (g)	Sat. Fat (g)	Sodium (mg)	Exchanges/Choices
Side Dish, Three-Cheese Potato (5.8 oz)	230	25	11	NA	410	1-1/2 carb., 1 med-fat meat, 1 fat
Side Dish, Ziti w/Marinara Sauce (6.3 oz)	220	25	9	NA	380	1-1/2 carb., 1 med-fat meat, 1 fat
Sirloin Beef in Herb Sauce (10 oz)	290	27	12	NA	770	2 carb., 2 med-fat meat
Slim Selects Beef Stroganoff (8.9 oz)	280	29	10	NA	560	2 carb., 2 med-fat meat
Slim Selects Cheese Ravioli (10 oz)	260	36	7	5	960	2-1/2 carb., 1 med-fat meat
Slim Selects Chicken Au Gratin (9.2 oz)	260	21	11	NA	820	1-1/2 carb., 2 med-fat meat
Slim Selects Chicken Enchilada Suiza (9 oz)	270	30	9	NA	1080	2 carb., 2 med-fat meat
Slim Selects Fettuccine w/Meat Sauce (10 oz)	290	34	10	NA	980	2 carb., 1 med-fat meat, 1 fat
Slim Selects Glazed Turkey (9 oz)	270	39	5	NA	760	2-1/2 carb., 1 med-fat meat
Slim Selects Lasagna w/Meat Sauce (10 oz)	290	32	10	NA	890	2 carb., 2 med-fat meat
Slim Selects Mandarin Chicken (10 oz)	290	40	6	NA	690	2-1/2 carb., 2 lean meat
Slim Selects Oriental Beef (10 oz)	290	36	9	NA	810	2-1/2 carb., 1 med-fat meat, 1 fat
Slim Selects Sirloin Enchilada Ranchero (9 oz)	290	20	15	NA	770	1 carb., 2 med-fat meat, 2 fat
Slim Selects Sirloin Salisbury Steak (9 oz)	280	31	8	NA	870	2 carb., 2 med-fat meat
Swedish Meatballs & Noodles (10 oz)	600	40	39	NA	1085	2-1/2 carb., 2 med-fat meat, 6 fat
Sweet & Sour Chicken & Rice (10 oz)	350	53	7	NA	640	3-1/2 carb., 1 med-fat meat

COMBINATION FOODS & FROZEN ENTREES

Products	Cal.	Carb. (g)	Fat (g)	Sat. Fat (g)	Sodium (mg)	Exchanges
Three-Cheese Lasagna (10 oz)	400	38	17	NA	760	2-1/2 carb., 2 med-fat meat, 1 fat
Turkey ala King w/Rice (10 oz)	390	36	18	NA	740	2-1/2 carb., 2 med-fat meat, 2 fat
CELESTE						
Pizza, Canadian Bacon (1/4)	329	28	17	5	976	2 carb., 2 med-fat meat, 1 fat
Pizza, Cheese (1/4)	317	28	17	7	770	2 carb., 1 med-fat meat, 2 fat
Pizza, Deluxe (1/4)	378	29	22	7	903	2 carb., 2 med-fat meat, 2 fat
Pizza, Pepperoni (1/4)	368	29	21	7	1000	2 carb., 1 med-fat meat, 3 fat
Pizza, Sausage (1/4)	376	30	22	7	907	2 carb., 1 med-fat meat, 3 fat
Pizza, Sausage Mushroom (1/4)	387	29	22	6	1033	2 carb., 2 med-fat meat, 2 fat
Pizza, Supreme (1/4)	381	29	24	7	1090	2 carb., 2 med-fat meat, 3 fat
Pizza-For-One, Canadian Bacon (7.9 oz)	541	50	26	NA	1593	3 carb., 3 med-fat meat, 2 fat
CHEF AMERICA						
Hot Pockets, Chicken Fajita (1)	260	36	8	3	770	2-1/2 carb., 1 med-fat meat, 1 fat
Hot Pockets, Ham/Cheese (1)	340	37	15	7	840	2-1/2 carb., 1 med-fat meat, 2 fat

COMBINATION FOODS & FROZEN ENTREES 105

Item	Cal	Carb	Fat		Sod	Exchanges
Hot Pockets, Pepperoni Pizza (1)	350	38	17	8	780	2-1/2 carb., 1 med-fat meat, 2 fat
Hot Pockets, Turkey/Broccoli/Cheese (1)	260	35	8	3	710	2 carb., 1 med-fat meat, 1 fat
CHEF BOYARDEE						
Beef Ravioli (1 cup)	220	36	5	2	1180	2-1/2 carb., 1 fat
Cheese Tortellini (1 cup)	240	50	<1	0	630	3 carb.
Spaghetti w/Meatballs (1 cup)	240	35	7	3	940	2 carb., 1 fat
CHEF MATE						
Italian Rotini & Meatballs Entree (1 cup)	270	28	11	4	1390	2 carb., 1 med-fat meat, 1 fat
Oriental Beef & Vegetables Entree (1 cup)	190	25	6	<1	1150	1-1/2 carb., 1 med-fat meat
Oriental Chicken & Vegetables Entree (1 cup)	210	24	8	2	1170	1-1/2 carb., 1 med-fat meat, 1 fat
Oriental Vegetables Entree (1 cup)	180	27	7	1	1410	2 carb., 1 fat
CHUN KING						
Chow Mein, Chicken (13 oz)	370	45	14	5	2010	3 carb., 1 med-fat meat, 2 fat
Crunchy Walnut Chicken (13 oz)	470	56	19	5	1820	4 carb., 1 med-fat meat, 3 fat
Egg Roll, Meat & Shrimp (6)	220	29	8	2	260	2 carb., 2 fat
Fried Rice w/Chicken (8 oz)	270	44	6	2	1330	3 carb., 1 fat

COMBINATION FOODS & FROZEN ENTREES

Products	Cal.	Carb. (g)	Fat (g)	Sat. Fat (g)	Sodium (mg)	Exchanges
Fried Rice w/Pork (8 oz)	290	48	6	2	1310	3 carb., 1 fat
Sweet & Sour Pork (13 oz)	450	86	6	3	1180	3 carb., 3 carb., 1 med-fat meat
DI GIORNO						
Cheese Tortellini (3/4 cup)	260	37	6	4	230	2-1/2 carb., 1 med-fat meat
Ravioli, Cheese & Garlic Light (1 cup)	270	45	2	1	580	3 carb., 1 lean meat
Ravioli, Italian Herb Cheese (1 cup)	350	44	13	8	610	3 carb., 1 med-fat meat, 2 fat
Ravioli w/Italian Sausage (3/4 cup)	340	41	12	5	630	3 carb., 1 med-fat meat, 1 fat
DINING LITE						
Cheese Cannelloni (9 oz)	310	38	9	NA	650	2-1/2 carb., 2 med-fat meat
Chicken a la King (9 oz)	240	30	7	NA	780	2 carb., 1 med-fat meat
Fettuccine (9 oz)	290	33	12	NA	1020	2 carb., 1 med-fat meat, 1 fat
Lasagna (9 oz)	240	36	5	NA	800	2-1/2 carb., 1 med-fat meat
Oriental Pepper Steak (9 oz)	260	33	6	NA	1050	2 carb., 2 lean meat
Salisbury Steak (9 oz)	200	14	8	NA	1000	1 carb., 2 med-fat meat

Food						Exchanges
Spaghetti w/Beef (9 oz)	220	25	8	NA	440	1-1/2 carb., 1 med-fat meat, 1 fat
Swedish Meatballs (9 oz)	280	34	10	NA	660	2 carb., 1 med-fat meat, 1 fat
FRANCO-AMERICAN						
Beef Ravioli w/Meat Sauce (7.9 oz)	250	36	7	4	1000	2-1/2 carb., 1 fat
Beefy Macaroni (7.6 oz)	230	30	8	4	1149	2 carb., 2 fat
CircusO's Pasta & Meatballs (1 cup)	260	31	11	5	1150	2 carb., 1 med-fat meat, 1 fat
Hearty Twists Pasta w/Meat (1 cup)	250	41	5	2	1159	3 carb., 1 fat
Macaroni & Cheese (1 cup)	200	29	7	3	1059	2 carb., 1 fat
Macaroni & Cheese, Elbow (7.6 oz)	190	25	6	3	880	1-1/2 carb., 1 med-fat meat
Spaghetti w/Beef & Tomato Sauce (7.6 oz)	230	30	9	4	1070	2 carb., 1 med-fat meat, 1 fat
Spaghetti w/Meatballs (7.4 oz)	220	28	8	4	870	2 carb., 1 med-fat meat, 1 fat
Spaghetti w/Meatballs & Sauce (1 cup)	270	35	10	5	1059	2 carb., 1 med-fat meat, 1 fat
Spaghetti w/Tomato & Cheese Sauce (1 cup)	210	41	2	1	1020	3 carb.
SpaghettiOs w/Franks (1 cup)	250	32	11	5	1210	2 carb., 1 med-fat meat, 1 fat
SpaghettiOs Garfield Beef (1 cup)	260	32	10	5	980	2 carb., 1 med-fat meat, 1 fat
SpaghettiOs Garfield Pizza (1 cup)	210	39	3	1	910	2-1/2 carb., 1 fat

COMBINATION FOODS & FROZEN ENTREES

Products	Cal.	Carb. (g)	Fat (g)	Sat. Fat (g)	Sodium (mg)	Exchanges
SpaghettiOs Tomato & Cheese Sauce (1 cup)	190	36	2	<1	990	2-1/2 carb.
GREAT STARTS						
Burrito, Sausage (3.5 oz)	240	24	12	4	500	1-1/2 carb., 1 med-fat meat, 1 fat
Burrito w/Scrambled Eggs (3.5 oz)	200	25	8	3	510	1-1/2 carb., 1 med-fat meat, 1 fat
Burrito w/Scrambled Eggs, Bacon (3.5 oz)	250	27	11	4	540	2 carb., 1 med-fat meat, 1 fat
Eggs & Silver Dollar Pancake (4.3 oz)	251	22	14	6	542	1-1/2 carb., 1 med-fat meat, 2 fat
French Toast, Cinnamon (5.6 oz)	440	34	28	12	580	2 carb., 1 med-fat meat, 5 fat
Muffin, Egg Bacon Cheese (4 oz)	290	25	15	6	750	1-1/2 carb., 1 med-fat meat, 2 fat
Pancake, Budget Silver Dollar (3.8 oz)	340	36	18	9	670	2-1/2 carb., 4 fat
Pancakes w/Bacon (4.6 oz)	400	42	20	7	1030	3 carb., 4 fat
Pancakes w/Sausage (6 oz)	490	52	25	11	950	3-1/2 carb., 1 med-fat meat, 4 fat
Sandwich, Egg & Cheese (4.3 oz)	360	35	19	8	950	2 carb., 1 med-fat meat, 3 fat
Scrambled Eggs & Bacon (5.3 oz)	290	17	19	9	700	1 carb., 1 med-fat meat, 3 fat
Scrambled Eggs & Sausage (6.3 oz)	360	21	26	10	800	1-1/2 carb., 1 med-fat meat, 5 fat

HEALTHY CHOICE

Beef & Peppers Cantonese (11.5 oz)	270	40	5	3	560	2-1/2 carb., 2 lean meat
Beef Pepper Steak Oriental (9.5 oz)	250	34	4	2	470	2 carb., 2 lean meat
Beef Stroganoff (11 oz)	310	44	6	3	440	3 carb., 2 lean meat
Cheddar Broccoli Potatoes (10.5 oz)	310	53	5	2	550	3-1/2 carb., 1 fat
Chicken & Vegetables Marsala (11.5 oz)	220	32	1	0	440	2 carb., 2 very lean meat
Chicken Broccoli Alfredo (12.1 oz)	370	53	8	3	470	3-1/2 carb., 2 med-fat meat
Chicken Dijon (11 oz)	280	41	4	2	410	3 carb., 2 lean meat
Chicken Fettuccine Alfredo (8.5 oz)	260	35	5	2	410	2 carb., 2 lean meat
Chicken Parmigiana (11.5 oz)	300	47	4	2	490	3 carb., 2 lean meat
Chicken Teriyaki (12.25 oz)	270	42	2	<1	420	3 carb., 2 very lean meat
Classics Beef Broccoli Bejing (12 oz)	330	55	3	1	500	3-1/2 carb., 1 lean meat
Classics Cacciatore Chicken (12.5 oz)	260	36	3	<1	510	2-1/2 carb., 2 very lean meat
Classics Chicken Francesca (12.5 oz)	360	51	5	2	500	3-1/2 carb., 2 lean meat
Classics Country Inn Roast Turkey (10 oz)	250	29	4	1	530	2 carb., 3 very lean meat
Classics Ginger Chicken Hunan (12.6 oz)	350	59	3	<1	430	4 carb., 2 lean meat

COMBINATION FOODS & FROZEN ENTREES

Products	Cal.	Carb. (g)	Fat (g)	Sat. Fat (g)	Sodium (mg)	Exchanges
Classics Mesquite Beef Barbeque (11 oz)	310	45	4	2	490	3 carb., 3 lean meat
Classics Pasta Shells Marinara (12 oz)	370	59	4	2	390	4 carb., 2 lean meat
Classics Salisbury Steak (11 oz)	260	32	6	3	500	2 carb., 2 lean meat
Classics Sesame Chicken Shanghai (12 oz)	310	42	5	1	460	3 carb., 2 lean meat
Classics Shrimp & Vegetables Maria (12.5 oz)	270	46	3	1	540	3 carb., 1 lean meat
Classics Traditional Swedish Meatballs (11.1 oz)	320	37	9	3	600	2-1/2 carb., 2 med-fat meat
Classics Turkey Fettuccine alla Crema (12.5 oz)	350	50	4	2	370	3 carb., 3 very lean meat
Country Glazed Chicken (8.5 oz)	200	30	2	<1	480	2 carb., 2 very lean meat
Country Herb Chicken (11.5 oz)	270	40	4	2	340	2-1/2 carb., 2 lean meat
Fiesta Chicken Fajitas (7 oz)	260	36	4	1	410	2-1/2 carb., 2 lean meat
French Bread Pizza, Cheese (1)	310	49	4	2	470	3 carb., 2 lean meat
French Bread Pizza, Pepperoni (6 oz)	360	48	9	4	580	3 carb., 2 med-fat meat
Honey Mustard Chicken (9.5 oz)	260	40	2	0	550	2-1/2 carb., 2 very lean meat

Food	Cal	Carb			Sod	Exchanges
Lasagna Roma (13.5 oz)	390	60	5	2	580	4 carb., 2 lean meat
Mesquite Chicken Barbeque (10.5 oz)	320	55	2	<1	290	3-1/2 carb., 2 very lean meat
Sesame Chicken (9.75 oz)	240	38	3	<1	600	2-1/2 carb., 1 lean meat
Southwestern Glazed Chicken (12.5 oz)	300	48	3	1	430	3 carb., 2 very lean meat
Three-Cheese Manicotti (11 oz)	310	41	9	5	450	3 carb., 1 med-fat meat, 1 fat
Traditional Beef Tips (11.25 oz)	260	32	5	2	390	2 carb., 2 lean meat
Traditional Meat Loaf Dinner (12 oz)	320	46	8	4	460	3 carb., 2 med-fat meat
Vegetable Pasta Italiano (10 oz)	240	48	1	0	480	3 carb.
Yankee Pot Roast (11 oz)	280	38	5	2	460	2-1/2 carb., 2 lean meat
HORMEL						
Kid's Kitchen Beans & Weiners (1 cup)	310	37	13	5	760	2-1/2 carb., 1 med-fat meat, 2 fat
Kid's Kitchen Beefy Mac (1 cup)	190	23	6	3	790	1-1/2 carb., 1 med-fat meat
Kid's Kitchen Cheezy Mac'n Cheese (1 cup)	260	30	11	6	660	2 carb., 1 med-fat meat, 1 fat
Kid's Kitchen Spaghetti & Mini Meatballs (1 cup)	220	28	7	4	950	2 carb., 1 med-fat meat

COMBINATION FOODS & FROZEN ENTREES

Products	Cal.	Carb. (g)	Fat (g)	Sat. Fat (g)	Sodium (mg)	Exchanges
KIDS CUISINE						
Big-League Hamburger Pizza (8.3 oz)	400	61	11	4	530	4 carb., 1 med-fat meat, 1 fat
Buckaroo Beef Patty Sandwich w/Cheese (8.5 oz)	410	58	15	5	540	4 carb., 1 med-fat meat, 2 fat
Cosmic Chicken Nuggets (9.1 oz)	440	54	16	5	1070	3-1/2 carb., 2 med-fat meat
Funtastic Fish Sticks (8.25 oz)	370	55	12	3	550	3-1/2 carb., 1 med-fat meat, 1 fat
High-Flying Fried Chicken (10.1 oz)	440	49	19	5	940	3 carb., 2 med-fat meat, 2 fat
Magical Macaroni & Cheese (10.6 oz)	420	68	12	5	920	4-1/2 carb., 1 med-fat meat, 1 fat
Pirate Pizza w/Cheese (8 oz)	430	71	11	3	440	5 carb., 1 med-fat meat, 1 fat
Raptor Ravioli w/Cheese (9.8 oz)	320	63	5	2	780	4 carb., 1 fat
Rip-Roaring Macaroni & Beef (9.6 oz)	370	58	9	4	900	4 carb., 1 med-fat meat, 1 fat
Super-Charging Chicken Sandwich (9.43 oz)	480	71	15	4	770	5 carb., 1 med-fat meat, 2 fat
LA CHOY						
Chicken Chow Mein Entree (1 cup)	80	6	4	1	1352	1/2 carb., 1 lean meat

Food						Exchanges
Noodles w/Vegetables & Beef Entree (1 cup)	156	27	4	2	1332	2 carb., 1 fat
Noodles w/Vegetables & Chicken Entree (1 cup)	163	24	3	1	858	1-1/2 carb., 1 med-fat meat
Noodles w/Vegetables Entree (1 cup)	131	27	1	<1	1311	2 carb.
Sweet & Sour Noodles w/Chicken Entree (1 cup)	256	49	3	1	697	3 carb., 1 fat
LARRY'S						
Potato, Deluxe Stuffed (5 oz)	200	27	9	NA	710	2 carb., 2 fat
Potato Stuffed w/Cheese (5 oz)	190	23	9	NA	620	1-1/2 carb., 2 fat
Potato Stuffed w/Chives (5 oz)	190	24	9	NA	495	1-1/2 carb., 2 fat
LEAN CUISINE						
Angel Hair Pasta (10 oz)	210	35	4	1	420	2 carb., 1 fat
Baked Chicken & Whipped Potatoes & Stuffing (8-5/8 oz)	250	30	6	<1	590	2 carb., 2 lean meat
Baked Fish w/Cheddar Shells (9 oz)	260	28	8	2	580	2 carb., 2 med-fat meat
Beef Pot Roast & Whipped Potatoes (9 oz)	210	21	7	2	570	1/2 carb., 2 lean meat

COMBINATION FOODS & FROZEN ENTREES

Products	Cal.	Carb. (g)	Fat (g)	Sat. Fat (g)	Sodium (mg)	Exchanges
Cafe Classics Bow Tie Pasta & Chicken (9-1/2 oz)	270	34	6	2	550	2 carb., 2 lean meat
Cafe Classics Calypso Chicken (8-1/2 oz)	280	42	6	2	590	3 carb., 1 med-fat meat
Cafe Classics Cheese Lasagna w/Chicken Scalopini (10 oz)	290	34	8	3	560	2 carb., 2 med-fat meat
Cafe Classics Chicken Breast in Wine Sauce (8-1/8 oz)	220	25	6	2	560	1-1/2 carb., 2 lean meat
Cafe Classics Chicken Carbonara (9 oz)	290	32	8	2	540	2 carb., 2 med-fat meat
Cafe Classics Chicken Mediterranean (10-7/8 oz)	250	35	4	1	570	2 carb., 2 lean meat
Cafe Classics Chicken Parmesan (10-7/8 oz)	240	25	7	3	580	1-1/2 carb., 2 lean meat
Cafe Classics Chicken Piccata (9 oz)	290	45	6	2	540	3 carb., 1 med-fat meat
Cafe Classics Glazed Turkey (9 oz)	250	36	6	2	590	2-1/2 carb., 1 med-fat meat
Cafe Classics Grilled Chicken Salsa (8-7/8 oz)	240	32	6	2	550	2 carb., 1 med-fat meat

Cafe Classics Grilled Fish w/Vegetables (8-7/8 oz)	170	14	5	1	520	1 carb, 2 lean meat
Cafe Classics Herb-Roasted Chicken (8 oz)	210	25	5	1	430	1-1/2 carb., 2 lean meat
Cafe Classics Honey Mustard Chicken (8 oz)	270	39	5	2	580	2-1/2 carb., 1 med-fat meat
Cafe Classics Mesquite Beef w/Rice (9 oz)	280	38	7	2	470	2-1/2 carb., 2 lean meat
Cafe Classics Sirloin Beef Peppercorn (8-1/2 oz)	210	24	7	2	480	2-1/2 carb., 1 med-fat meat
Cheddar Bake w/Pasta (9 oz)	220	29	6	2	560	2 carb., 1 med-fat meat
Cheese Cannelloni (9-1/8 oz)	240	29	5	3	590	2 carb., 1 med-fat meat
Cheese Ravioli (8-1/2 oz)	240	34	7	3	590	2 carb., 1 med-fat meat
Chicken & Vegetables (10-1/2 oz)	240	30	5	1	520	2 carb., 2 lean meat
Chicken a l'Orange (9 oz)	260	40	3	<1	260	2-1/2 carb., 2 very lean meat
Chicken Chow Mein w/Rice (9 oz)	210	28	5	1	510	2 carb., 1 med-fat meat
Chicken Enchilada Suiza w/Mexican-Style Rice (9 oz)	290	48	5	2	538	3 carb., 1 med-fat meat
Chicken Fettuccine (9 oz)	270	33	6	3	580	2 carb., 2 lean meat

COMBINATION FOODS & FROZEN ENTREES

Products	Cal.	Carb. (g)	Fat (g)	Sat. Fat (g)	Sodium (mg)	Exchanges
Chicken in Peanut Sauce (9 oz)	280	33	6	1	590	2 carb., 2 lean meat
Chicken Italiano w/Fettuccine & Vegetables (9 oz)	270	31	6	2	560	2 carb., 2 lean meat
Chicken Oriental w/Vegetables & Vermicelli (9 oz)	260	30	6	1	530	1 carb., 2 lean meat
Chicken Pie (9-1/2 oz)	320	39	10	3	590	2-1/2 carb., 1 med-fat meat, 1 fat
Country Vegetables & Beef (9 oz)	220	32	4	1	570	2 carb., 1 med-fat meat
Deluxe Cheddar Potato (10-3/8 oz)	230	32	6	3	570	2 carb., 1 med-fat meat
Fettuccine Alfredo (9 oz)	270	38	7	3	590	2-1/2 carb., 1 med-fat meat
Fettuccine Primavera (10 oz)	260	33	8	3	580	2 carb., 1 med-fat meat, 1 fat
Fiesta Chicken w/Rice & Vegetables (8-1/2 oz)	260	35	5	<1	550	2 carb., 2 lean meat
French Bread Pizza, Cheese (6 oz)	350	48	8	4	400	3 carb., 2 med-fat meat
French Bread Pizza, Deluxe (6-1/8 oz)	330	45	6	3	560	3 carb., 3 lean meat
French Bread Pizza, Pepperoni (5-1/4 oz)	330	46	7	3	590	3 carb., 2 med-fat meat

Item						Exchanges
Glazed Chicken w/Vegetable Rice (8-1/2 oz)	240	24	6	1	460	1-1/2 carb, 3 lean meat
Homestyle Turkey (9-3/8 oz)	230	26	6	2	590	2 carb, 2 lean meat
Lasagna, Classic Cheese (11-1/2 oz)	290	38	6	3	560	2-1/2 carb, 2 lean meat
Lasagna, Vegetable (10-1/2 oz)	270	35	7	3	540	2 carb, 1 med-fat meat
Lasagna w/Meat Sauce (10-1/2 oz)	290	35	8	4	560	2 carb, 2 med-fat meat
Lunch Express Broccoli & Cheddar Baked Potato (10 oz)	220	30	6	5	580	2 carb, 1 med-fat meat
Lunch Express Macaroni & Cheese & Broccoli (9-3/4 oz)	240	35	6	3	460	2 carb, 1 med-fat meat
Lunch Express Mandarin Chicken (9-3/4 oz)	270	41	6	1	520	3 carb., 1 med-fat meat
Lunch Express Mexican-Style Rice w/Chicken (9 oz)	270	39	8	2	590	2-1/2 carb., 1 med-fat meat, 1 fat
Lunch Express Pasta & Chicken Marinara (9-1/8 oz)	270	38	6	2	540	2-1/2 carb., 1 med-fat meat
Lunch Express Pasta & Tuna Casserole (9-5/8 oz)	280	39	6	2	590	2-1/2 carb., 1 med-fat meat

COMBINATION FOODS & FROZEN ENTREES

Products	Cal.	Carb. (g)	Fat (g)	Sat. Fat (g)	Sodium (mg)	Exchanges
Lunch Express Pasta & Turkey Dijon (9-7/8 oz)	270	37	6	2	570	2-1/2 carb., 1 med-fat meat
Lunch Express Rice & Chicken Stir-Fry (9 oz)	280	39	9	1	590	2-1/2 carb., 1 med-fat meat, 1 fat
Lunch Express Teriyaki Stir-Fry (9 oz)	260	39	5	1	550	2-1/2 carb., 1 med-fat meat
Macaroni & Beef (10 oz)	270	39	7	4	550	2-1/2 carb., 1 med-fat meat
Marinara Twist (10 oz)	240	42	3	1	440	3 carb.
Meat Loaf & Whipped Potatoes (9-3/8 oz)	250	25	7	2	570	1-1/2 carb., 3 lean meat
Oriental Beef (9 oz)	250	30	8	3	480	2 carb., 1 med-fat meat, 1 fat
Rigatoni (9 oz)	180	25	4	2	560	1-1/2 carb., 1 med-fat meat
Roasted Turkey Breast & Stuffing & Cinnamon Apples (9-3/4 oz)	290	48	4	1	530	3 carb., 2 lean meat
Salisbury Steak w/Macaroni & Cheese (9-1/2 oz)	270	27	8	4	590	2 carb., 3 lean meat
Spaghetti w/Meat Sauce (11-1/2 oz)	290	45	6	2	550	3 carb., 1 med-fat meat
Spaghetti w/Meatballs (9-1/2 oz)	290	40	7	2	520	2-1/2 carb., 2 lean meat

Stuffed Cabbage w/Whipped Potatoes (9-1/2 oz)	220	27	7	2	460	2 carb., 1 med-fat meat
Swedish Meatballs w/Pasta (9-1/8 oz)	290	32	3	3	590	2 carb., 2 med-fat meat
Three-Bean Chili w/Rice (9 oz)	210	32	6	2	460	2 carb., 1 fat
Turkey Pie (9-1/2 oz)	300	34	9	2	590	2 carb., 2 med-fat meat
MORTON						
Breaded Chicken Patty Meal (6.75 oz)	280	24	15	3	840	1-1/2 carb., 1 med-fat meat, 2 fat
Chicken Nuggets Meal (7 oz)	320	30	17	4	460	2 carb., 1 med-fat meat, 2 fat
Chili Gravy w/Beef Enchilada & Tamale (10 oz)	260	40	7	3	1000	2-1/2 carb., 1 fat
Fried Chicken Meal (9 oz)	420	30	25	8	1000	2 carb., 2 med-fat meat, 3 fat
Gravy & Charbroiled Beef Patty Meal (9 oz)	290	26	16	7	1210	2 carb., 1 med-fat meat, 2 fat
Gravy & Salisbury Steak Meal (9 oz)	210	23	9	4	950	1-1/2 carb., 1 med-fat meat, 1 fat
Gravy & Turkey w/Dressing Meal (9 oz)	230	27	8	3	1090	2 carb., 1 med-fat meat, 1 fat
Macaroni & Cheese (6.5 oz)	200	35	3	2	600	2 carb., 1 fat
Meat Loaf w/Tomato Sauce (9 oz)	250	24	13	4	1110	1-1/2 carb., 1 med-fat meat, 2 fat
Spaghetti w/Meat Sauce (8.5 oz)	170	30	3	1	600	2 carb., 1 fat

COMBINATION FOODS & FROZEN ENTREES

Products	Cal.	Carb. (g)	Fat (g)	Sat. Fat (g)	Sodium (mg)	Exchanges
Veal Parmigiana w/Tomato Sauce (8.75 oz)	280	30	13	4	950	2 carb., 3 fat
Vegetable Pot Pie w/Beef (7 oz)	310	34	17	8	1380	2 carb., 3 fat
Vegetable Pot Pie w/Chicken (7 oz)	320	32	18	7	1020	2 carb., 3 fat
Vegetable Pot Pie w/Turkey (7 oz)	300	29	18	9	1060	2 carb., 3 fat
MRS. PAUL'S						
Cod Fillets, Premium (1)	250	24	11	3	510	1-1/2 carb., 1 med-fat meat, 1 fat
Corn Fritters (1)	130	16	7	2	310	2 carb., 1 fat
Deviled Crab Miniatures (6)	240	27	11	3	540	2 carb., 2 fat
Deviled Crabs (3 oz)	180	19	9	3	540	1 carb., 1 med-fat meat, 1 fat
Fish Fillets, Batter Dip (1)	170	16	10	3	420	1 carb., 1 med-fat meat, 1 fat
Fish Fillets, Crispy Crunchy Breaded (2)	220	21	10	3	490	1-1/2 carb., 1 med-fat meat, 1 fat
Fish Fillets, Crunchy Battered (2)	250	23	13	3	680	1-1/2 carb., 1 med-fat meat, 2 fat
Fish Sticks (2)	210	25	8	2	740	1-1/2 carb., 1 med-fat meat, 1 fat
Fish Sticks, Battered (6)	270	27	15	4	670	2 carb., 3 fat

OLD EL PASO

						Exchanges/Choices
Burrito, Bean & Cheese (1)	290	44	9	5	840	3 carb., 1 med-fat meat, 1 fat
Burrito, Beef/Bean, Medium (1)	320	46	10	4	800	3 carb., 1 med-fat meat, 1 fat
Chimichanga, Beef (1)	370	37	20	5	470	2-1/2 carb., 4 fat
Chimichanga, Chicken (1)	350	39	16	4	540	2-1/2 carb., 1 med-fat meat, 2 fat
Pizza Burrito, Cheese (1)	320	27	9	4	430	2 carb., 1 med-fat meat, 1 fat
Pizza Burrito, Pepperoni (1)	260	31	10	5	510	2 carb., 1 med-fat meat, 1 fat
Pizza Burrito, Sausage (1)	260	32	9	4	420	2 carb., 1 med-fat meat, 1 fat

ORE IDA

						Exchanges/Choices
Baked BBQ Sauce w/Beef Pocket (5 oz)	350	48	11	3	580	3 carb., 1 med-fat meat, 1 fat
Chicken Broccoli Cheese Pocket (5 oz)	330	43	11	3	590	3 carb., 1 med-fat meat, 1 fat
Chicken Fajita Pocket (4 oz)	250	35	8	2	390	2 carb., 1 med-fat meat, 1 fat
Fried Shredded Beef Cheddar Pocket (6 oz)	430	45	19	7	550	3 carb., 2 med-fat meat, 2 fat
Ham & Cheese Pocket (5 oz)	370	46	15	6	880	3 carb., 1 med-fat meat, 2 fat
Pepperoni Pizza Pocket (6 oz)	510	50	26	7	1040	3 carb., 1 med-fat meat, 4 fat
Pizza Deluxe Pocket (5 oz)	400	39	19	7	590	2-1/2 carb., 2 med-fat meat, 2 fat

COMBINATION FOODS & FROZEN ENTREES

Products	Cal.	Carb. (g)	Fat (g)	Sat. Fat (g)	Sodium (mg)	Exchanges
Turkey Swiss Broccoli Pocket (6 oz)	380	49	14	5	690	3 carb., 1 med-fat meat, 2 fat
OSCAR MAYER						
Lunchables Bologna/American (4.5-oz pkg)	470	22	35	17	1670	1-1/2 carb., 2 med-fat meat, 5 fat
Lunchables Deluxe Chicken/Turkey (5.1-oz pkg)	390	25	23	11	1830	1-1/2 carb., 2 med-fat meat, 3 fat
Lunchables Deluxe Turkey/Ham (5.1-oz pkg)	370	25	21	10	1940	1-1/2 carb., 2 med-fat meat, 2 fat
Lunchables Fun Pack Bologna w/Wild Cherry (1 pkg)	530	60	28	14	1180	4 carb., 1 med-fat meat, 5 fat
Lunchables Fun Pack Ham w/Fruit Punch (1 pkg)	440	54	20	9	1270	3-1/2 carb., 2 med-fat meat, 2 fat
Lunchables Fun Pack Mozzarella Pizza w/Fruit Punch (1 pkg)	450	61	15	9	740	4 carb., 1 med-fat meat, 2 fat
Lunchables Fun Pack Pepperoni Pizza w/Orange (1 pkg)	450	62	16	8	850	4 carb., 1 med-fat meat, 2 fat

Food						Exchanges
Lunchables Fun Pack Turkey w/Pacific Cooler Juice Drink (1 pkg)	450	54	20	10	1340	3-1/2 carb., 2 med-fat meat, 2 fat
Lunchables Ham/Cheddar (4.5-oz pkg)	360	21	22	11	1750	1-1/2 carb., 2 med-fat meat, 2 fat
Lunchables Ham/Swiss (4.5-oz pkg)	340	20	20	10	1780	1 carb., 3 med-fat meat, 1 fat
Lunchables Low-Fat Turkey w/Pacific Cooler Juice Drink (1 pkg)	360	56	9	5	1190	4 carb., 1 med-fat meat, 1 fat
Lunchables Low-Fat Ham w/Fruit Punch (1 pkg)	350	50	10	5	1150	3 carb., 2 med-fat meat
Lunchables Low-Fat Ham w/Surfer Cooler Juice Drink (1 pkg)	390	58	11	5	1350	4 carb., 2 med-fat meat
Lunchables Pizza, 2-Cheese (4.5-oz pkg)	300	29	13	7	710	2 carb., 1 med-fat meat, 2 fat
Lunchables Pizza, Pepperoni/Mozzarella (4.5-oz pkg)	330	32	15	7	850	2 carb., 1 med-fat meat, 2 fat
Lunchables Salami/American (4.5-oz pkg)	430	21	30	15	1610	1-1/2 carb., 2 med-fat meat, 4 fat
Lunchables Turkey/Cheddar (4.5-oz pkg)	350	22	20	11	1760	1-1/2 carb., 3 med-fat meat, 1 fat
Lunchables Turkey/Monterey Jack (4.5-oz pkg)	350	20	21	11	1690	1-1/2 carb., 2 med-fat meat, 2 fat

COMBINATION FOODS & FROZEN ENTREES

Products	Cal.	Carb. (g)	Fat (g)	Sat. Fat (g)	Sodium (mg)	Exchanges
PAPPALO'S						
Pizza-For-One, Pepperoni (7.8 oz)	569	52	27	13	1277	3-1/2 carb., 3 med-fat meat, 2 fat
Pizza-For-One, Three-Cheese (7.3 oz)	492	50	20	10	957	3 carb., 3 med-fat meat, 1 fat
PATIO						
Enchilada Dinner, Beef (12 oz)	350	52	10	4	1700	3-1/2 carb., 1 med-fat meat, 1 fat
Enchilada Dinner, Cheese (12 oz)	330	52	8	3	1570	3-1/2 carb., 1 med-fat meat, 1 fat
Enchilada Dinner, Chicken (12 oz)	380	58	9	3	1470	4 carb., 1 med-fat meat, 1 fat
Fiesta Dinner (12 oz)	340	51	9	4	1760	3-1/2 carb., 1 med-fat meat, 1 fat
Mexican-Style Dinner (13.25 oz)	430	59	15	6	1840	4 carb., 1 med-fat meat, 2 fat
Ranchera Dinner (13 oz)	410	55	15	6	2400	3-1/2 carb., 1 med-fat meat, 2 fat
Salisbury Con Queso (11 oz)	390	33	20	11	1570	2 carb., 2 med-fat meat, 2 fat
PROGRESSO						
Ravioli, Beef (1 cup)	260	45	5	2	940	3 carb., 1 fat
Ravioli, Cheese (1 cup)	220	43	2	1	930	3 carb.

RED BARON

Pizza Pouches, Chicken Fajita (1)	240	35	7	2	540	2 carb., 1 med-fat meat
Pizza Pouches, Ham & Cheese (1)	320	33	15	5	980	2 carb., 1 med-fat meat, 2 fat
Pizza Pouches, Pepperoni (1)	340	33	17	6	740	2 carb., 1 med-fat meat, 2 fat
Pizza Pouches, Taco (1)	310	34	14	6	650	2 carb., 1 med-fat meat, 2 fat

SPAGO

Pizza, 5-Grain, Whole-Wheat, Artichoke Hearts (2.7 oz)	170	19	7	NA	12	1 carb., 1 med-fat meat
Pizza, 5-Grain, Whole-Wheat, Spicy Chicken (2.7 oz)	180	18	8	NA	320	1 carb., 1 med-fat meat, 1 fat

STOUFFER'S

Baked Potato, Broccoli Cheese (10.3 oz)	320	30	15	6	770	2 carb., 1 med-fat meat, 1 fat
Baked Potato, Cheese Bacon (9.5 oz)	380	31	22	8	900	2 carb., 1 med-fat meat, 3 fat
Beef Pie (10 oz)	450	36	26	9	1140	2-1/2 carb., 2 med-fat meat, 3 fat
Beef Stroganoff (9.9 oz)	380	30	20	7	1100	2 carb., 2 med-fat meat, 2 fat
Cheese Manicotti (9 oz)	340	32	16	7	810	2 carb., 2 med-fat meat, 1 fat

COMBINATION FOODS & FROZEN ENTREES

Products	Cal.	Carb. (g)	Fat (g)	Sat. Fat (g)	Sodium (mg)	Exchanges
Cheese Pasta Shell & Tomato Sauce (9.4 oz)	340	29	16	7	920	2 carb., 2 med-fat meat, 1 fat
Cheese Tortellini & Tomato Sauce (9.4 oz)	290	40	6	5	740	2-1/2 carb., 2 lean meat
Chicken Divan (8 oz)	210	10	10	4	570	1/2 carb., 3 lean meat
Chicken Oriental (9 oz)	260	30	6	1	530	2 carb., 2 lean meat
Cream Chipped Beef & Biscuit (9 oz)	460	40	28	7	1650	2-1/2 carb., 2 med-fat meat, 4 fat
Creamed Chipped Beef (9 oz)	150	6	11	3	690	1/2 carb., 1 med-fat meat, 1 fat
Enchilada, Cheese (10 oz)	370	48	14	5	890	3 carb., 1 med-fat meat. 2 fat
Enchilada, Chicken (10 oz)	370	45	14	4	970	3 carb., 1 med-fat meat, 2 fat
Green Pepper Steak (10.6 oz)	330	45	9	3	650	3 carb., 1 med-fat meat, 1 fat
Green Peppers, Stuffed (10 oz)	200	24	8	2	900	1-1/2 carb., 1 med-fat meat, 1 fat
Ham w/Asparagus Bake (9.6 oz)	520	32	36	14	1040	2 carb., 2 med-fat meat, 5 fat
Homestyle Baked Chicken (9 oz)	270	19	12	3	750	1 carb., 3 med-fat meat
Homestyle Beef & Potatoes (8.2 oz)	270	25	10	3	900	1-1/2 carb., 2 med-fat meat
Homestyle Beef Pot Roast (9 oz)	270	25	10	3	640	1-1/2 carb., 2 med-fat meat

						Exchanges/Choices
Homestyle Chicken Fettuccine (10.6 oz)	380	32	15	4	1250	2 carb., 4 lean meat
Homestyle Chicken Monterey (9.5 oz)	410	35	20	9	700	2 carb., 2 med-fat meat, 2 fat
Homestyle Chicken Parmigiana (11 oz)	320	30	10	2	890	2 carb., 2 med-fat meat
Homestyle Chicken Tenders (6.7 oz)	380	33	18	3	1060	2 carb., 2 med-fat meat, 2 fat
Homestyle Fish & Macaroni & Cheese (9 oz)	430	37	21	5	930	2-1/2 carb., 1 med-fat meat, 2 fat
Homestyle Fried Chicken (7.2 oz)	330	29	16	4	780	2 carb., 2 med-fat meat, 1 fat
Homestyle Meat Loaf (10 oz)	380	24	24	8	910	1-1/2 carb., 2 med-fat meat, 3 fat
Homestyle Roast Turkey (8 oz)	280	25	11	3	950	1-1/2 carb., 2 med-fat meat
Homestyle Salisbury Steak & Vegetable (9.9 oz)	370	26	19	NA	1220	1-1/2 carb., 1 vegetable, 2 med-fat meat, 2 fat
Homestyle Veal Parmigana (12 oz)	420	43	19	4	1200	3 carb., 2 med-fat meat, 2 fat
Lasagna, Vegetable (10.6 oz)	370	31	19	5	820	2 carb., 2 med-fat meat, 2 fat
Lasagna, Four-Cheese (10.9 oz)	410	37	19	10	840	2-1/2 carb., 2 med-fat meat, 2 fat
Lasagna w/Meat Sauce (7.7 oz)	260	24	10	4	560	1-1/2 carb., 2 med-fat meat
Pizza, French Bread Cheeseburger (6 oz)	440	31	26	9	1110	2 carb., 2 med-fat meat, 3 fat
Pizza, French Bread Double Cheese (6 oz)	420	44	19	7	790	3 carb., 2 med-fat meat, 2 fat

COMBINATION FOODS & FROZEN ENTREES

Products	Cal.	Carb. (g)	Fat (g)	Sat. Fat (g)	Sodium (mg)	Exchanges
Pizza, French Bread Garden Vegetable (6.4 oz)	340	45	12	4	540	3 carb., 2 fat
Pizza, Lunch Express Pepperoni (5.8 oz)	440	39	23	8	960	2-1/2 carb., 2 med-fat meat, 2 fat
Macaroni & Cheese (12 oz)	330	31	17	6	940	2 carb., 1 med-fat meat, 2 fat
Macaroni w/Beef (11.6 oz)	340	40	12	5	1530	2-1/2 carb., 2 med-fat meat
Noodles Romanoff (12 oz)	460	48	25	6	1400	3 carb., 1 med-fat meat, 4 fat
Ravioli, Beef (9.6 oz)	370	43	14	4	680	3 carb., 1 med-fat meat, 2 fat
Ravioli & Tomato Sauce, Cheese (9.6 oz)	360	42	14	5	720	3 carb., 1 med-fat meat, 2 fat
Side Dish, Potatoes Au Gratin (4.7 oz)	130	15	6	3	590	1 carb., 1 fat
Side Dish, Scalloped Potatoes (4.6 oz)	130	17	6	1	450	1 carb., 1 fat
Spaghetti & Meatballs (12.6 oz)	420	51	15	4	680	3-1/2 carb., 1 med-fat meat, 2 fat
Swedish Meatballs (9.4 oz)	440	36	23	8	840	2-1/2 carb., 2 med-fat meat, 3 fat
Tuna-Noodle Casserole (10 oz)	330	31	14	2	1130	2 carb., 1 med-fat meat, 1 fat
Turkey Pie (10 oz)	530	36	33	9	1040	2-1/2 carb., 2 med-fat meat, 5 fat
Turkey Tetrazzini (10 oz)	360	28	19	3	1140	2 carb., 2 med-fat meat, 2 fat

SWANSON

Food						Exchanges
3-Compartment Noodles & Chicken (10.6 oz)	288	37	11	3	786	2-1/2 carb., 1 med-fat meat, 1 fat
4-Compartment Beef Dinner (11.4 oz)	333	38	8	NA	790	2-1/2 carb., 3 lean meat
4-Compartment Beef Enchilada (14 oz)	475	55	21	NA	1343	3-1/2 carb., 1 med-fat meat, 3 fat
Battered Fish & Chips Dinner (10 oz)	480	55	20	4	1040	3-1/2 carb., 1 med-fat meat, 1 fat
Beef & Gravy Dinner (11 oz)	330	37	9	5	660	2-1/2 carb., 3 lean meat
Beef Enchilada Dinner (14 oz)	480	56	21	12	1350	4 carb., 1 med-fat meat, 3 fat
Beef Pie (7 oz)	364	36	19	5	705	2-1/2 carb., 1 med-fat meat, 3 fat
Beef Pot Pie (7 oz)	380	39	19	8	730	2-1/2 carb., 1 med-fat meat, 3 fat
Budget Breaded Fish Sticks Meal (7 oz)	370	51	13	6	610	2-1/2 carb., 3 fat
Budget Chicken Parmigiana Meal (10 oz)	340	33	18	8	760	2 carb., 1 med-fat meat, 3 fat
Budget Macaroni & Cheese (10.4 oz)	320	43	11	7	960	3 carb., 2 fat
Budget Meat Loaf Meal (9.4 oz)	350	29	21	10	870	2 carb., 1 med-fat meat, 3 fat
Budget Mexican-Style Meal (10.6 oz)	400	52	16	7	1349	3-1/2 carb., 1 med-fat meat, 2 fat
Budget Pasta & Chicken Meal (9 oz)	250	30	11	6	660	2 carb., 1 med-fat meat, 1 fat
Budget Spaghetti & Meatballs (10 oz)	300	36	13	6	1040	2-1/2 carb., 1 med-fat meat, 2 fat

COMBINATION FOODS & FROZEN ENTREES

Products	Cal.	Carb. (g)	Fat (g)	Sat. Fat (g)	Sodium (mg)	Exchanges
Burrito, Hot & Spicy (3.5 oz)	220	30	7	3	490	2 carb., 1 fat
Chicken & Noodles Entree (9 oz)	314	31	15	4	1000	2 carb., 1 med-fat meat, 2 fat
Chicken & Noodles w/Vegetables (9 oz)	320	32	15	8	980	2 carb., 1 med-fat meat, 2 fat
Chicken & Noodles w/Vegetables in Cream (9 oz)	320	32	15	8	980	2 carb., 1 med-fat meat, 2 fat
Chicken Nibbles (3 oz)	290	19	18	5	660	1 carb., 1 med-fat meat, 3 fat
Chicken Nibbles (4.3 oz)	340	31	20	9	730	2 carb., 1 med-fat meat, 3 fat
Chicken Nibbles w/Fries (4.3 oz)	322	27	19	NA	715	2 carb., 1 med-fat meat, 3 fat
Chicken Parmigiana Dinner (11.6 oz)	400	43	19	7	1150	3 carb., 1 med-fat meat, 3 fat
Chicken Pot Pie (7 oz)	410	45	22	8	810	3 carb., 4 fat
Chicken Tenders Platter (8 oz)	320	39	12	3	790	2-1/2 carb., 1 med-fat meat, 1 fat
Fish'n Chips (5.6 oz)	310	38	12	5	620	2-1/2 carb., 1 med-fat meat, 1 fat
Fried Chicken Dark Portion Meal (9.6 oz)	420	36	22	8	1040	2-1/2 carb., 2 med-fat meat, 2 fat
Fried Chicken Dinner, Dark Meat (9.9 oz)	560	56	28	11	1139	4 carb., 1 med-fat meat, 5 fat

Fried Chicken Dinner, White Meat (10.4 oz)	550	60	26	11	1409	4 carb., 2 med-fat meat, 3 fat
Fried Chicken w/Whipped Potatoes (7 oz)	400	34	21	8	1120	2 carb., 2 med-fat meat, 2 fat
Hot Roast Beef Sandwich Dinner (10.4 oz)	380	46	13	4	500	3 carb., 1 med-fat meat, 2 fat
Hungry Man Beef Pie (14 oz)	620	65	29	14	1370	4 carb., 4 med-fat meat, 4 fat
Hungry Man Boneless Chicken Dinner (17.5 oz)	700	76	28	11	1379	5 carb., 3 med-fat meat, 3 fat
Hungry Man Chicken Pie (14 oz)	650	64	35	14	1470	4 carb., 1 med-fat meat, 6 fat
Hungry Man Fried Chicken, Mostly White Meat (16.7 oz)	810	77	40	14	2060	5 carb., 3 med-fat meat, 5 fat
Hungry Man Fried Chicken Dinner, Dark Meat (14.4 oz)	810	76	41	14	1710	5 carb., 3 med-fat meat, 5 fat
Hungry Man Grilled Chicken Patty Dinner (17.2 oz)	580	67	19	8	1350	4-1/2 carb., 3 med-fat meat, 1 fat
Hungry Man Meat Loaf Dinner (16.7 oz)	620	57	31	16	1639	4 carb., 2 med-fat meat, 4 fat
Hungry Man Mexican-Style Dinner (20 oz)	780	86	36	16	2120	6 carb., 1 med-fat meat, 6 fat
Hungry Man Salisbury Steak Dinner (16.5 oz)	610	45	34	17	1459	3 carb., 3 med-fat meat, 4 fat

COMBINATION FOODS & FROZEN ENTREES

Products	Cal.	Carb. (g)	Fat (g)	Sat. Fat (g)	Sodium (mg)	Exchanges
Hungry Man Turkey Dinner, Mostly White Meat (16.7 oz)	490	59	13	8	1419	4 carb., 3 med-fat meat
Hungry Man Turkey Pie (14 oz)	650	65	34	13	1449	4 carb., 1 med-fat meat, 6 fat
Hungry Man Sirloin Beef Tips Dinner (16 oz)	450	49	16	6	870	3 carb., 3 med-fat meat
Hungry Man Veal Parmigiana Dinner (18.5 oz)	590	58	25	14	1750	4 carb., 3 med-fat meat, 2 fat
Hungry Man Yankee Pot Roast Dinner (16.2 oz)	400	47	11	3	910	3 carb., 3 lean meat
Kid Breakfast, French Toast Stick (3.8 oz)	310	41	14	4	300	3 carb., 2 fat
Kids Fun Feast Roarin' Ravioli (11 oz)	420	69	11	5	500	4-1/2 carb., 1 fat
Macaroni & Cheese Entree (9 oz)	280	36	10	5	1050	2-1/2 carb., 1 med-fat meat, 1 fat
Meat Loaf Dinner (11.4 oz)	410	44	18	9	1060	3 carb., 1 med-fat meat, 1 fat
Pizza w/Cheese & Pepperoni (3.5 oz)	240	28	9	3	410	2 carb., 1 med-fat meat, 1 fat
Plump & Juicy Fried Chicken (3 oz)	240	15	14	5	610	1 carb., 2 med-fat meat, 2 fat
Rib-Shaped Pork Patty Dinner (10 oz)	510	57	23	8	1139	4 carb., 2 med-fat meat, 3 fat
Salisbury Steak Dinner (10.6 oz)	390	42	18	7	880	3 carb., 1 med-fat meat, 3 fat

Item						Exchanges
Sirloin Beef Tip Noodles & Gravy (10 oz)	290	32	11	5.01	490	2 carb., 2 med-fat meat
Sirloin Beef Tips & Noodles (9 oz)	410	39	22	8	1009	2-1/2 carb., 1 med-fat meat, 3 fat
Turkey Breast Meat w/Pasta (11.4 oz)	290	31	8	4	700	2 carb., 2 med-fat meat
Turkey Dinner, Mostly White Meat (11.6 oz)	310	42	7	2	970	3 carb., 3 lean meat
Turkey Pot Pie (7 oz)	440	44	24	9	750	3 carb., 5 fat
Turkey w/Gravy & Dressing (9 oz)	280	30	10	5	860	2 carb., 2 med-fat meat
Veal Parmigiana (10 oz)	310	33	12	5	970	2 carb., 2 med-fat meat
Veal Parmigiana Dinner (11.6 oz)	400	40	18	8	1060	2-1/2 carb., 2 med-fat meat, 2 fat
Yankee Pot Roast Dinner (11.6 oz)	270	36	7	4	660	2-1/2 carb., 1 med-fat meat
TOMBSTONE						
Pizza-For-One, Cheese & Pepperoni (7 oz)	580	41	35	15	1170	3 carb., 2 med-fat meat, 5 fat
Pizza-For-One, Sausage & Pepperoni (7 oz)	590	40	37	15	1200	2-1/2 carb., 3 med-fat meat, 4 fat
Pizza-For-One, Supreme (7.7 oz)	570	41	34	14	1130	3 carb., 2 med-fat meat, 5 fat
TOTINO'S						
Microwave Pizza-For-One, For One (4.25 oz)	284	25	16	4	558	1-1/2 carb., 1 med-fat meat, 2 fat
Microwave Pizza-For-One, Supreme (4.3 oz)	290	25	17	4	679	1-1/2 carb., 1 med-fat meat, 2 fat

COMBINATION FOODS & FROZEN ENTREES

Products	Cal.	Carb. (g)	Fat (g)	Sat. Fat (g)	Sodium (mg)	Exchanges
Party Pizza, Combination, Family (1/4)	306	28	16	4	738	2 carb., 1 med-fat meat, 2 fat
Party Pizza, Canadian Bacon (1/2)	320	33	15	3	900	2 carb., 1 med-fat meat, 2 fat
Party Pizza, Cheese (1/2)	320	33	14	5	630	2 carb., 1 med-fat meat, 2 fat
Party Pizza, Pepperoni (1/2)	380	33	21	5	920	2 carb., 1 med-fat meat, 3 fat
Party Pizza, Sausage, Family (1/4)	307	29	16	4	727	2 carb., 1 med-fat meat, 2 fat
Party Pizza, Three-Meat (1/2)	360	33	19	4	910	2 carb., 1 med-fat meat, 3 fat
Pizza Pops, Pepperoni (4 oz)	320	30	16	6	794	2 carb., 1 med-fat meat, 2 fat
Pizza Pops, Supreme (4 oz)	299	30	15	5	676	2 carb., 1 med-fat meat, 2 fat
Pizza Rolls, Pepperoni & Cheese (10)	358	37	17	5	580	2-1/2 carb., 1 med-fat meat, 2 fat
Pizza Rolls, Three-Cheese (10)	362	42	15	6	609	3 carb., 1 med-fat meat, 2 fat
Pizza Rolls, Three-Meat (10)	347	37	15	5	629	2-1/2 carb., 1 med-fat meat, 2 fat
Select Pizza, Supreme (1/3)	347	29	18	7	772	2 carb., 2 med-fat meat, 2 fat
Select Pizza, Two-Cheese & Pepperoni (1/3)	363	30	20	8	823	2 carb., 2 med-fat meat, 2 fat

VAN DE KAMP

	Cal.	Carb.	Fat	Sat. Fat	Sod.	Exchanges/Choices
Battered Fish Portions (2)	350	26	22	4	710	2 carb., 1 med-fat meat, 3 fat
Enchilada, Cheese (7.6 oz)	300	31	15	NA	980	2 carb., 1 med-fat meat, 2 fat
Enchilada, Shredded Beef (5.6 oz)	360	40	14	NA	1010	2-1/2 carb., 2 med-fat meat, 1 fat

WEIGHT WATCHERS

	Cal.	Carb.	Fat	Sat. Fat	Sod.	Exchanges/Choices
Angel Hair Pasta (9 oz)	180	33	2	<1	230	2 carb.
Barbecue-Glazed Chicken (7.5 oz)	190	22	4	1	340	1-1/2 carb., 2 lean meat
Broccoli & Cheese Baked Potato Entree (10 oz)	230	34	7	2	510	2 carb., 1 med-fat meat
Chicken Chow Mein (9 oz)	200	34	2	<1	430	2 carb., 1 lean meat
Chicken Cordon Bleu (9 oz)	220	27	6	2	500	2 carb., 2 lean meat
Chicken Enchiladas Suiza Entree (9 oz)	250	28	8	3	570	2 carb., 1 med-fat meat, 1 fat
Chicken Fettuccine Entree (8.4 oz)	280	25	9	3	590	1-1/2 carb., 3 lean meat
Chicken Marsala Entree (9 oz)	150	22	2	<1	500	1-1/2 carb., 1 lean meat
Chicken Mirabella (9.3 oz)	170	26	2	<1	410	2 carb., 1 lean meat
Chicken Parmigiana (9.2 oz)	230	25	6	3	470	1-1/2 carb., 2 lean meat
English Muffin Sandwich (4 oz)	220	31	7	2	380	2 carb., 1 med-fat meat

COMBINATION FOODS & FROZEN ENTREES

Products	Cal.	Carb. (g)	Fat (g)	Sat. Fat (g)	Sodium (mg)	Exchanges
Fettuccine Alfredo w/Broccoli (8.6 oz)	220	24	6	3	540	1-1/2 carb., 2 lean meat
Fiesta Chicken (8.6 oz)	220	38	2	<1	480	2-1/2 carb., 1 lean meat
Fried Fillet of Fish (7.8 oz)	230	25	8	3	450	1-1/2 carb., 2 med-fat meat
Garden Omelet Sandwich (3.6 oz)	220	31	6	2	440	2 carb., 1 med-fat meat
Grilled Salisbury Beef Steak (8.6 oz)	250	24	9	3	590	1-1/2 carb., 2 med-fat meat
Ham & Cheese Omelet (4 oz)	230	30	6	3	470	2 carb., 1 med-fat meat
Honey Dijon Turkey Pretzel Sandwich (4 oz)	230	36	4	2	500	2-1/2 carb., 1 med-fat meat
Honey Mustard Chicken (8.6 oz)	200	33	2	<1	340	2 carb., 1 lean meat
Lasagna, Garden (11 oz)	230	30	5	1	460	2 carb., 2 lean meat
Lasagna Curls w/Italian Vegetables (9.6 oz)	170	33	2	<1	390	2 carb., 1 vegetable
Lasagna Entree, Italian Cheese (11 oz)	300	28	8	3	560	2 carb., 3 lean meat
Lasagna Florentine (10 oz)	210	35	2	<1	420	2 carb., 1 lean meat
Lasagna w/Meat Sauce Entree (10.4 oz)	290	34	7	3	580	2 carb., 3 lean meat
Lemon Herb Chicken Piccata (8.6 oz)	190	32	2	<1	590	2 carb., 1 lean meat

Food	Calories	Carb (g)	Fat (g)	Sat Fat (g)	Sodium (mg)	Exchanges
Macaroni & Beef (9-1/2 oz)	220	32	5	2	560	2 carb., 1 med-fat meat
Macaroni & Cheese (9 oz)	260	43	6	2	550	3 carb., 1 med-fat meat
Nacho Grande Chicken Enchiladas (9 oz)	290	42	8	3	560	3 carb., 1 med-fat meat, 1 fat
Penne Pasta w/Sun-Dried Tomatoes (10 oz)	290	48	9	3	550	3 carb., 1 med-fat meat, 1 fat
Pizza, Extra Cheese (5.8 oz)	390	49	12	4	590	3 carb., 2 med-fat meat
Pizza, Pepperoni (6.2 oz)	427	50	13	4	712	3 carb., 2 med-fat meat
Pocket Sandwich, Deluxe Pizza (5 oz)	300	46	7	3	490	3 carb., 1 med-fat meat
Pocket Sandwich, Ham & Cheese (5 oz)	240	32	7	3	480	2 carb., 1 med-fat meat
Ravioli Florentine (8.6 oz)	200	37	2	<1	480	2-1/2 carb.
Roast Glazed Chicken (9 oz)	200	25	5	3	510	1-1/2 carb., 2 lean meat
Roast Turkey Medallions (8.6 oz)	190	34	2	<1	530	2 carb., 1 lean meat
Sausage Biscuit (3 oz)	230	20	11	4	560	1 carb., 1 med-fat meat, 1 fat
Shrimp Marinara (9 oz)	190	35	2	<1	400	2 carb., 1 lean meat
Southern Fried Chicken (8 oz)	280	25	11	5	590	1-1/2 carb., 2 med-fat meat
Spaghetti w/Meat Sauce Entree (10 oz)	250	24	6	2	470	1-1/2 carb., 2 lean meat
Swedish Meatballs (9 oz)	280	35	8	3	510	2 carb., 2 med-fat meat

COMBINATION FOODS & FROZEN ENTREES

Products	Cal.	Carb. (g)	Fat (g)	Sat. Fat (g)	Sodium (mg)	Exchanges
Tex-Mex Chicken (8.4 oz)	260	35	4	2	430	2 carb., 2 lean meat
Tuna-Noodle Casserole (9.6 oz)	240	30	7	3	580	2 carb., 1 med-fat meat

DESSERTS

Products	Cal.	Carb. (g)	Fat (g)	Sat. Fat (g)	Sodium (mg)	Exchanges
Angel Food Cake (1 piece)	137	31	<1	<1	397	2 carb.
Apple Brown Betty (3/4 cup)	294	51	9	5	329	3-1/2 carb., 2 fat
Apple Turnover (1)	289	36	15	4	262	2-1/2 carb., 3 fat
Bread Pudding w/Raisins (1/2 cup)	212	31	7	3	291	2 carb., 1 fat
Brownie (1 small)	115	18	5	1	88	1 carb., 1 fat
Brownie w/Nuts (2-inch square)	140	20	7	1	83	1 carb., 1 fat
Cake, Chocolate w/Chocolate Icing (1 piece)	253	38	11	3	230	2-1/2 carb., 2 fat
Cake, Frosted (2-inch square)	175	29	6	2	194	2 carb., 1 fat
Cake, German Chocolate w/Icing (1 slice)	404	55	21	5	369	3-1/2 carb., 4 fat
Cake, Pound w/Butter (1 piece)	113	14	6	1	115	1 carb., 1 fat
Cake, Unfrosted (2-inch square)	97	16	3	<1	168	1 carb., 1 fat
Cake, White w/White Icing (1 piece)	266	45	10	4	166	3 carb., 2 fat

DESSERTS

Products	Cal.	Carb. (g)	Fat (g)	Sat. Fat (g)	Sodium (mg)	Exchanges
Cake, Yellow w/Chocolate Icing (1 piece)	262	38	14	3	233	2-1/2 carb., 3 fat
Cake/Wafer Ice Cream Cone (1)	17	3	<1	<1	6	free
Cheesecake (1/12)	295	24	21	11	190	1-1/2 carb., 4 fat
Chocolate Chips, Semisweet (1/4 cup)	203	27	13	8	5	2 carb., 3 fat
Cobbler, Apple (3 x 3-inch piece)	199	35	6	1	304	2 carb., 1 fat
Cobbler, Cherry (3 x 3-inch piece)	198	34	6	1	311	2 carb., 1 fat
Cobbler, Peach (3 x 3-inch piece)	204	37	6	1	308	2-1/2 carb., 1 fat
Coconut Macaroons (1, 2-inch)	97	17	3	3	59	1 carb., 1 fat
Coffee Cake, Cinnamon w/Crumb Topping (1 piece)	263	29	15	3	221	2 carb., 3 fat
Cookies (1, 3-inch)	142	19	7	2	103	1 carb., 1 fat
Cookies, Chocolate Chip (1)	78	9	5	1	55	1/2 carb., 1 fat
Cookies, Fat-Free (2)	68	16	<1	0	51	1 carb.
Cookies, Fortune (2)	61	13	<1	<1	44	1 carb.
Cookies, Lady Fingers (4)	161	26	4	1	65	2 carb., 1 fat

Cookies, Oatmeal (1)	81	12	3	<1	69	1 carb., 1 fat
Cookies, Peanut Butter (1)	72	9	4	2	62	1/2 carb., 1 fat
Cookies, Sandwich w/Creme Filling (2)	94	14	4	<1	120	1 carb., 1 fat
Cookies, Shortbread (4)	161	21	8	2	146	1-1/2 carb., 2 fat
Cookies, Snickerdoodle (1)	81	12	4	2	68	1 carb., 1 fat
Cookies, Soft Raisin (1)	60	10	2	<1	51	1/2 carb.
Cookies, Sugar (1)	72	10	3	2	54	1/2 carb., 1 fat
Crepe, Chocolate-Filled (1)	119	15	5	2	148	1 carb., 1 fat
Crepe, Fruit-Filled (1)	131	21	4	1	124	1-1/2 carb., 1 fat
Crisp, Apple, Homemade (1/2 cup)	230	46	5	1	257	3 carb., 1 fat
Crisp, Cherry (3 x 3-inch piece)	158	28	5	<1	73	2 carb., 1 fat
Crisp, Peach (3 x 3-inch piece)	166	30	5	<1	69	2 carb., 1 fat
Cupcake, Chocolate w/Chocolate Icing (1)	154	23	7	2	140	1-1/2 carb., 1 fat
Cupcake, Frosted (1 small)	172	28	6	NA	161	2 carb., 1 fat
Custard, Homemade (1/2 cup)	148	15	7	3	109	1 carb., 1 fat
Fruit Juice Bar, Frozen, w/Cream (1)	87	19	1	<1	20	1 carb.

DESSERTS

Products	Cal.	Carb. (g)	Fat (g)	Sat. Fat (g)	Sodium (mg)	Exchanges
Fruit Juice Bar, Frozen, 100% Juice (1, 3 oz)	75	19	<1	0	3	1 carb.
Frozen Yogurt, Fat-Free (1/3 cup)	60	12	0	0	58	1 carb.
Frozen Yogurt, Low-Fat (1/3 cup)	66	14	1	<1	26	1 carb.
Gelatin, Mandarin Orange (1/2 cup)	90	20	0	0	70	1 carb.
Gelatin Snacks, Grape (1)	80	18	0	0	45	1 carb.
Gelatin Snacks, Orange (1)	80	18	0	0	45	1 carb.
Gingersnaps (3)	87	16	2	<1	137	1 carb.
Ice Cream (1/2 cup)	133	16	7	7	53	1 carb., 1 fat
Ice Cream, Fat-Free (1/2 cup)	90	20	0	0	65	1 carb.
Ice Cream, Light (1/2 cup)	100	14	4	3	35	1 carb., 1 fat
Ice Cream, No Sugar Added (1/2 cup)	100	13	4	3	45	1 carb., 1 fat
Ice Cream Bar, Creamsicle/Dreamsicle (1)	92	18	2	1	43	1 carb.
Ice Cream Bar, Drumstick (1)	157	18	9	4	48	1 carb., 2 fat
Ice Cream Bar, Fudgesicle (1)	91	19	<1	<1	55	1 carb.

Food						Exchanges
Ice Cream Sandwich (1)	144	22	6	3	36	1-1/2 carb., 1 fat
Ice Pops/Popsicles, Double Stick (1)	92	24	0	0	15	1-1/2 carb.
Marshmallows (4 large)	90	23	<1	0	13	1-1/2 carb.
Parfait, Lime (1/2 cup)	120	21	3	3	105	1-1/2 carb., 1 fat
Pie, Fruit, 2-Crust (1/6)	290	43	13	2	300	3 carb., 3 fat
Pie, Pumpkin or Custard (1/8)	168	19	4	1	209	1 carb., 2 fat
Pudding, Chocolate w/Whole Milk, Homemade (1/2 cup)	221	40	6	3	137	2-1/2 carb., 1 fat
Pudding, Regular (1/2 cup)	144	27	3	2	201	2 carb., 1 fat
Pudding, Rice w/Raisins, Homemade (1/2 cup)	217	40	4	3	85	2-1/2 carb., 1 fat
Pudding, Sugar-Free (1/2 cup)	90	13	2	2	420	1 carb.
Pudding, Tapioca w/2% Milk (1/2 cup)	147	28	2	2	172	2 carb.
Pudding, Tapioca w/Whole Milk, Homemade (1/2 cup)	103	14	4	2	157	1 carb., 1 fat
Pudding, Vanilla w/Whole Milk, Homemade (1/2 cup)	130	20	4	3	113	1 carb., 1 fat

DESSERTS

Products	Cal.	Carb. (g)	Fat (g)	Sat. Fat (g)	Sodium (mg)	Exchanges
Pudding Pop, Chocolate (1)	72	12	2	2	78	1 carb.
Pudding Pop, Vanilla (1)	75	13	2	2	50	1 carb.
Sherbet, Orange (1/2 cup)	132	29	2	1	44	2 carb.
Sorbet, Citrus Fruit (1/2 cup)	92	23	0	0	8	1-1/2 carb.
Sorbet, Non-Citrus Fruit (1/2 cup)	70	17	<1	<1	46	1 carb.
Sugar/Rolled Ice Cream Cone (1)	40	8	<1	<1	32	1/2 carb.
Topping, Butterscotch (2 Tbsp)	103	27	<1	<1	143	2 carb.
Topping, Hot Fudge Chocolate (2 Tbsp)	74	13	3	1	28	1 carb., 1 fat
Topping, Marshmallow Creme (2 Tbsp)	118	30	<1	0	18	2 carb.
Topping, Whipped (2 Tbsp)	24	2	2	1	0	free
Topping, Whipped, Light (2 Tbsp)	19	2	1	<1	0	free
ARCHWAY						
Coconut Macaroons (5)	90	14	5	4	55	1 carb., 1 fat
Cookie Jar Hermits (1)	115	20	3	1	140	1 carb., 1 fat

Cookies, Apple-Filled (1)	110	19	4	1	118	1 carb., 1 fat
Cookies, Apple N' Raisin (1)	130	20	5	1	105	1 carb., 1 fat
Cookies, Blueberry-Filled (1)	110	19	4	1	118	1 carb., 1 fat
Cookies, Chocolate Chip & Toffee (1)	140	19	7	2	120	1 carb., 1 fat
Cookies, Chocolate Chip (3)	130	17	7	2	70	1 carb., 1 fat
Cookies, Cinnamon Honey Heart, Fat-Free (3)	100	24	0	0	115	1-1/2 carb.
Cookies, Cinnamon Snaps (5)	150	20	7	2	120	1 carb., 1 fat
Cookies. Dark Molasses (1)	110	20	4	<1	150	1 carb., 1 fat
Cookies, Date-Filled Oatmeal (1)	90	19	2	0	110	1 carb.
Cookies, Dutch Cocoa (1)	120	19	4	1	108	1 carb., 1 fat
Cookies, Frosty Lemon (1)	120	19	5	1	110	1 carb., 1 fat
Cookies, Frosty Orange (1)	115	20	4	1	140	1 carb., 1 fat
Cookies, Fruit & Honey Bar (f)	110	19	4	1	118	1 carb., 1 fat
Cookies, Fruit Bar, Fat-Free (1)	100	22	0	0	110	1-1/2 carb.
Cookies, Fruit Bar, No-Fat (1)	90	21	0	0	95	1-1/2 carb.
Cookies, Fudge Nut Bar (1)	110	17	5	1	120	1 carb., 1 fat

DESSERTS

Products	Cal.	Carb. (g)	Fat (g)	Sat. Fat (g)	Sodium (mg)	Exchanges
Cookies, Granola, Fat-Free (1)	100	20	0	0	120	1 carb.
Cookies, Iced Gingerbread (3)	140	23	5	1	130	1-1/2 carb., 1 fat
Cookies, Iced Molasses (1)	110	19	4	1	170	1 carb., 1 fat
Cookies, Lemon Snaps (5)	150	20	7	2	115	1 carb., 1 fat
Cookies, Mini Fun Chip (12)	140	21	6	1	100	1-1/2 carb., 1 fat
Cookies, Mini Oatmeal (12)	150	19	8	2	130	1 carb., 2 fat
Cookies, Molasses, Plain/Iced (1)	115	20	4	1	140	1 carb., 1 fat
Cookies, New Orleans Cake (1)	110	19	4	2	98	1 carb., 1 fat
Cookies, Oatmeal (1)	110	20	3	1	100	1 carb., 1 fat
Cookies, Oatmeal Pecan (1)	120	18	5	2	100	1 carb., 1 fat
Cookies, Oatmeal Raisin (1)	110	19	4	1	115	1 carb., 1 fat
Cookies, Oatmeal Raisin, Fat-Free (1)	100	24	0	0	170	1-1/2 carb.
Cookies, Oatmeal Raisin, No-Fat (1)	100	23	0	0	170	1-1/2 carb.
Cookies, Oatmeal Raisin Bran (1)	110	19	4	1	100	1 carb., 1 fat

Cookies, Old-Fashioned Molasses (1)	115	20	3	1	140	1 carb., 1 fat
Cookies, Old-Fashioned Windmill (1)	100	15	4	<1	95	1 carb., 1 fat
Cookies, Peanut Butter (1)	140	16	7	2	125	1 carb., 1 fat
Cookies, Peanut Butter Nougat (3)	160	18	9	2	140	1 carb., 2 fat
Cookies, Pecan Crunch (6)	150	18	8	2	120	1 carb., 2 fat
Cookies, Pfeffernousse (2)	140	32	1	0	100	2 carb.
Cookies, Pineapple-Filled (1)	110	17	4	1	65	1 carb., 1 fat
Cookies, Raspberry-Filled (1)	110	17	4	1	65	1 carb., 1 fat
Cookies, Raspberry Oatmeal, No-Fat (1)	100	24	0	0	170	1-1/2 carb.
Cookies, Ruth's Golden Oatmeal (1)	120	19	4	1	108	1 carb., 1 fat
Cookies, Soft Sugar (1)	110	18	4	1	110	1 carb., 1 fat
Cookies, Soft Sugar Drop (1)	110	19	4	1	118	1 carb., 1 fat
Cookies, Strawberry/Cherry-Filled (1)	110	19	4	2	98	1 carb., 1 fat
Cookies, Sugar (1)	120	20	4	1	190	1 carb., 1 fat
Cookies, Vanilla Wafer (5)	130	22	4	1	130	1-1/2 carb., 1 fat
Cookies, Wedding Cake (3)	160	20	8	2	45	1 carb., 2 fat

DESSERTS

Products	Cal.	Carb. (g)	Fat (g)	Sat. Fat (g)	Sodium (mg)	Exchanges
BANQUET						
Pie, Apple (1/5)	300	41	13	6	370	3 carb., 3 fat
Pie, Banana (1/3)	350	39	21	5	290	2-1/2 carb., 4 fat
Pie, Blackberry (1/5)	300	45	12	5	430	3 carb., 2 fat
Pie, Blueberry (1/5)	260	36	12	5	400	2-1/2 carb., 2 fat
Pie, Cherry (1/5)	290	39	14	6	310	2-1/2 carb., 3 fat
Pie, Chocolate (1/3)	360	43	20	5	240	3 carb., 4 fat
Pie, Coconut (1/3)	350	39	20	6	250	2-1/2 carb., 4 fat
Pie, Lemon (1/3)	360	43	20	5	240	3 carb., 4 fat
Pie, Mincemeat (1/5)	310	46	13	6	430	3 carb., 3 fat
Pie, Peach (1/5)	260	36	12	5	340	2-1/2 carb., 2 fat
Pie, Pumpkin (1/5)	250	40	8	3	340	2-1/2 carb., 2 fat
Pie, Strawberry (1/3)	340	44	17	4	240	3 carb., 3 fat

BEN & JERRY'S

	Calories	Carb.	Fat	Sat. Fat	Sodium	Exchanges
Frozen Yogurt, Cappucino, No-Fat (1/2 cup)	140	32	0	0	85	2 carb.
Frozen Yogurt, Cherry Garcia (1/2 cup)	170	31	3	2	70	2 carb., 1 fat
Frozen Yogurt, Chocolate Fudge Brownie (1/2 cup)	190	36	3	1.5	115	2-1/2 carb., 1 fat
Frozen Yogurt, Chocolate Raspberry (1/2 cup)	200	40	3	2	75	2-1/2 carb., 1 fat
Frozen Yogurt, Coffee Almond Fudge (1/2 cup)	200	30	7	2	85	2 carb., 1 fat
Frozen Yogurt, English Toffee Crunch (1/2 cup)	190	32	6	3	110	2 carb., 1 fat
Ice Cream, Aztec Harvest Coffee (1/2 cup)	230	22	16	10	55	1-1/2 carb., 3 fat
Ice Cream, Butter Pecan (1/2 cup)	310	20	25	11	125	1 carb., 5 fat
Ice Cream, Cherry Garcia (1/2 cup)	240	25	16	10	60	1-1/2 carb., 3 fat
Ice Cream, Chocolate Chip Cookie Dough (1/2 cup)	270	30	17	9	95	2 carb., 3 fat
Ice Cream, Chocolate Fudge Brownie (1/2 cup)	250	33	14	8	90	2 carb., 3 fat
Ice Cream, Chubby Hubby (1/2 cup)	350	31	23	11	160	2 carb., 5 fat
Ice Cream, Coffee Toffee Crunch (1/2 cup)	280	28	19	10	120	2 carb., 4 fat
Ice Cream, Deep Dark Chocolate (1/2 cup)	260	32	15	9	55	2 carb., 3 fat
Ice Cream, Double Chocolate Fudge Swirl (1/2 cup)	260	33	15	9	55	2 carb., 3 fat

DESSERTS

Products	Cal.	Carb. (g)	Fat (g)	Sat. Fat (g)	Sodium (mg)	Exchanges
Ice Cream, Mint Chocolate Cookie (1/2 cup)	260	27	17	10	120	2 carb., 3 fat
Ice Cream, Mocha Fudge (1/2 cup)	270	30	18	10	65	2 carb., 3 fat
Ice Cream, New York Fudge Crunch (1/2 cup)	290	28	20	11	55	2 carb., 4 fat
Ice Cream, No-Fat Strawberry (1/2 cup)	140	31	0	0	65	2 carb.
Ice Cream, No-Fat Vanilla Fudge (1/2 cup)	150	32	0	0	80	2 carb.
Ice Cream, Peanut Butter Cup (1/2 cup)	340	30	26	12	140	2 carb., 5 fat
Ice Cream, Vanilla (1/2 cup)	230	21	17	10	55	1-1/2 carb., 3 fat
Ice Cream, Vanilla Bean (1/2 cup)	230	21	17	10	55	1-1/2 carb., 3 fat
Ice Cream, Vanilla Carmel Fudge Swirl (1/2 cup)	280	33	17	10	75	2 carb., 3 fat
Ice Cream, Wavy Gravy (1/2 cup)	330	29	24	10	95	2 carb., 5 fat
Ice Cream, White Russian (1/2 cup)	220	21	16	9	45	1-1/2 carb., 3 fat
BIRD'S EYE						
Cool Whip Topping, Extra Creamy (2 Tbsp)	30	2	2	2	5	free
Cool Whip Topping, Lite (2 Tbsp)	20	2	1	1	0	free

Food	Cal.	Carb.	Fat	Sat. Fat	Sodium	Exchanges
Cool Whip Topping, Regular (2 Tbsp)	25	2	2	2	0	free
BREYERS LIGHT						
Premium Ice Milk, Chocolate (1/2 cup)	123	19	4	3	46	1 carb., 1 fat
Premium Ice Milk, Strawberry (1/2 cup)	123	19	4	3	63	1 carb., 1 fat
Premium Ice Milk, Vanilla (1/2 cup)	123	19	4	3	63	1 carb., 1 fat
BREYERS						
Ice Cream, Chocolate (1/2 cup)	160	20	8	5	30	1 carb., 2 fat
Ice Cream, Strawberry (1/2 cup)	130	16	6	4	40	1 carb., 1 fat
Ice Cream, Vanilla (1/2 cup)	150	15	8	5	50	1 carb., 2 fat
DANNON						
Frozen Yogurt, All Flavors, Nonfat (1/2 cup)	95	22	<1	<1	53	1-1/2 carb.
Frozen Yogurt, Chocolate (1/2 cup)	122	23	2	NA	64	1-1/2 carb.
Frozen Yogurt, Fruit (1/2 cup)	104	18	2	NA	52	1 carb.
Frozen Yogurt, Variety (1/2 cup)	105	18	2	1	53	1 carb.
DOLE						
Fruit 'N Cream, Strawberry (1)	80	17	1	0	25	1 carb.

DESSERTS

Products	Cal.	Carb. (g)	Fat (g)	Sat. Fat (g)	Sodium (mg)	Exchanges
Fruit 'N Juice Bar, Strawberry (1)	70	17	0	0	5	1 carb.
Juice Bar, Strawberry (1)	45	11	0	0	5	1 carb.
Juice Bar, Strawberry, No Sugar Added (1)	25	6	0	0	5	1/2 carb.
DOVE						
Ice Cream Bar, Chocolate w/Chocolate Coating (1)	339	36	23	14	56	2-1/2 carb., 5 fat
ENTENMANN'S						
Cake, All-Butter French Crumb (1 slice)	210	29	10	6	240	2 carb., 2 fat
Cake, All-Butter Loaf (1 slice)	220	31	10	6	290	2 carb., 2 fat
Cake, Banana Crunch (1 slice)	220	32	9	2	280	2 carb., 2 fat
Cake, Carrot (1 slice)	290	35	16	4	240	2 carb., 3 fat
Cake, Chocolate Fudge (1 slice)	310	47	14	5	260	3 carb., 3 fat
Cake, Fat-Free Cholesterol-Free Apple Spice Crumb (1 slice)	107	25	0	0	115	1-1/2 carb.

Cake, Fat-Free Cholesterol-Free Banana Crunch (1 slice)	140	33	0	0	150	2 carb.
Cake, Fat-Free Cholesterol-Free Banana Loaf (1 slice)	108	25	0	0	137	1-1/2 carb.
Cake, Fat-Free Cholesterol-Free Blueberry Crunch (1 slice)	140	32	0	0	200	2 carb.
Cake, Fat-Free Cholesterol-Free Carrot (1 slice)	170	40	0	0	230	2-1/2 carb.
Cake, Fat-Free Cholesterol-Free Chocolate Crunch (1 slice)	130	32	0	0	170	2 carb.
Cake, Fat-Free Cholesterol-Free Chocolate Loaf (1 slice)	130	30	0	0	250	2 carb.
Cake, Fat-Free Cholesterol-Free Fudge Chocolate (1 slice)	210	51	0	0	270	3-1/2 carb.
Cake, Fat-Free Cholesterol-Free Fudge Gold (1 slice)	220	52	0	0	200	3-1/2 carb.

DESSERTS

Products	Cal.	Carb. (g)	Fat (g)	Sat. Fat (g)	Sodium (mg)	Exchanges
Cake, Fat-Free Cholesterol-Free Gold Chocolate Chip (1 slice)	130	31	0	0	220	2 carb.
Cake, Fat-Free Cholesterol-Free Gold French Crumb (1 slice)	140	35	0	0	150	2 carb.
Cake, Fat-Free Cholesterol-Free Gold Loaf (1 slice)	120	28	0	0	160	2 carb.
Cake, Fat-Free Cholesterol-Free Marble Loaf (1 slice)	130	29	0	0	190	2 carb.
Cake, Fat-Free Cholesterol-Free Raisin Loaf (1 slice)	140	33	0	0	150	2 carb.
Cake, Louisana Crunch (1 slice)	310	45	13	4	290	3 carb., 3 fat
Cake, Marble Loaf (1 slice)	200	25	10	6	230	1-1/2 carb., 2 fat
Cake, Marshmallow-Iced Devil's Food (1 slice)	350	45	18	5	290	3 carb., 4 fat
Cake, Raisin Loaf (1 slice)	220	32	9	2	200	2 carb., 2 fat
Cake, Thick Fudge Golden (1 slice)	330	48	16	4	270	2 carb., 3 fat
Coffee Cake, Cheese (1 slice)	190	24	8	4	160	1-1/2 carb., 2 fat
Coffee Cake, Cheese-Filled Crumb (1 slice)	210	25	10	4	190	1-1/2 carb., 2 fat

Food	Cal	Carb	Fat	Sat Fat	Sod	Exchanges
Coffee Cake, Crumb (1 slice)	250	33	12	3	210	2 carb., 2 fat
Coffee Cake, Fat-Free Cholesterol-Free Cinnamon Apple (1 slice)	130	29	0	0	110	2 carb.
Pie, Coconut Custard (1 slice)	340	35	19	8	310	2 carb., 4 fat
Pie, Fat-Free Cholesterol-Free Cherry Behive (1 slice)	270	64	0	0	310	4 carb.
Pie, Homestyle Apple (1 slice)	300	42	14	4	300	3 carb., 3 fat
Pie, Lemon (1 slice)	340	45	17	5	420	3 carb., 3 fat
ESKIMO PIE						
Ice Cream Bar, Original (1)	160	12	12	8	30	1 carb., 2 fat
Ice Cream Bar, Pecan (1)	190	12	15	8	80	1 carb., 3 fat
Ice Cream Bar, Reduced-Fat (1)	120	13	8	6	10	1 carb., 2 fat
ESTEE						
Cookies, Chocolate Chip (4)	150	21	7	2	30	1-1/2 carb., 1 fat
Cookies, Coconut (4)	140	19	6	2	25	1 carb., 1 fat
Cookies, Fudge (4)	150	19	7	2	45	1 carb., 1 fat

DESSERTS

Products	Cal.	Carb. (g)	Fat (g)	Sat. Fat (g)	Sodium (mg)	Exchanges
Cookies, Oatmeal Raisin (4)	130	19	5	1	25	1 carb., 1 fat
Cookies, Sandwich, Chocolate (3)	160	24	6	2	60	1-1/2 carb., 1 fat
Cookies, Sandwich, Original (3)	160	24	6	2	45	1-1/2 carb., 1 fat
Cookies, Sandwich, Peanut Butter (3)	160	22	7	1	55	1-1/2 carb., 1 fat
Cookies, Sandwich, Vanilla (3)	160	25	5	1	35	1-1/2 carb., 1 fat
Cookies, Shortbread (4)	130	22	4	1	150	1-1/2 carb., 1 fat
Cookies, Vanilla or Lemon (4)	140	19	6	1	25	1 carb., 1 fat
Creme Wafers, Vanilla & Chocolate (7)	150	20	9	2	0	1-1/2 carb., 2 fat
Fig Bars, All Flavors (2 bars)	100	22	1	0	23	1-1/2 carb.
Topping, Choco-Syp (2 Tbsp)	50	11	0	0	15	1 carb.
FROOKIE						
Cookies, Fat-Free Apple Spice (2)	95	22	0	0	165	1-1/2 carb.
Cookies, Fat-Free Banana (2)	95	22	0	0	165	1-1/2 carb.
Cookies, Fat-Free Cranberry Orange (2)	90	20	0	0	150	1 carb.

Food						Exchanges
Cookies, Fat-Free Fruitins Fig (2)	90	21	0	0	75	1-1/2 carb.
Cookies, Fat-Free Oatmeal Raisin (2)	95	22	0	0	165	1-1/2 carb.
HAAGEN DAZS						
Frozen Yogurt, 98% Fat-Free, Orange Tango (1/2 cup)	130	26	<1	<1	25	2 carb.
Frozen Yogurt, 98% Fat-Free, Raspberry Rendezvous (1/2 cup)	130	26	2	<1	25	2 carb.
Frozen Yogurt, Vanilla (1/2 cup)	170	26	4	2	50	2 carb., 1 fat
Frozen Yogurt Bar, Peach (1)	100	19	<1	0	20	1 carb.
Frozen Yogurt Bar, Raspberry (1)	100	19	<1	0	20	1 carb.
Frozen Yogurt Classics, Chocolate (1/2 cup)	160	26	3	2	60	2 carb., 1 fat
Frozen Yogurt Classics, Coffee (1/2 cup)	160	26	3	2	55	2 carb., 1 fat
Frozen Yogurt Classics, Vanilla (1/2 cup)	160	26	3	2	55	2 carb., 1 fat
Frozen Yogurt Crunch Bar, Vanilla Chocolate (1)	210	23	11	2	45	1-1/2 carb., 2 fat
Ice Cream, Chocolate (1/2 cup)	269	24	17	8	50	1-1/2 carb., 3 fat
Ice Cream, Vanilla (1/2 cup)	259	23	17	8	55	1-1/2 carb., 3 fat

DESSERTS

Products	Cal.	Carb. (g)	Fat (g)	Sat. Fat (g)	Sodium (mg)	Exchanges
HEALTH VALLEY						
Cookies, Fat-Free Apple Spice (3)	100	24	0	0	50	1-1/2 carb.
Cookies, Fat-Free Bakes Apple (1)	70	18	0	0	30	1 carb.
Cookies, Fat-Free Bakes Blueberry Apple (1)	110	26	0	0	25	2 carb.
Cookies, Fat-Free Bakes Date (1)	70	18	0	0	30	1 carb.
Cookies, Fat-Free Bakes Raisin (1)	70	18	0	0	30	1 carb.
Cookies, Fat-Free Bakes Raspberry (1)	110	26	0	0	25	2 carb.
Cookies, Fat-Free Bakes Strawberry (1)	110	26	0	0	25	2 carb.
Cookies, Fat-Free Date Delight (3)	100	24	0	0	50	1-1/2 carb.
Cookies, Fat-Free Hawaiian (3)	100	24	0	0	50	1-1/2 carb.
Cookies, Fat-Free Oatmeal Raisin (3)	100	24	0	0	50	1-1/2 carb.
Breakfast Bar Cookie, Fat-Free Apple (1)	110	26	0	0	25	2 carb.
Breakfast Bar Cookie, Fat-Free Apricot (1)	110	26	0	0	25	2 carb.
Breakfast Bar Cookie, Fat-Free Blueberry (1)	110	26	0	0	25	2 carb.

Breakfast Bar Cookie, Fat-Free Cherry (1)	110	26	0	0	25	2 carb.
Breakfast Bar Cookie, Fat-Free Chocolate (1)	110	26	0	0	30	2 carb.
Breakfast Bar Cookie, Fat-Free Raspberry (1)	110	26	0	0	25	2 carb.
Breakfast Bar Cookie, Fat-Free Strawberry (1)	110	26	0	0	25	2 carb.
Brownie Bar Cookie, Fat-Free Caramel Top (1)	110	26	0	0	30	2 carb.
Brownie Bar Cookie, Fat-Free FudgeTop (1)	110	26	0	0	30	2 carb.
Fruit Bar Cookie, Fat-Free Apple (1)	140	35	0	0	0	2 carb.
Fruit Bar Cookie, Fat-Free Apricot (1)	140	35	0	0	5	2 carb.
Fruit Bar Cookie, Fat-Free Date (1)	140	34	0	0	5	2 carb.
Fruit Bar Cookie, Fat-Free Raisin (1)	140	35	0	0	5	2 carb.
Fruit Center Cookie, Fat-Free Apple Raisin (1)	70	18	0	0	20	1 carb.
Fruit Center Cookie, Fat-Free Date (1)	70	18	0	0	20	1 carb.
Granola Bar, Fat-Free Chocolate Chip (1)	140	35	0	0	5	2 carb.
Granola Bar, Fat-Free Strawberry (1)	140	35	0	0	5	2 carb.
Granola Bar, Fat-Free Raspberry (1)	140	35	0	0	5	2 carb.
Healthy Chips Cookies, Fat-Free Double Fudge (3)	100	24	0	0	20	1-1/2 carb.

DESSERTS

Products	Cal.	Carb. (g)	Fat (g)	Sat. Fat (g)	Sodium (mg)	Exchanges
Healthy Chips Cookies, Fat-Free Old-Fashioned (3)	100	24	0	0	20	1-1/2 carb.
Healthy Chocolate Cookies, Fat-Free Fudge Center (2)	70	17	0	0	20	1 carb.
Healthy Chocolate Cookies, Fat-Free Caramel Center (2)	70	17	0	0	20	1 carb.
Healthy Tarts, Fat-Free Baked Apple Cinnamon (1)	150	35	0	0	30	2 carb.
Healthy Tarts, Fat-Free California Strawberry (1)	150	35	0	0	30	2 carb.
Healthy Tarts, Fat-Free Chocolate Fudge (1)	150	35	0	0	30	2 carb.
Healthy Tarts, Fat-Free Cranberry Apple (1)	150	35	0	0	30	2 carb.
Healthy Tarts, Fat-Free Mountain Blueberry (1)	150	35	0	0	30	2 carb.
Healthy Tarts, Fat-Free Red Cherry (1)	150	35	0	0	30	2 carb.
Healthy Tarts, Fat-Free Red Raspberry (1)	150	35	0	0	30	2 carb.
Jumbo Fruit Cookie, Fat-Free Raisin (1)	80	19	0	0	35	1 carb.
Marshmallow Bar, Fat-Free Chocolate (1)	90	22	0	0	0	1-1/2 carb.

Marshmallow Bar, Fat-Free Old-Fashioned (1)	90	22	0	0	0	1-1/2 carb.
Marshmallow Bar, Fat-Free Tropical Fruit (1)	90	22	0	0	0	1-1/2 carb.
Sandwich Bar, Fat-Free Chocolate Caramel Creme (1)	150	26	0	0	35	2 carb.
Sandwich Bar, Fat-Free Chocolate Peanut Creme (1)	150	26	0	0	35	2 carb.
Sandwich Bar, Fat-Free Chocolate Vanilla Creme (1)	150	26	0	0	35	2 carb.

HEALTHY CHOICE

Ice Cream, Low-Fat Bordeax Cherry (1/2 cup)	110	19	2	2	55	1 carb.
Ice Cream, Low-Fat Brownie (1/2 cup)	120	22	2	1	55	1-1/2 carb.
Ice Cream, Low-Fat Butter Pecan (1/2 cup)	120	22	2	1	60	1-1/2 carb.
Ice Cream, Low-Fat Chocolate Chip (1/2 cup)	120	21	2	1	50	1-1/2 carb.
Ice Cream, Low-Fat Cookies & Cream (1/2 cup)	120	21	2	2	90	1-1/2 carb.
Ice Cream, Low-Fat Praline & Cream (1/2 cup)	130	25	2	<1	70	1-1/2 carb.
Ice Cream, Low-Fat Vanilla (1/2 cup)	100	18	2	<1	50	1 carb.
Ice Cream, Low-Fat Vanilla Fudge (1/2 cup)	120	21	2	2	50.1	1-1/2 carb.
Ice Cream, Triple Chocolate Chunk (1/2 cup)	110	21	2	1	60	1-1/2 carb.
Sorbet, Strawberry & Cream (1/2 cup)	90	17	2	1	50	1 carb.

DESSERTS

Products	Cal.	Carb. (g)	Fat (g)	Sat. Fat (g)	Sodium (mg)	Exchanges
HEALTHY INDULGENCE						
Ice Cream, Low-Fat Butter Pecan (1/2 cup)	120	22	2	1	75	1-1/2 carb.
Ice Cream, Low-Fat Delectable Chocolate (1/2 cup)	100	20	1	<1	80	1 carb.
Ice Cream, Low-Fat Vanilla (1/2 cup)	100	20	2	1	70	1 carb.
HEATH						
Ice Cream Bar, English Toffee (1)	206	17	15	12	43	1 carb., 3 fat
HOSTESS						
Twinkies (1)	153	27	5	2	153	2 carb., 1 fat
HUNT'S						
Pudding, Snack Pack, Chocolate (1)	167	25	6	2	173	1-1/2 carb., 1 fat
Pudding, Snack Pack, Fat-Free Chocolate (1/2 cup)	96	21	<1	0	212	1-1/2 carb.
Pudding, Snack Pack, Fat-Free Vanilla (1/2 cup)	93	21	<1	0	167	1-1/2 carb.
Pudding, Snack Pack, Vanilla (1)	163	25	6	1	167	1-1/2 carb., 1 fat

JELL-O

Frozen Gelatin Pops/Bars (1)	31	7	<1	NA	20	1/2 carb.
Gelatin Dessert (1/2 cup)	80	19	0	0	57	1 carb.
Gelatin Dessert, Sugar-Free (1/2 cup)	8	<1	0	0	56	free
Gelatin Snacks, Berry Blue (1)	80	18	0	0	45	1 carb.
Gelatin Snacks, Cherry (1)	80	18	0	0	45	1 carb.
Gelatin Snacks, Strawberry (1)	80	18	0	0	45	1 carb.
Gelatin Snacks, Strawberry Banana (1)	80	18	0	0	45	1 carb.
Pudding Snacks, Chocolate (1)	160	28	5	2	190	2 carb., 1 fat
Pudding Snacks, Chocolate Caramel Swirl (1)	160	27	5	2	180	2 carb., 1 fat
Pudding Snacks, Fat-Free, Chocolate (1)	100	23	0	0	190	1-1/2 carb.
Pudding Snacks, Fat-Free, Chocolate Vanilla Swirl (1)	100	23	0	0	210	1-1/2 carb.
Pudding Snacks, Fat-Free, Vanilla Chocolate Swirl (1)	100	23	0	0	220	1-1/2 carb.
Pudding Snacks, Tapioca (1)	140	26	4	1.5	160	2 carb., 1 fat

DESSERTS

Products	Cal.	Carb. (g)	Fat (g)	Sat. Fat (g)	Sodium (mg)	Exchanges
Pudding Snacks, Vanilla (1)	160	25	5	2	170	2 carb., 1 fat
Pudding Snacks, Vanilla Chocolate Swirl (1)	160	26	5	2	180	2 carb., 1 fat
KEEBLER						
Apple Cinnamon Graham (8)	123	21	4	<1	NA	1-1/2 carb., 1 fat
Chips Deluxe (1)	80	9	5	2	60	1/2 carb., 1 fat
Chips Deluxe, Reduced-Fat (1)	70	11	3	1	70	1 carb.
Chips Deluxe, Soft 'n' Chewy (1)	80	11	4	1	60	1 carb., 1 fat
Cinnamon Crisp (8)	123	22	3	<1	NA	1-1/2 carb., 1 fat
Cinnamon Graham Stick, Low-Fat (16)	111	24	1	<1	NA	1-1/2 carb.
Deluxe Grahams (3)	140	19	7	5	105	1 carb., 1 fat
Deluxe Grahams, Reduced-Fat (3)	120	19	5	2	130	1 carb., 1 fat
E.L. Fudge, Chocolate (2)	120	17	6	1	90	1 carb., 1 fat
Fudge Shoppe (3)	160	21	8	5	140	1-1/2 carb., 2 fat
Fudge Shoppe, Reduced-Fat (3)	130	20	5	2	160	1 carb., 1 fat

Graham Selects (8)	123	22	3	<1	NA	1-1/2 carb., 1 fat
Pecan Sandies (1)	80	9	5	1	75	1/2 carb., 1 fat
Soft Batch, Chocolate Chip (1)	80	10	4	1	70	1/2 carb., 1 fat
KLONDIKE						
Ice Cream Bar, Vanilla (1)	290	24	20	14	65	1-1/2 carb., 4 fat
Ice Cream Sandwich, Big Bear (1)	200	31	7	3	130	2 carb., 1 fat
KRAFT						
Marshmallow Creme (1 oz)	93	23	0	0	23	1-1/2 carb.
Marshmallows, Jet Puffed (5)	110	27	0	0	40	2 carb.
Marshmallows, Miniature (1/2 cup)	100	25	0	0	30	1-1/2 carb.
Topping, Caramel (2 Tbsp)	120	28	0	0	90	2 carb.
Topping, Chocolate-Flavored (2 Tbsp)	110	26	0	0	30	2 carb.
Topping, Pineapple (2 Tbsp)	110	28	0	0	15	2 carb.
Topping, Real Cream (2 Tbsp)	20	1	2	1	0	free
Topping, Strawberry (2 Tbsp)	110	29	0	0	15	2 carb.
Topping, Whipped (2 Tbsp)	20	1	2	1	0	free

DESSERTS

Products	Cal.	Carb. (g)	Fat (g)	Sat. Fat (g)	Sodium (mg)	Exchanges
LA CHOY						
Cookies, Fortune (4)	112	26	<1	<1	11	2 carb.
LIBBY'S						
Pie Filling, Apple (1/3 cup)	80	20	0	0	10	1 carb.
Pie Filling, Blueberry (1/3 cup)	80	19	0	0	0	1 carb.
Pie Filling, Cherry (1/3 cup)	90	22	0	0	0	1-1/2 carb.
MOCHA MIX						
Mocha Mix, Nondairy, Neopolitan (3/4 cup)	207	26	11	2	119	2 carb., 2 fat
Mocha Mix, Nondairy, Vanilla (3/4 cup)	209	26	11	2	117	2 carb., 2 fat
Mocha Mix, Nondairy, Vanilla Chocolate Almond (3/4 cup)	234	27	13	4	171	2 carb., 3 fat
MRS. SMITH'S						
Pie, Natural Juice Cherry (1/7)	410	59	18	NA	380	4 carb., 4 fat
Pie, Old-Fashioned Apple (1/8)	530	69	27	NA	670	4-1/2 carb., 5 fat

Item					Exchanges
Pie, Old-Fashioned Apple Raisin (1/8)	560	74	28	NA	705	5 carb, 6 fat
Pie, Old-Fashioned Blueberry 1/8)	460	72	17	NA	455	5 carb, 3 fat
Pie, Old-Fashioned Cherry (1/8)	460	67	19	NA	515	4-1/2 carb., 4 fat
Pie, Old-Fashioned Peach (1/8)	460	67	19	5	470	4-1/2 carb., 4 fat
Pie, Ready-To-Bake Apple (1/8)	390	56	17	4	590	4 carb., 3 fat
Pie, Ready-To-Bake Berry (1/8)	400	62	16	NA	470	4 carb., 3 fat
Pie, Ready-To-Bake Blueberry (1/8)	380	54	17	NA	535	3-1/2 carb., 3 fat
Pie, Ready-To-Bake Cherry (1/8)	400	60	16	4	445	4 carb., 3 fat
Pie, Ready-To-Bake Coconut Custard (1/8)	330	40	15	NA	550	2-1/2 carb., 3 fat
Pie, Ready-To-Bake Dutch Apple (1/8)	420	72	13	NA	420	5 carb., 3 fat
Pie, Ready-To-Bake Egg Custard (1/8)	300	45	9	NA	490	3 carb., 2 fat
Pie, Ready-To-Bake Peach (1/8)	365	53	16	4	435	3-1/2 carb., 3 fat
Pie, Ready-To-Bake Pumpkin Custard (1/8)	310	46	11	NA	495	3 carb., 2 fat
Pie, Ready-To-Bake Red Raspberry (1/8)	390	61	15	NA	460	4 carb., 3 fat
Pie, Ready-To-Bake Strawberry Rhubarb (1/8)	410	60	17	NA	490	4 carb., 3 fat
Pie, Thaw 'N Serve Apple Lattice (1/8)	280	44	11	NA	425	3 carb., 2 fat

DESSERTS

Products	Cal.	Carb. (g)	Fat (g)	Sat. Fat (g)	Sodium (mg)	Exchanges
Pie, Thaw 'N Serve Banana Cream (1/8)	240	31	12	NA	180	2 carb., 2 fat
Pie, Thaw 'N Serve Blueberry Lattice (1/8)	290	45	11	NA	310	3 carb., 2 fat
Pie, Thaw 'N Serve Cherry Lattice (1/8)	300	50	10	NA	305	3 carb., 2 fat
Pie, Thaw 'N Serve Lemon Meringue (1/8)	290	58	6	2	250	4 carb., 1 fat
Pie, Thaw 'N Serve Peach Lattice (1/8)	300	44	12	NA	285	3 carb., 2 fat
Pie Shells (1/8)	130	14	8	NA	270	1 strch, 2 fat
NABISCO						
Beach Bears (22)	120	22	4	<1	150	1-1/2 carb., 1 fat
Bugs Bunny Graham Crackers (10)	120	22	4	<1	140	1-1/2 carb., 1 fat
Chips Ahoy! Chocolate Chip Cookies (2)	142	19	7	2	98	1 carb., 1 fat
Chocolate Chip Snaps (6)	140	22	4	<1	110	1-1/2 carb., 1 fat
Chocolate Snaps (8)	120	20	4	2	160	1 carb., 1 fat
Famous Chocolate Wafers (5)	124	21	4	1	204	1-1/2 carb., 1 fat
Fat-Free Apple Newtons (2)	90	20	0	0	50	1 carb.

Food	Cal.	Carb.	Fat	Sat. Fat	Sod.	Exchanges
Fat-Free Fig Newtons (2)	100	23	0	0	115	1-1/2 carb.
Fat-Free Raspberry Newtons (2)	100	23	0	0	115	1-1/2 carb.
Fat-Free Strawberry Newtons (2)	100	23	0	0	115	1-1/2 carb.
Fig Newtons (2)	107	18	3	<1	107	1 carb., 1 fat
Holiday Bears (22)	120	22	4	<1	150	1-1/2 carb., 1 fat
Homestyle Chocolate Chip Cookies (2)	150	21	7	2	90	1-1/2 carb., 1 fat
Homestyle Oatmeal Cookies (2)	120	18	5	1	120	1 carb., 1 fat
Homestyle Sugar Cookies (2)	130	19	5	1	140	1 carb., 1 fat
Lorna Doone Shortbread (4)	140	19	7	2	130	1 carb., 1 fat
Nilla Wafers (7)	124	21	4	<1	89	1-1/2 carb., 1 fat
Nutter Butters (2)	130	19	6	1	110	1 carb., 1 fat
Old-Fashioned Ginger Snaps (4)	122	22	3	<1	172	1-1/2 strch, 1 fat
Oreo Sandwich Cookies (2)	138	20	6	1	189	1 carb., 1 fat
Oreo Sandwich Cookies, Reduced-Fat (3)	130	25	4	1	210	1-1/2 carb., 1 fat
Snackwell's Chocolate Chip Cookies (13)	130	22	4	2	170	1-1/2 carb., 1 fat
Snackwell's Cinnamon Graham Snacks (20)	100	26	0	0	90	2 carb.

DESSERTS

Products	Cal.	Carb. (g)	Fat (g)	Sat. Fat (g)	Sodium (mg)	Exchanges
Snackwell's Creme Sandwich Cookies (2)	110	21	3	<1	100	1-1/2 carb., 1 fat
Snackwell's Devil's Food Cookie Cakes (1)	50	13	0	0	25	1 carb.
Snackwell's Fudge Brownie Bars (1)	130	26	2	2	80	2 carb.
Snackwell's Fudge Cookies, Fat-Free (1)	53	12	<1	<1	71	1 carb.
Snackwell's Ice Cream Sandwich (1)	90	18	2	1	85	1 carb.
Snackwell's Low-Fat Ice Cream, Praline Carmel Fudge (1/2 cup)	140	28	2	1	90	2 carb.
Snackwell's Low-Fat Ice Cream, Rocky Road (1/2 cup)	130	27	2	1	25	2 carb.
Snackwell's Low-Fat Ice Cream, Vanilla (1/2 cup)	100	18	2	2	5	1 carb.
Social Tea Biscuit (6)	140	22	4	<1	110	1-1/2 carb., 1 fat
Teddy Grahams, Chocolate (22)	120	22	4	<1	170	1-1/2 carb., 1 fat
Teddy Grahams, Cinnamon (22)	120	22	4	<1	170	1-1/2 carb., 1 fat
Teddy Grahams, Honey (22)	120	22	4	<1	170	1-1/2 carb., 1 fat

Teddy Grahams, Vanilla Snack (22)	120	22	4	<1	130	1-1/2 carb., 1 fat
Vanilla & Chocolate Rockin' Bear (22)	120	22	4	<1	150	1-1/2 carb., 1 fat
Vanilla Wafers (8)	140	24	5	1	105	1-1/2 carb., 1 fat
Vanilla Wafers, Reduced-Fat (8)	120	24	2	<1	105	1-1/2 carb.
NESTLE						
Crunch Bar (1)	200	17	14	11	40	1 carb., 3 fat
Drumstick (1)	340	35	19	11	90	2 carb., 4 fat
ORVAL KENT						
Dessert, Chocolate Chip Amaretto (1/2 cup)	310	31	20	16	230	2 carb., 4 fat
Dessert, Pistachio Creme (1/2 cup)	170	29	5	5	135	2 carb., 1 fat
Parfait, Wild Strawberry (1/2 cup)	130	22	3	3	105	1-1/2 carb., 1 fat
Pudding, Chocolate (1/2 cup)	160	27	4	2	110	2 carb., 1 fat
Pudding, Pearl Tapioca (1/2 cup)	150	25	4	2	95	1-1/2 carb., 1 fat
Pudding, Rice (1/2 cup)	130	21	3	2	75	1-1/2 carb., 1 fat
PEPPERIDGE FARM						
Biscuit, Esprits Noir (Dark Chocolate) (1)	90	10	5	4	50	1/2 carb., 1 fat

DESSERTS

Products	Cal.	Carb. (g)	Fat (g)	Sat. Fat (g)	Sodium (mg)	Exchanges
Cake, All-Butter Pound (1/5)	290	39	13	7	280	2-1/2 carb., 3 fat
Cake, Large Chocolate Fudge Layer (1/6)	300	38	16	5	230	2-1/2 carb., 3 fat
Cake, Large Coconut Layer (1/6)	300	41	14	4	200	3 carb., 3 fat
Cake, Large Devil's Food Layer (1/6)	290	40	14	5	220	2-1/2 carb., 3 fat
Cake, Large German Chocolate Layer (1/6)	300	37	16	4	280	2-1/2 carb., 3 fat
Cake, Large Strawberry Stripe Layer (1/6)	310	47	13	4	150	3 carb., 3 fat
Cake, Special Recipe Boston Creme (1/8)	260	42	9	3	120	3 carb., 2 fat
Cake, Special Recipe Chocolate Mousse (1/8)	250	35	10	3	120	2 carb., 2 fat
Cake, Special Recipe Deluxe Carrot (1/8)	310	39	16	4	320	2-1/2 carb., 3 fat
Cake, Special Recipe Lemon Mousse (1/8)	250	34	12	4	100	2 carb., 2 fat
Cake, Special Recipe Strawberry Cream w/Coconut (1/9)	230	38	9	3	115	2-1/2 carb., 2 fat
Cookies, Beacon Hill Chocolate Chocolate Walnut (1)	115	14	6	2	89	1 carb., 1 fat
Cookies, Charleston (1)	130	16	7	3	110	1 carb., 1 fat

Cookies, Cherry Cobbler Fruit (1)	70	11	3	1	45	1 carb., 1 fat
Cookies, Chesapeake Chocolate Chunk Pecan (1)	124	13	7	1	89	1 carb., 1 fat
Cookies, Distinctive Bordeaux (2)	66	10	3	1	48	1/2 carb., 1 fat
Cookies, Distinctive Brussels (2)	100	13	5	2	53	1 carb., 1 fat
Cookies, Distinctive Brussels Mint (2)	128	15	7	2	67	1 carb., 1 fat
Cookies, Distinctive Caramel Pecan (1)	127	16	7	2	55	1 carb., 1 fat
Cookies, Distinctive Chessman (2)	80	12	2	2	53	1 carb.
Cookies, Distinctive Chocolate Chocolate Walnut (1)	128	16	6	2	44	1 carb., 1 fat
Cookies, Distinctive Double Chocolate Milano (2)	152	17	8	3	71	1 carb., 2 fat
Cookies, Distinctive Geneva (2)	107	13	6	2	64	1 carb., 1 fat
Cookies, Distinctive Hazelnut Milano (2)	128	15	7	2	64	1 carb., 1 fat
Cookies, Distinctive Lido (2)	175	21	9	3	87	1-1/2 carb., 2 fat
Cookies, Distinctive Milano (2)	120	14	7	2	53	1 carb., 1 fat
Cookies, Distinctive Milk Chocolate Macadamia (1)	128	16	6	3	54	1 carb., 1 fat
Cookies, Distinctive Milk Chocolate Milano (3)	180	21	10	4	80	1-1/2 carb., 2 fat
Cookies, Distinctive Mint Milano (2)	142	16	8	4	71	1 carb., 2 fat

DESSERTS

Products	Cal.	Carb. (g)	Fat (g)	Sat. Fat (g)	Sodium (mg)	Exchanges
Cookies, Distinctive Orange Milano (2)	142	17	8	3	71	1 carb., 2 fat
Cookies, Mini Chocolate Chip (5)	160	22	7	2	110	1-1/2 carb., 1 fat
Cookies, Nantucket Chocolate Chunk (1)	115	14	6	3	66	1 carb., 1 fat
Cookies, Oatmeal Raisin (1)	110	17	4	1	85	1 carb., 1 fat
Cookies, Old-Fashioned Chocolate Chip (2)	108	12	5	2	44	1 carb., 1 fat
Cookies, Old-Fashioned Gingerman (2)	60	11	2	<1	25	1 carb.
Cookies, Old-Fashioned Hazelnut (2)	108	14	5	1	91	1 carb., 1 fat
Cookies, Old-Fashioned Lemon Nut Crunch (2)	114	12	6	1	40	1 carb., 1 fat
Cookies, Old-Fashioned Molasses Crisps (2)	61	8	2	<1	57	1/2 carb.
Cookies, Old-Fashioned Oatmeal Raisin (2)	107	15	4	1	100	1 carb., 1 fat
Cookies, Old-Fashioned Pecan Shortbread (1)	70	7	5	1	43	1/2 carb., 1 fat
Cookies, Old-Fashioned Sugar (2)	93	13	4	<1	60	1 carb., 1 fat
Cookies, Peach Tart Fruit (2)	120	23	3	1	115	1-1/2 carb., 1 fat
Cookies, Santa Fe Oatmeal Raisin (1)	106	16	4	<1	97	1 carb., 1 fat

Cookies, Sausalito Milk Chocolate Macadamia (1)	124	14	6	2	97	1 carb., 1 fat
Cookies, Soft-Baked Chocolate Chunk (1)	128	16	6	3	34	1 carb., 1 fat
Cookies, Soft-Baked Oatmeal Raisin (1)	108	17	4	<1	59	1 carb., 1 fat
Cookies, Tahoe American Collection (1)	130	16	7	3	110	1 carb., 1 fat
Cookies, Wholesome Choice Raspberry Tart (1)	59	11	2	<1	57	1 carb.
PET						
Topping, Whipped (2 Tbsp)	30	2	2	2	0	free
PILLSBURY						
Bar Mixes, Deluxe Fudge Swirl Cookie (1/20)	180	25	8	2	110	1-1/2 carb., 2 fat
Bar Mixes, Deluxe Lemon Cheesecake (1/24)	180	20	10	4	50	1 carb., 2 fat
Brownie Mix, Deluxe Chocolate Deluxe (1/20)	180	28	7	2	110	2 carb., 1 fat
Brownie Mix, Deluxe Lovin' Lites Fudge (1/16)	160	29	4	1	5	2 carb., 1 fat
Cake Mix, Bundt Double Hot Fudge (1/16)	280	32	16	5	220	2 carb., 3 fat
Cake Mix, Moist Supreme French Vanilla (1/10)	300	42	13	3	350	3 carb., 3 fat
Cake Mix, Moist Supreme Chocolate (1/12)	250	35	11	5	280	2 carb., 2 fat
Cake Mix, Moist Supreme Lovin' Lites White (1/10)	230	42	5	8	15	3 carb., 1 fat

DESSERTS

Products	Cal.	Carb. (g)	Fat (g)	Sat. Fat (g)	Sodium (mg)	Exchanges
Cookies, Chocolate Chip (1 oz)	130	17	6	2	85	1 carb., 1 fat
Cookies, Oatmeal Chocolate Chip (1 oz)	120	16	6	2	95	1 carb., 1 fat
Cookies, Sugar (2)	130	19	5	2	125	1 carb., 1 fat
Frosting Supreme, Chocolate (2 Tbsp)	140	21	6	2	75	1-1/2 carb., 1 fat
Frosting Supreme, French Vanilla (2 Tbsp)	160	26	6	2	75	2 carb., 1 fat
Sweet Rolls, Caramel (1)	170	25	7	2	330	1-1/2 carb., 1 fat
Sweet Rolls, Cinnamon w/Icing (1)	140	21	5	2	330	1-1/2 carb., 1 fat
Turnovers, Apple (2)	350	45	17	4	660	3 carb., 3 fat
SUNSHINE						
Cookies, Fig Bar (2)	110	20	3	<1	60	1 carb., 1 fat
Cookies, Lemon Coolers (5)	140	21	6	2	100	1-1/2 carb., 1 fat
Crackers, Animal (14)	140	24	4	1	125	1-1/2 carb., 1 fat
ULTRA SLIM FAST						
Pudding, Butterscotch (4 oz)	100	21			230	1-1/2 carb.

Pudding, Chocolate (4 oz)	100	21			240	1-1/2 carb.
Pudding, Vanilla (4 oz)	100	21			230	1-1/2 carb.

WEIGHT WATCHERS

Apple Raisin Cookie Bar (1)	70	14	2	<1	60	1 carb.
Chocolate Cookies (3)	80	13	3	1	70	1 carb., 1 fat
Chocolate Eclair (1)	150	24	5	2	150	1-1/2 carb., 1 fat
Chocolate Mocha Pie (1 slice)	170	31	4	1	125	2 carb., 1 fat
Chocolate Mousse Bar (2)	70	18	1	<1	80	1 carb.
Light Ice Cream, Cookie Dough Craze (1/2 cup)	140	24	4	2	85	1-1/2 carb., 1 fat
Light Ice Cream, Oh! So Very Vanilla (1/2 cup)	120	20	3	2	65	1 carb., 1 fat
Light Ice Cream, Positive Praline Crunch (1/2 cup)	140	25	3	2	105	1-1/2 carb., 1 fat
Light Ice Cream, Reckless Rocky Road (1/2 cup)	140	23	3	2	75	1-1/2 carb., 1 fat
Light Ice Cream, Triple Chocolate Tornado (1/2 cup)	150	26	4	2	80	2 carb., 1 fat
Smart Snackers Chocolate Chip Cookies (2)	140	22	5	2	90	1-1/2 carb., 1 fat
Smart Snackers Fruit Cookies, Fig (1)	70	16	0	0	50	1 carb.
Smart Snackers Fruit Cookies, Raspberry (2)	70	16	0	0	45	1 carb.

DESSERTS

Products	Cal.	Carb. (g)	Fat (g)	Sat. Fat (g)	Sodium (mg)	Exchanges
Smart Snackers Oatmeal Raisin Cookies (2)	120	22	2	0	90	1-1/2 carb.
Smart Snackers Sandwich Cookies, Chocolate (2)	140	23	4	1	160	1-1/2 carb., 1 fat
Smart Snackers Sandwich Cookies, Vanilla (2)	140	25	3	1	80	1-1/2 carb., 1 fat
Vanilla Sandwich Bar (1)	160	30	4	2	180	2 carb., 1 fat
YOPLAIT						
Frozen Yogurt, Chocolate (1/2 cup)	133	23	3	2	53	1-1/2 carb., 1 fat
Frozen Yogurt, Coffee/Vanilla (1/2 cup)	120	21	3	NA	53	1-1/2 carb., 1 fat
Frozen Yogurt, Fruit (1/2 cup)	120	21	3	2	53	1-1/2 carb., 1 fat
Frozen Yogurt, Vanilla/Chocolate Chip (1/2 cup)	133	23	4	NA	53	1-1/2 carb., 1 fat

EGGS AND EGG DISHES

Products	Cal.	Carb. (g)	Fat (g)	Sat. Fat (g)	Sodium (mg)	Exchanges
1-Egg Omelet, Plain (1)	90	<1	7	2	159	1 med-fat meat
1-Egg Omelet, Spanish (1)	125	7	9	2	251	1 vegetable, 1 med-fat meat, 1 fat
1-Egg Omelet w/Cheese & Ham (1)	142	<1	11	4	368	1 med-fat meat, 1 fat
1-Egg Omelet w/Chicken (1)	149	<1	10	3	222	2 med-fat meat
1-Egg Omelet w/Fish (1)	132	<1	9	3	277	2 med-fat meat
1-Egg Omelet w/Mushroom (1)	91	1	7	2	158	1 med-fat meat
1-Egg Omelet w/Onion, Pepper, Tomato, Mushroom (1)	125	7	9	2	251	1 vegetable, 1 med-fat meat, 1 fat
1-Egg Omelet w/Sausage & Mushroom (1)	172	1	13	4	454	2 med-fat meat, 1 fat
1-Egg Omelet w/Spinach (1)	95	2	7	2	201	1 med-fat meat
Deviled Egg (1/2 egg + filling)	63	<1	5	1	94	1 med-fat meat

EGGS AND EGG DISHES

Products	Cal.	Carb. (g)	Fat (g)	Sat. Fat (g)	Sodium (mg)	Exchanges
Egg, Boiled/Cooked (1 extra large)	90	<1	6	2	72	1 med-fat meat
Egg, Boiled/Cooked (1 jumbo)	99	<1	7	2	79	1 med-fat meat
Egg, Boiled/Cooked (1 large)	78	<1	5	2	62	1 med-fat meat
Egg, Boiled/Cooked (1 medium)	68	<1	5	1	55	1 med-fat meat
Egg, Boiled/Cooked (1 small)	57	<1	4	1	46	1 med-fat meat
Egg, Fried in Margarine (1 large)	92	<1	7	2	162	1 high-fat meat
Egg, Scrambled, w/Milk & Margarine (1 large)	101	1	7	2	171	1 high-fat meat
Egg Substitute (1/4 cup)	35	2	0	0	110	1 very lean meat
Egg Whites (2)	34	<1	0	0	110	1 very lean meat
Eggs, Scrambled, Plain (2)	155	1	11	3	124	2 med-fat meat
Souffle, Cheese (1 cup)	207	6	16	8	346	1/2 reduced-fat milk, 1 med-fat meat, 1 fat
Souffle, Spinach (1 cup)	218	3	18	7	763	1/2 reduced-fat milk, 1 med-fat meat, 2 fat

FLEISCHMANN'S						
Egg Beaters (1/4 cup)	30	1	0	0	100	1 very lean meat
Egg Beaters w/Cheez (1/2 cup)	130	3	6	0	440	2 lean meat
Whole Eggs (1/4 cup)	70	1	5	1.5	65	1 med-fat meat
LAND O'LAKES						
Egg Substitute, Country Morning (1/2 cup)	173	1	12	NA	180	2 med-fat meat
Scramblend (1/2 cup)	143	3	9	NA	173	2 med-fat meat
MORNINGSTAR						
Scramblers (1/4 cup)	58	3	2	<1	94	1 lean meat
NABISCO						
Royal Break-O-Morn Eggs (1/4 cup)	60	1	4	2	160	1 med-fat meat
Royal Egg Eze (1/4 cup)	70	1	5	2	95	1 med-fat meat

FAST FOODS

FAST FOODS

ARBY'S

ROAST BEEF SANDWICHES

Products	Cal.	Carb. (g)	Fat (g)	Sat. Fat (g)	Sodium (mg)	Exchanges
Arby-Q (1)	431	48	18	6	1321	3 carb., 2 med-fat meat, 2 fat
Arby's Melt w/Cheddar (1)	368	36	18	6	937	2-1/2 carb., 2 med-fat meat, 1 fat
Bac'n Cheddar Deluxe (1)	539	38	34	10	1140	2-1/2 carb., 2 med-fat meat, 5 fat
Beef'n Cheddar (1)	487	40	28	9	1216	2-1/2 carb., 3 med-fat meat, 3 fat
Roast Beef, Giant (1)	555	43	28	11	1561	3 carb., 4 med-fat meat, 2 fat
Roast Beef, Junior (1)	324	35	14	5	779	2 carb., 2 med-fat meat, 1 fat
Roast Beef, Regular (1)	388	33	19	7	1009	2 carb., 2 med-fat meat, 2 fat
Roast Beef, Super (1)	523	50	27	9	1189	3 carb., 2 med-fat meat, 3 fat

CHICKEN

Products	Cal.	Carb. (g)	Fat (g)	Sat. Fat (g)	Sodium (mg)	Exchanges
Breaded Chicken Fillets (1)	536	38	28	5	1016	3 carb., 3 med-fat meat, 3 fat
Chicken Fingers (2)	290	20	16	2	677	1-1/2 carb., 2 med-fat meat, 1 fat

Grilled Chicken BBQ (1)	388	47	13	3	1002	3 carb., 2 med-fat meat, 1 fat
Grilled Chicken Deluxe (1)	430	41	20	4	848	3 carb., 2 med-fat meat, 2 fat
Roast Chicken Club (1)	546	37	31	9	1103	2-1/2 carb., 3 med-fat meat, 3 fat

SUB ROLL SANDWICHES

French Dip (1)	475	40	22	8	1411	2-1/2 carb., 3 med-fat meat, 2 fat
Philly Beef 'n Swiss (1)	755	48	47	15	2025	3 carb., 4 med-fat meat, 5 fat
Sub, Italian (1)	675	46	36	13	2089	3 carb., 3 med-fat meat, 4 fat
Sub, Roast Beef (1)	700	44	42	14	2034	3 carb., 4 med-fat meat, 4 fat
Sub, Turkey (1)	550	47	27	7	2084	3 carb., 3 med-fat meat, 2 fat

LIGHT MENU

Light Roast Beef Deluxe (1)	296	33	10	3	826	2 carb., 2 med-fat meat
Light Roast Chicken Deluxe (1)	276	33	6	2	777	2 carb., 2 lean meat
Light Roast Turkey Deluxe (1)	260	33	7	2	1262	2 carb., 2 lean meat
Salad, Garden (1)	61	12	<1	0	40	2 vegetable
Salad, Roast Chicken (1)	149	12	2	<1	418	3 very lean meat, 2 vegetable
Salad, Side (1)	23	4	<1	0	15	1 vegetable

FAST FOODS

Products	Cal.	Carb. (g)	Fat (g)	Sat. Fat (g)	Sodium (mg)	Exchanges
OTHER SANDWICHES						
Fish Fillet (1)	529	50	27	7	864	3 carb., 2 med-fat meat, 3 fat
Ham'n Cheese Sandwich (1)	359	34	14	5	1283	2 carb., 3 med-fat meat
POTATOES						
Baked Potato, Broccoli 'n Cheddar (1)	571	89	20	5	565	6 carb., 3 fat
Baked Potato, Deluxe (1)	736	86	36	16	499	6 carb., 6 fat
Baked Potato, Margarine & Sour Cream (1)	578	85	24	9	209	5-1/2 carb., 4 fat
Baked Potato, Plain (1)	355	82	<1	0	26	5-1/2 carb.
Curly Fries (3.5 oz)	300	38	15	3	853	2-1/2 carb., 3 fat
Curly Fries, Cheddar (4.25 oz)	333	40	18	4	1016	2-1/2 carb., 4 fat
French Fries (2.5 oz)	246	30	13	3	114	2 carb., 3 fat
Potato Cakes (3 oz)	204	20	12	2	397	2 carb., 2 fat
DESSERTS						
Cheesecake, Plain (1)	320	23	23	14	240	1-1/2 carb., 5 fat

	Cal.	Carb.	Fat	Sat. Fat	Sod.	Exchanges
Chocolate Chip Cookie(1)	125	16	6	2	85	1 carb., 1 fat
Peanut Butter Cup Polar Swirl (1)	517	61	24	8	385	4 carb., 4 fat
Turnover, Apple (1)	330	48	14	7	180	3 carb., 3 fat
Turnover, Cherry (1)	320	46	13	5	190	3 carb., 3 fat

BOSTON MARKET

ENTREES

	Cal.	Carb.	Fat	Sat. Fat	Sod.	Exchanges
1/4 Dark Meat Chicken w/o skin (1)	210	1	10	2.5	320	4 lean meat
1/4 Dark Meat Chicken w/skin (1)	330	2	22	6	460	4 med-fat meat
1/4 White Meat Chicken w/o skin (1)	160	0	3.5	1	350	4 very lean meat
1/4 White Meat Chicken w/skin (1)	330	2	17	4.5	530	6 lean meat
1/2 Chicken w/skin (1)	630	2	37	19	960	11 lean meat
Chunky Chicken Salad (1)	390	3	30	5	790	4 med-fat meat, 2 fat
Ham w/Cinnamon Apples (1)	350	35	13	4.5	1750	4 lean meat, 2 fruit
Meat Loaf & Brown Gravy (1)	390	19	22	8	1040	1 carb., 4 med-fat meat
Meat Loaf & Chunky Tomato Sauce (1)	370	22	18	8	1170	1-1/2 carb., 4 med-fat meat
Original Chicken Pot Pie (1)	750	78	34	9	2380	5 carb., 3 med-fat meat, 4 fat

FAST FOODS

Products	Cal.	Carb. (g)	Fat (g)	Sat. Fat (g)	Sodium (mg)	Exchanges
Skinless Rotisserie Turkey Breast (1)	170	1	1	.5	850	5 very lean meat
SOUPS, SALADS, AND SANDWICHES						
Salad, Caesar w/o Dressing (1)	240	14	13	7	780	2 med-fat meat, 2 vegetable, 1 fat
Salad, Chicken Caesar (1)	670	16	47	13	1860	1 carb., 6 med-fat meat, 3 fat
Sandwich, Chicken Salad (1)	680	63	33	4	1350	4 carb., 4 med-fat meat, 3 fat
Sandwich, Chicken w/Cheese & Sauce (1)	760	71	32	11	1810	5 carb., 4 med-fat meat, 2 fat
Sandwich, Chicken w/o Sauce & Cheese (1)	430	61	4	1	860	4 carb., 4 very lean meat
Sandwich, Ham & Turkey Club w/Cheese & Sauce (1)	890	79	43	20	2310	5 carb., 5 med-fat meat, 4 fat
Sandwich, Ham & Turkey Club w/o Cheese & Sauce (1)	430	64	6	2	1330	4 carb., 2 lean meat
Sandwich, Ham w/Cheese & Sauce (1)	760	71	35	13	1880	5 carb., 3 med-fat meat, 4 fat
Sandwich, Ham w/o Cheese & Sauce (1)	450	66	9	3	1600	4-1/2 carb., 2 med-fat meat
Sandwich, Meat Loaf w/Cheese (1)	860	95	33	16	2270	6 carb., 4 med-fat meat, 3 fat

Sandwich, Meat Loaf w/o Cheese (1)	690	86	21	7	1610	6 carb., 3 med-fat meat, 1 fat
Sandwich, Turkey w/Cheese & Sauce (1)	710	68	28	10	1390	4-1/2 carb., 5 med-fat meat, 1 fat
Sandwich, Turkey w/o Cheese & Sauce (1)	400	61	4	1	1070	4 carb., 3 very lean meat
Soup, Chicken (6 oz)	80	4	3	1	470	1 lean meat, 1 vegetable
Soup, Chicken Tortilla (8 oz)	220	19	11	4	1470	1 strch, 1 med-fat meat, 1 fat

HOT SIDE DISHES

BBQ Baked Beans (1 order)	330	53	9	3	630	3-1/2 carb., 2 fat
Buttered Corn (1 order)	190	39	4	1	130	2-1/2 carb., 1 fat
Butternut Squash (1 order)	160	25	6	4	580	1-1/2 carb., 1 fat
Chicken Gravy (1 order)	15	2	1	0	170	free
Creamed Spinach (1 order)	300	13	24	15	790	1 med-fat meat, 2 vegetable, 4 fat
Homestyle Mashed Potatoes & Gravy (1 order)	200	27	9	5	560	2 carb., 2 fat
Hot Cinnamon Apples (1 order)	250	56	5	<1	45	4 fruit, 1 FAT(OTHER CHO) ?
Macaroni & Cheese (1 order)	280	36	10	6	760	2-1/2 carb., 1 med-fat meat, 1 fat
Potatoes, Mashed (1 order)	180	25	8	5	390	1-1/2 carb., 2 fat
Potatoes, New (1 order)	140	25	3	<1	100	1-1/2 carb., 1 fat

FAST FOODS

Products	Cal.	Carb. (g)	Fat (g)	Sat. Fat (g)	Sodium (mg)	Exchanges
Rice Pilaf (1 order)	180	32	5	1	600	2 carb., 1 fat
Steamed Vegetables (1 order)	35	7	<1	0	35	1 vegetable
Stuffing (1 order)	310	44	12	2	1140	3 strch., 2 fat
Zucchini Marinara (1 order)	80	10	4	<1	470	2 vegetable, 1 fat
COLD SIDE DISHES						
Coleslaw (1 order)	280	32	16	3	520	2 carb., 3 fat
Cranberry Relish (1 order)	370	84	5	<1	5	5-1/2 carb., 1 fat
Salad, Caesar Side (1)	210	6	17	5	560	1 med-fat meat, 1 vegetable , 2 fat
Salad, Fruit (1 order)	70	17	<1	0	10	1 fruit
Salad, Mediterranean Pasta (1 order)	170	16	10	3	490	1 strch, 2 fat
Salad, Tortellini (1 order)	380	29	24	5	530	2 strch, 1 med-fat meat, 4 fat
BAKED DISHES						
Brownie (1)	450	47	27	7	190	3 carb., 5 fat
Chocolate Chip Cookie (1)	340	48	17	6	240	3 carb., 3 fat

Oatmeal Raisin Cookie (1)	320	48	13	3	260	3 carb., 3 fat
Corn Bread (1 loaf)	200	33	6	2	390	2 strch, 1 fat

BURGER KING

BURGERS

Cheeseburger (1)	380	28	19	9	770	2 carb., 2 med-fat meat, 1 fat
Cheeseburger, Double (1)	600	28	36	17	1060	2 carb., 5 med-fat meat, 2 fat
Cheeseburger, Double w/Bacon (1)	640	28	39	18	1240	2 carb., 5 med-fat meat, 3 fat
Hamburger (1)	330	28	15	6	530	2 carb., 2 med-fat meat, 1 fat
Whopper Jr. Sandwich (1)	420	29	24	8	530	2 carb., 2 med-fat meat, 3 fat
Whopper Jr. Sandwich w/Cheese (1)	460	29	28	10	770	2 carb., 2 med-fat meat, 4 fat
Whopper Sandwich (1)	640	45	39	11	870	3 carb., 3 med-fat meat, 5 fat
Whopper Sandwich, Double (1)	870	45	56	19	940	3 carb., 5 med-fat meat, 5 fat
Whopper Sandwich w/Cheese (1)	730	46	46	16	1350	3 carb., 3 med-fat meat, 6 fat
Whopper Sandwich w/Cheese, Double (1)	960	46	63	24	1420	3 carb., 6 med-fat meat, 7 fat

SANDWICHES/SIDE ORDERS

Chicken Tenders (6)	230	14	12	3	530	1 carb., 2 med-fat meat

FAST FOODS

Products	Cal.	Carb. (g)	Fat (g)	Sat. Fat (g)	Sodium (mg)	Exchanges
French Fries, Salted (1 medium order)	370	43	20	5	240	3 carb., 4 fat
Onion Rings (1 order)	310	41	14	2	810	3 carb., 2 fat
Pie, Dutch Apple (1)	300	39	15	3	230	2-1/2 carb., 3 fat
Salad, Broiled Chicken, w/o dressing (1)	200	7	10	4	110	3 lean meat, 1 vegetable
Salad, Garden, w/o dressing (1)	100	7	5	3	110	1 med-fat meat, 1 vegetable
Salad, Side, w/o dressing (1)	60	4	3	2	55	1 vegetable, 1 fat
Sandwich, BK Broiler Chicken (1)	550	41	29	6	480	3 carb., 3 med-fat meat, 3 fat
Sandwich, BK Big Fish (1)	700	56	41	6	980	4 carb., 2 med-fat meat, 6 fat
Sandwich, Chicken (1)	710	54	43	9	1400	3-1/2 carb., 2 med-fat meat, 7 fat
DRINKS						
Orange Juice, Tropicana (1)	140	33	0	0	0	2 fruit
Shake, Chocolate (1 medium)	320	54	7	4	230	3-1/2 carb., 1 fat
Shake, Chocolate, Syrup Added (1 medium)	440	84	7	4	260	5-1/2 carb., 1 fat
Shake, Strawberry, Syrup Added (1 medium)	420	83	6	4	260	5-1/2 carb., 1 fat

	Calories				Sodium	Exchanges
Shake, Vanilla (1 medium)	300	53	6	4	230	3-1/2 carb., 1 fat

BREAKFAST

Biscuit w/Bacon, Egg, Cheese (1)	510	39	31	10	1530	2-1/2 carb., 2 med-fat meat, 4 fat
Biscuit w/Sausage (1)	590	41	40	13	1390	2-1/2 carb., 2 med-fat meat, 6 fat
Croissan'wich w/Sausage, Egg & Cheese (1)	600	25	46	16	1140	1-1/2 carb., 3 med-fat meat, 3 fat
French Toast Sticks (1 order)	500	60	27	7	490	4 carb., 5 fat
Hash Browns (1)	220	25	12	3	320	2 carb., 2 fat
Jam, a.m. Express Grape (1 pkt)	30	7	0	0	0	1/2 carb.
Jam, a.m. Express Strawberry (1 pkt)	30	8	0	0	5	1/2 carb.

CONDIMENTS

a.m. Express Dip (1 pkt)	80	21	0	0	20	1-1/2 carb.
BBQ Sauce, Bull's Eye (1 pkt)	20	5	0	0	140	free
Dipping Sauce, Barbeque (1 pkt)	35	9	0	0	400	1/2 carb.
Dipping Sauce, Honey (1 pkt)	90	23	0	0	10	1-1/2 carb.
Dipping Sauce, Ranch (1 pkt)	170	2	17	3	200	3 fat
Dipping Sauce, Sweet & Sour (1 pkt)	45	11	0	0	50	1 carb.

FAST FOODS

DAIRY QUEEN

SANDWICHES

Products	Cal.	Carb. (g)	Fat (g)	Sat. Fat (g)	Sodium (mg)	Exchanges
Cheese Dog (1)	290	20	18	8	950	1 carb., 1 med-fat meat, 3 fat
Chicken Strip Basket w/Gravy (1)	860	88	42	11	1820	6 carb., 2 med-fat meat, 6 fat
Chili Dog (1)	280	21	16	6	870	1-1/2 carb., 1 med-fat meat, 2 fat
Chili N' Cheese Dog (1)	330	22	21	9	1090	1-1/2 carb., 1 med-fat meat, 3 fat
Cheeseburger, Homestyle (1)	340	29	17	8	850	2 carb., 2 med-fat meat, 1 fat
Cheeseburger, Homestyle Bacon Double (1)	610	31	36	18	1380	2 carb., 5 med-fat meat, 2 fat
Cheeseburger, Homestyle Deluxe Double (1)	540	31	31	16	1130	2 carb., 4 med-fat meat, 2 fat
Cheeseburger, Homestyle Double (1)	540	30	31	16	1130	2 carb., 4 med-fat meat, 2 fat
Hamburger, Homestyle (1)	290	29	12	5	630	2 carb., 2 med-fat meat
Hot Dog (1)	240	19	14	5	730	1 carb., 1 med-fat meat, 2 fat
Sandwich, Breaded Chicken Fillet (1)	430	37	20	4	760	2-1/2 carb., 2 med-fat meat, 2 fat
Sandwich, Breaded Chicken Fillet w/Cheese (1)	480	38	25	7	980	2-1/2 carb., 3 med-fat meat, 2 fat

	Calories	Carb. (g)	Fat (g)	Sat. Fat (g)	Sodium (mg)	Exchanges
Sandwich, Fish Fillet (1)	370	39	16	3.5	630	2-1/2 carb., 1 med-fat meat, 2 fat
Sandwich, Fish Fillet w/Cheese (1)	420	40	21	6	850	2-1/2 carb., 2 med-fat meat, 2 fat
Sandwich, Grilled Chicken Fillet (1)	310	30	10	2.5	1040	2 carb., 3 med-fat meat

SIDE ITEMS

	Calories	Carb. (g)	Fat (g)	Sat. Fat (g)	Sodium (mg)	Exchanges
French Fries (1 regular order)	300	40	14	4	160	2-1/2 carb., 3 fat
Onion Rings (1 regular order)	240	29	12	2.5	135	2 carb., 2 fat

SOFT-SERVE ICE CREAM AND TREATS

	Calories	Carb. (g)	Fat (g)	Sat. Fat (g)	Sodium (mg)	Exchanges
Banana Split (1)	510	96	12	8	180	6-1/2 carb., 2 fat
Buster Bar (1)	450	41	28	12	280	3 carb., 6 fat
Chocolate Dilly Bar (1)	210	21	13	7	75	1-1/2 carb., 3 fat
Ice Cream Cake, Frozen, 10-inch Round (1/12)	360	55	12	8	260	3-1/2 carb., 2 fat
Ice Cream Cone, Chocolate (1 regular)	360	56	11	8	180	4 carb., 2 fat
Ice Cream Cone, Dipped (1 regular)	510	63	25	13	200	4 carb., 5 fat
Ice Cream Cone, Queen's Choice Vanilla Big Scoop (1)	250	27	14	9	100	2 carb., 3 fat
Ice Cream Cone, Vanilla (1 regular)	350	57	10	7	170	4 carb., 2 fat

FAST FOODS

Products	Cal.	Carb. (g)	Fat (g)	Sat. Fat (g)	Sodium (mg)	Exchanges
Ice Cream Sandwich (1)	150	24	5	2	115	1-1/2 carb., 1 fat
Ice Cream Sundae, Chocolate (1 regular)	410	73	10	6	210	5 carb., 2 fat
Mr. Misty (1 regular)	250	63	0	0	10	4 carb.
Misty Slush (1 regular)	290	74	0	0	30	5 carb.
Peanut Buster Parfait (1)	730	99	31	17	400	6-1/2 carb., 6 fat
Strawberry-Banana DQ Treatzza Pizza (1/8)	180	29	6	3	140	2 carb., 1 fat
MALTS, SHAKES, AND BLIZZARDS						
Blizzard, Chocolate Chip Cookie Dough (1 regular)	950	143	36	19	660	9-1/2 carb., 7 fat
Blizzard, Strawberry (1 regular)	570	95	16	11	260	6 carb., 3 fat
Malt, Chocolate (1 regular)	880	153	22	14	500	10 carb., 4 fat
Malt, Vanilla (1 regular)	610	106	14	8	230	7 carb., 3 fat
Shake, Chocolate (1 regular)	770	130	20	13	420	8-1/2 carb., 4 fat
Shake, Vanilla (1 regular)	520	88	14	8	230	6 carb., 3 fat

NONFAT FROZEN YOGURT

Frozen Yogurt Cone (1 regular)	280	59	1	.5	170	4 carb.
Frozen Yogurt Strawberry Breeze (1 regular)	460	99	1	1	270	6-1/2 carb.
Frozen Yogurt Strawberry Sundae (1 regular)	300	66	.5	.5	180	4-1/2 carb.

DOMINO'S

12-INCH HAND-TOSSED PIZZA

Cheese (2 slices)	349	49	11	5	673	3 carb., 1 med-fat meat, 1 fat
Ham (2 slices)	367	50	11	5	835	3 carb., 1 med-fat meat, 1 fat
Italian Sausage (2 slices)	404	51	15	6	844	3-1/2 carb., 1 med-fat meat, 2 fat
Pepperoni (2 slices)	412	49	11	7	872	3 carb., 1 med-fat meat, 1 fat
Veggie (2 slices)	373	52	12	5	746	3-1/2 carb., 1 med-fat meat, 1 fat

12-INCH THIN-CRUST PIZZA

Cheese (1/4)	273	30	12	5	759	2 carb., 1 med-fat meat, 1 fat
Ham (1/4)	291	30	12	5	921	2 carb., 1 med-fat meat, 1 fat
Italian Sausage (1/4)	328	32	16	7	930	2 carb., 1 med-fat meat, 2 fat
Pepperoni (1/4)	335	30	17	7	958	2 carb., 1 med-fat meat, 2 fat

FAST FOODS

Products	Cal.	Carb. (g)	Fat (g)	Sat. Fat (g)	Sodium (mg)	Exchanges
Veggie (1/4)	297	33	13	5	832	2 carb., 1 med-fat meat, 2 fat
12-INCH DEEP-DISH PIZZA						
Cheese (2 slices)	467	52	21	8	998	3-1/2 carb., 1 med-fat meat, 3 fat
Ham (2 slices)	484	52	22	8	1161	3-1/2 carb., 1 med-fat meat, 3 fat
Italian Sausage (2 slices)	522	53	26	10	1169	3-1/2 carb., 1 med-fat meat, 4 fat
Pepperoni (2 slices)	529	52	27	10	1197	3-1/2 carb., 2 med-fat meat, 3 fat
Veggie (2 slices)	490	54	23	8	1071	3-1/2 carb., 1 med-fat meat, 4 fat
BREADSTICKS						
Breadsticks (2)	155	21	7	1	317	1-1/2 carb., 1 fat
Cheesy Bread (2)	206	22	11	4	363	1-1/2 carb., 2 fat
BUFFALO WINGS						
Barbeque Wings (10)	501	16	24	7	1753	1 carb., 7 lean meat, 1 fat
Hot Wings (10)	449	5	24	7	3544	8 lean meat

HARDEE'S

BREAKFAST

Big Country Breakfast, Bacon (1)	820	62	49	15	1870	4 carb., 3 med-fat meat, 6 fat
Big Country Breakfast, Sausage (1)	1000	62	66	38	2310	4 carb., 4 med-fat meat, 9 fat
Biscuit, Bacon & Egg (1)	570	45	33	11	1400	3 carb., 2 med-fat meat, 5 fat
Biscuit, Bacon, Egg, & Cheese (1)	610	45	37	13	1630	3 carb., 2 med-fat meat, 5 fat
Biscuit, Country Ham (1)	430	45	22	6	1930	3 carb., 1 med-fat meat, 3 fat
Biscuit, Ham (1)	400	47	20	6	1340	3 carb., 1 med-fat meat, 3 fat
Biscuit, Ham, Egg, & Cheese (1),	540	48	30	11	1660	3 carb., 2 med-fat meat, 4 fat
Biscuit 'N' Gravy (1)	510	55	28	9	1500	3-1/2 carb., 6 fat
Biscuit, Rise 'N' Shine (1)	390	44	21	6	1000	3 carb., 4 fat
Biscuit, Sausage & Egg (1)	630	45	40	22	1480	3 carb., 2 med-fat meat, 6 fat
Biscuit, Sausage (1)	510	44	31	10	1360	3 carb., 1 med-fat meat, 5 fat
Biscuit, Ultimate Omelet (1)	570	45	33	12	1370	3 carb., 2 med-fat meat, 5 fat
Frisco Breakfast Sandwich, Ham (1)	500	46	25	9	1370	3 carb., 2 med-fat meat, 3 fat
Hash Rounds, Regular (16)	230	24	14	3	560	1-1/2 carb., 3 fat

FAST FOODS

Products	Cal.	Carb. (g)	Fat (g)	Sat. Fat (g)	Sodium (mg)	Exchanges
Three Pancakes (1 order)	280	56	2	1	890	4 carb.
SANDWICHES						
Burger, Frisco (1)	720	43	46	16	1340	3 carb., 3 med-fat meat, 6 fat
Burger, Mushroom 'N' Swiss (1)	490	39	25	12	1100	3-1/2 carb., 3 med-fat meat, 2 fat
Burger, The Boss (1)	570	42	33	12	910	3 carb., 3 med-fat meat, 3 fat
Burger, The Works (1)	530	41	30	12	1030	3 carb., 2 med-fat meat, 4 fat
Cheeseburger (1)	310	30	14	6	890	2 carb., 1 med-fat meat, 2 fat
Cheeseburger, Cravin' Bacon (1)	690	38	46	15	1150	2-1/2 carb., 2 med-fat meat, 7 fat
Cheeseburger, Mesquite Bacon (1)	370	32	18	7	970	2 carb., 2 med-fat meat, 2 fat
Cheeseburger, Quarter Pound Double (1)	470	31	25	11	1290	2 carb., 3 med-fat meat, 2 fat
Fisherman's Fillet (1)	560	54	27	7	1330	3-1/2 carb., 2 med-fat meat, 3 fat
Hamburger (1)	270	29	11	3	670	2 carb., 1 med-fat meat, 1 fat
Hot Ham 'N' Cheese (1)	310	34	12	6	1410	2 carb., 1 med-fat meat, 1 fat
Sandwich, Big Roast Beef (1)	460	35	24	9	1230	2 carb., 3 med-fat meat, 2 fat

Item						Exchanges
Sandwich, Chicken Fillet (1)	480	54	18	3	1280	3-1/2 carb., 2 med-fat meat, 2 fat
Sandwich, Grilled Chicken (1)	350	38	11	2	950	2-1/2 carb., 3 lean meat
Sandwich, Regular Roast Beef (1)	320	26	16	6	820	2 carb., 2 med-fat meat, 1 fat
FRIED CHICKEN/SIDES						
Baked Beans (5 oz, small)	170	32	1	0	600	2 carb.
Chicken Breast (1 serving)	370	29	15	4	1190	2 carb., 3 med-fat meat
Chicken Leg (1 serving)	170	15	7	2	570	1 carb., 1 med-fat meat, 1 fat
Chicken Thigh (1 serving)	330	30	15	4	1000	2 carb., 2 med-fat meat, 1 fat
Chicken Wing (1 serving)	200	23	8	2	740	1-1/2 carb., 1 med-fat meat, 1 fat
Coleslaw (1/2 cup)	240	13	20	3	340	2 vegetable, 4 fat
Gravy (1-1/2 oz)	20	3	<1	<1	260	free
Potatoes, Mashed (1/2 cup)	70	14	<1	<1	330	1 carb.
SALADS/FRIES						
French Fries (1 medium order)	350	49	15	4	150	3 carb., 3 fat
Salad, Garden (1)	220	11	13	9	350	1 med-fat meat, 2 vegetable, 2 fat
Salad, Grilled Chicken (1)	150	11	3	1	610	2 very lean meat, 2 vegetable

FAST FOODS

Products	Cal.	Carb. (g)	Fat (g)	Sat. Fat (g)	Sodium (mg)	Exchanges
Salad, Side (1)	25	4	<1	<1	45	1 vegetable
SHAKES/DESSERTS						
Big Cookie (1)	280	41	12	4	150	3 carb., 2 fat
Cool Twist Cone, Vanilla/Chocolate (1)	180	34	2	1	120	2 carb.
Shake, Strawberry (1)	420	83	4	3	270	5-1/2 carb., 1 fat
Shake, Vanilla (1)	350	65	5	3	300	4 carb., 1 fat
Sundae, Hot Fudge (1)	290	51	6	3	310	3-1/2 carb., 1 fat

JACK IN THE BOX

BURGERS

Products	Cal.	Carb. (g)	Fat (g)	Sat. Fat (g)	Sodium (mg)	Exchanges
Burger, Grilled Sourdough (1)	670	39	43	16	1180	2-1/2 carb., 4 med-fat meat, 5 fat
Cheeseburger (1)	320	32	15	6	670	2 carb., 1 med-fat meat, 2 fat
Cheeseburger, Double (1)	450	35	24	12	970	2 carb., 3 med-fat meat, 2 fat
Cheeseburger, Ultimate (1)	1030	30	79	26	1200	2 carb., 6 med-fat meat, 10 fat
Hamburger (1)	280	31	11	4	470	2 carb., 1 med-fat meat, 1 fat

Hamburger, Jumbo Jack (1)	560	41	32	10	740	3 carb., 3 med-fat meat, 3 fat
Hamburger, Jumbo Jack w/Cheese (1)	650	42	40	14	1150	3 carb., 3 med-fat meat, 5 fat
Hamburger, Quarter Pound (1)	510	39	27	10	1080	2-1/2 carb., 3 med-fat meat, 2 fat

SANDWICHES

Chicken (1)	400	38	18	4	1290	2-1/2 carb., 2 med-fat meat, 2 fat
Chicken Caesar (1)	520	44	26	6	1050	3 carb., 3 med-fat meat, 2 fat
Chicken Fajita Pita (1)	290	29	8	3	700	2 carb., 3 lean meat
Chicken Supreme (1)	620	48	36	11	1520	3 carb., 2 med-fat meat, 5 fat
Grilled Chicken Fillet (1)	430	36	19	5	1070	2-1/2 carb., 3 med-fat meat, 1 fat
Spicy Crispy Chicken (1)	560	55	27	5	1020	3-1/2 carb., 2 med-fat meat, 2 fat

SALADS

Garden Chicken (1)	200	8	9	4	420	3 lean meat, 1 vegetable
Side (1)	70	3	4	5	80	1 vegetable, 1 fat

MEXICAN FOODS

Taco (1)	190	15	11	4	410	1 carb., 1 med-fat meat, 1 fat
Taco, Monster (1)	283	22	17	6	760	1-1/2 carb., 1 med-fat meat, 2 fat

FAST FOODS

Products	Cal.	Carb. (g)	Fat (g)	Sat. Fat (g)	Sodium (mg)	Exchanges
TERIYAKI BOWLS						
Chicken (1)	580	115	2	<1	1220	7 carb., 1 lean meat, 2 vegetable
FINGER FOODS						
Bacon & Cheddar Potato Wedges (1)	800	49	58	16	1470	3 carb., 2 med-fat meat, 10 fat
Chicken Strips (4)	290	18	15	3	700	1 carb., 3 med-fat meat
Egg Rolls (3)	440	54	24	7	960	3 carb., 5 fat, 1 vegetable
Stuffed Jalapeños (7)	420	29	27	12	1620	2 carb., 1 med-fat meat, 4 fat
SIDES						
Seasoned Curly Fries (1 regular order)	360	39	20	5	1070	2-1/2 carb., 4 fat
Potato French Fries (1 regular order)	350	45	17	4	190	3 carb., 3 fat
Onion Rings (1 order)	380	38	23	6	450	2-1/2 carb., 5 fat
BREAKFAST						
Breakfast Jack (1)	300	30	12	5	890	2 carb., 2 med-fat meat
Breakfast Sandwich, Sourdough (1)	380	31	20	7	1120	2 carb., 2 med-fat meat, 2 fat

Item	Cal	Carb	Fat	Sat Fat	Sodium	Exchanges
Breakfast Sandwich, Ultimate (1)	620	39	35	11	1800	2-1/2 carb., 4 med-fat meat, 3 fat
Croissant, Sausage (1)	670	39	48	19	940	2-1/2 carb., 2 med-fat meat, 8 fat
Croissant, Supreme (1)	570	39	36	15	1240	2-1/2 carb., 2 med-fat meat, 5 fat
Hash Browns (1 order)	160	14	11	3	310	1 carb., 2 fat
Pancake Platter (1)	400	59	12	3	980	4 carb., 2 fat
Pancake Syrup (1 pkt)	120	30	0	0	5	2 carb.
Scrambled Egg Pocket (1)	430	31	21	8	1060	2 carb., 3 med-fat meat, 1 fat

KFC

TENDER ROAST CHICKEN

Item	Cal	Carb	Fat	Sat Fat	Sodium	Exchanges
Breast w/o skin (1)	169	1	4	1	797	4 very lean meat
Breast w/skin (1)	251	1	11	3	830	5 lean meat
Drumstick w/o skin (1)	67	<1	2	<1	259	2 very lean meat
Drumstick w/skin (1)	97	<1	4	1	271	2 lean meat
Thigh w/o skin (1)	106	<1	6	2	312	2 lean meat
Thigh w/skin (1)	207	<2	12	4	504	3 med-fat meat
Wing w/skin (1)	121	1	8	2	331	2 med-fat meat

FAST FOODS

Products	Cal.	Carb. (g)	Fat (g)	Sat. Fat (g)	Sodium (mg)	Exchanges
ORIGINAL RECIPE CHICKEN						
Breast (1)	400	16	24	6	1116	1 carb., 4 med-fat meat, 1 fat
Drumstick (1)	140	4	9	2	422	2 med-fat meat
Thigh (1)	250	6	18	5	747	1/2 carb., 2 med-fat meat, 2 fat
Whole Wing (1)	140	5	10	3	414	1 med-fat meat, 1 fat
EXTRA TASTY CRISPY CHICKEN						
Breast (1)	470	25	28	7	930	1-1/2 carb., 4 med-fat meat, 2 fat
Drumstick (1)	190	8	11	3	260	1/2 carb., 2 med-fat meat
Thigh (1)	370	18	25	6	540	1 carb., 2 med-fat meat, 3 fat
Whole Wing (1)	200	10	13	4	290	1/2 carb., 1 med-fat meat, 2 fat
HOT AND SPICY CHICKEN						
Breast (1)	530	23	35	8	1110	1-1/2 carb., 4 med-fat meat, 3 fat
Drumstick (1)	190	10	11	3	300	1/2 carb., 2 med-fat meat
Thigh (1)	370	13	27	7	570	1 carb., 2 med-fat meat, 3 fat

Whole Wing (1)	210	9	15	4	340	1/2 carb., 1 med-fat meat, 2 fat

OTHER CHICKEN CHOICES

Colonel's Crispy Strips (3)	261	10	16	4	658	1/2 carb., 3 med-fat meat
Hot Wings (6)	471	18	33	8	1230	1 carb., 3 med-fat meat, 4 fat
Kentucky Nuggets (6)	284	15	18	4	865	1 carb., 2 med-fat meat, 2 fat
Pot Pie, Chunky Chicken (1)	770	69	42	13	2160	4-1/2 carb., 2 med-fat meat, 6 fat
Sandwich, Original Recipe Chicken (1)	497	46	22	5	1213	3 carb., 3 med-fat meat, 1 fat
Sandwich, Value BBQ-Flavored (1)	256	28	8	1	782	2 carb., 2 med-fat meat

SIDE CHOICES

BBQ Baked Beans (1 order)	190	33	3	1	760	2 carb., 1 fat
Biscuit (1)	180	20	10	3	560	1 carb., 2 fat
Coleslaw (1 order)	180	21	9	2	280	1/2 carb., 2 fat
Corn Bread (1 piece)	228	25	13	2	194	1-1/2 carb., 3 fat
Corn On The Cob (1)	190	34	3	<1	20	2 carb., 1 fat
Garden Rice (1 order)	120	23	2	0	890	1-1/2 carb.
Green Beans (1 order)	45	7	2	<1	730	1 vegetable

FAST FOODS

Products	Cal.	Carb. (g)	Fat (g)	Sat. Fat (g)	Sodium (mg)	Exchanges
Macaroni & Cheese (1 order)	180	21	8	3	860	1-1/2 carb., 2 fat
Mean Greens (1 order)	70	11	3	1	650	2 vegetables, 1 fat
Potato Salad (1 order)	230	23	14	2	540	1-1/2 carb., 3 fat
Potato Wedges (1 order)	280	28	13	4	750	2 carb., 3 fat
Potatoes, Mashed, w/Gravy (1 order)	120	17	6	1	440	1 carb., 1 fat
Red Beans & Rice (1 order)	130	21	3	1	360	1-1/2 carb., 1 fat

LITTLE CAESAR'S

PIZZA

Products	Cal.	Carb. (g)	Fat (g)	Sat. Fat (g)	Sodium (mg)	Exchanges
Crazy Bread (1 piece)	106	16	3	<1	114	1 carb., 1 fat
Crazy Sauce (6 oz)	74	14	<1	0	381	3 vegetable
Pan!Pan!, Cheese (1 slice)	181	22	6	3	379	1-1/2 carb., 1 med-fat meat
Pan!Pan!, Pepperoni (1 slice)	199	22	8	4	452	1-1/2 carb., 1 med-fat meat
Pizza!Pizza!, Cheese (1 slice)	201	24	7	4	281	1-1/2 carb., 1 med-fat meat
Pizza!Pizza!, Pepperoni (1 slice)	220	24	9	4	358	1-1/2 carb., 1 med-fat meat, 1 fat

SALADS

Item					Exchanges
Salad, Antipasto (1)	176	7	12	2	542	1 med-fat meat, 1 vegetable, 1 fat
Salad, Caesar (1)	140	14	5	3	372	1/2 carb., 1 med-fat meat, 1 vegetable
Salad, Greek (1)	168	12	10	<1	653	1 med-fat meat, 1 vegetable, 1 fat
Salad, Tossed (1)	116	19	3	<1	170	1 carb., 1 vegetable, 1 fat

SALAD DRESSINGS

Item					Exchanges
1000 Island (1 pkt)	183	6	17	3	542	1/2 carb., 3 fat
Blue Cheese (1 pkt)	160	8	14	2	600	1/2 carb., 3 fat
Caesar (1 pkt)	255	3	27	4	404	5 fat
French (1 pkt)	166	6	16	2	553	1/2 carb., 3 fat
Greek (1 pkt)	268	<1	30	8	202	6 fat
Italian (1 pkt)	200	3	21	3	468	4 fat
Italian, Fat-Free (1 pkt)	15	3	0	0	420	free
Ranch (1 pkt)	221	5	22	3	340	4 fat

FAST FOODS

Products	Cal.	Carb. (g)	Fat (g)	Sat. Fat (g)	Sodium (mg)	Exchanges
HOT OVEN-BAKED SANDWICHES						
Cheeser (1)	822	75	39	20	2244	5 carb., 4 med-fat meat, 4 fat
Meatsa (1)	1036	75	56	24	3302	5 carb., 6 med-fat meat, 5 fat
Pepperoni (1)	899	74	47	23	2428	5 carb., 4 med-fat meat, 5 fat
Supreme (1)	894	77	46	21	2367	5 carb., 4 med-fat meat, 5 fat
Veggie (1)	669	79	24	14	1534	5 carb., 2 med-fat meat, 3 fat
COLD DELI-STYLE SANDWICHES						
Ham & Cheese (1)	728	71	35	13	1602	5 carb., 2 med-fat meat, 5 fat
Italian (1)	740	71	37	12	1831	5 carb., 2 med-fat meat, 5 fat
Veggie (1)	647	74	29	13	1195	5 carb., 1 med-fat meat, 5 fat
LONG JOHN SILVER'S						
SANDWICHES						
Batter-Dipped Fish, No Sauce (1)	320	40	13	4	800	2-1/2 carb., 1 med-fat meat, 2 fat
Ultimate Fish (1)	430	44	21	7	1340	3 carb., 1 med-fat meat, 3 fat

POPCORN

Chicken (1 order)	250	17	14	4	590	1 carb., 2 med-fat meat, 1 fat
Fish (1 order)	290	27	14	4	1090	2 carb., 1 med-fat meat, 2 fat
Shrimp (1 order)	280	27	15	4	920	2 carb., 1 med-fat meat, 2 fat

FISH, SEAFOOD, AND CHICKEN

Chicken, Batter-Dipped (1 piece)	120	11	6	2	400	1 carb., 1 med-fat meat
Clams (3 oz)	300	31	17	4	670	2 carb., 1 med-fat meat, 2 fat
Fish, Batter-Dipped (1 piece)	170	12	11	3	470	1 carb., 1 med-fat meat, 1 fat
Shrimp, Batter-Dipped (1 piece)	35	2	3	<1	95	1 fat

SIDE ITEMS

Cheese Sticks (1 order)	160	12	9	4	360	1 carb., 2 fat
Coleslaw (1 order)	140	20	6	NA	260	1 carb., 1 fat
Corn Cobbette w/butter (1)	140	19	8	2	0	1 carb., 2 fat
Corn Cobbette w/o butter (1)	80	3	<1	0	0	1 carb.
Fries (1 order)	250	28	15	3	500	2 carb., 3 fat
Green Beans (1 order)	30	5	<1	0	310	1 vegetable

FAST FOODS

Products	Cal.	Carb. (g)	Fat (g)	Sat. Fat (g)	Sodium (mg)	Exchanges
Hush Puppy (1)	60	9	3	0	25	1/2 carb., 1 fat
Potato, Baked (1)	210	49	0	0	10	3 carb.
Rice Pilaf (1 order)	140	26	3	1	210	2 carb., 1 fat
Salad, Side (1)	25	4	0	0	15	1 vegetable
CONDIMENTS						
Sauce, Honey Mustard (1 pkt)	20	5	0	0	60	free
Sauce, Shrimp (1 pkt)	15	3	0	0	180	free
Sauce, Sweet 'N' Sour (1 pkt)	20	5	0	0	45	free
Sauce, Tartar (1 pkt)	35	5	2	NA	35	1 fat
DRESSINGS						
French, Fat-Free (1 pkt)	50	14	0	0	360	1 carb.
Italian (1 pkt)	130	2	14	2	280	3 fat
Ranch (1 pkt)	170	1	18	3	260	3 fat
Ranch, Fat-Free (1 pkt)	50	13	0	0	380	1 carb.

Thousand Island (1 pkt)	110	5	10	2	280	2 fat

MCDONALD'S

SANDWICHES

Arch Deluxe (1)	570	43	31	11	1110	3 carb., 3 med-fat meat, 3 fat
Arch Deluxe w/cheese (1)	610	43	34	12	1250	3 carb., 3 med-fat meat, 4 fat
Big Mac (1)	530	47	28	10	880	3 carb., 2 med-fat meat, 4 fat
Cheeseburger (1)	320	35	14	6	770	2 carb., 1 med-fat meat, 2 fat
Filet-O-Fish (1)	360	40	16	4	690	2-1/2 carb., 1 med-fat meat, 2 fat
Hamburger (1)	270	34	10	3.5	530	2 carb., 1 med-fat meat, 1 fat
McChicken Sandwich (1)	510	44	30	5	820	3 carb., 1 med-fat meat, 5 fat
McGrilled Chicken Classic (1)	260	33	4	1	500	2 carb., 3 very lean meat
Quarter Pounder (1)	430	37	21	8	730	2-1/2 carb., 2 med-fat meat, 2 fat
Quarter Pounder w/Cheese (1)	530	38	30	13	1200	2-1/2 carb., 3 med-fat meat, 3 fat

FRENCH FRIES

French Fries (1 large order)	450	57	22	4	290	4 carb., 4 fat
French Fries (1 small order)	210	26	10	1.5	135	2 carb., 2 fat

FAST FOODS

Products	Cal.	Carb. (g)	Fat (g)	Sat. Fat (g)	Sodium (mg)	Exchanges
CHICKEN NUGGETS/SAUCES						
Chicken Nuggets (6-piece)	290	15	17	3.5	510	1 carb., 2 med-fat meat, 3 fat
Sauce, Barbecue (1 pkt)	45	10	0	0	250	1/2 carb.
Sauce, Honey Mustard (1 pkt)	50	3	4.5	0.5	85	1 fat
Sauce, Hot Mustard (1 pkt)	60	7	3.5	0	240	1/2 carb., 1 fat
Sauce, Sweet 'N Sour (1 pkt)	50	11	0	0	140	1 carb.
SALADS						
Bacon Bits (1 pkt)	15	0	1	0	90	free
Croutons (1 pkt)	50	7	1.5	0	125	1/2 carb.
Salad, Chef (1)	206	9	11	4	727	2 med-fat meat, 2 vegetable
Salad, Chunky Chicken (1)	164	8	5	1	318	3 very lean meat, 2 vegetable
Salad, Fajita Chicken (1)	160	9	6	2	400	2 lean meat, 2 vegetable
Salad, Garden (1)	80	7	4	1	60	1 med-fat meat, 1 vegetable
Salad, Side (1)	46	4	2	1	33	1 vegetable

SALAD DRESSINGS

Item						Exchanges
1000 Island (1 pkt)	190	16	13	2	510	1 carb., 3 fat
Bleu Cheese (1 pkt)	190	8	17	3	650	1/2 carb., 3 fat
Lite Vinaigrette (1 pkt)	50	9	2	0	240	1/2 carb.
Ranch (1 pkt)	230	10	21	3	550	1/2 carb., 4 fat
Red French, Reduced-Calorie (1 pkt)	160	23	8	1	490	1-1/2 carb., 2 fat

BREAKFAST

Item						Exchanges
Biscuit (1)	260	32	13	3	840	2 carb., 3 fat
Biscuit, Bacon, Egg, & Cheese (1)	440	33	26	8	1310	2 carb., 2 med-fat meat, 3 fat
Biscuit, Sausage (1)	430	32	29	9	1130	2 carb., 1 med-fat meat, 5 fat
Biscuit, Sausage w/Egg (1)	520	33	35	10	1220	2 carb., 1 med-fat meat, 6 fat
Breakfast Burrito (1)	320	23	20	7	600	1-1/2 carb., 1 med-fat meat, 3 fat
English Muffin (1)	140	25	2	0	220	1-1/2 carb.
Hash Browns (1)	130	14	8	1.5	330	1 carb., 2 fat
Hotcakes, Plain (1 order)	310	53	7	1.5	610	3-1/2 carb., 1 fat
McMuffin, Egg (1)	290	27	13	4.5	730	2 carb., 2 med-fat meat, 1 fat

FAST FOODS

Products	Cal.	Carb. (g)	Fat (g)	Sat. Fat (g)	Sodium (mg)	Exchanges
McMuffin, Sausage (1)	360	26	23	8	750	2 carb., 1 med-fat meat, 3 fat
McMuffin, Sausage w/Egg (1)	440	27	29	10	820	2 carb., 2 med-fat meat, 4 fat
Scrambled Eggs (1 order)	170	1	12	3.5	190	2 med-fat meat
Sausage (1)	170	0	16	5	190	1 med-fat meat, 2 fat
MUFFINS/DANISH						
Danish, Apple (1)	360	51	16	5	290	3-1/2 carb., 3 fat
Danish, Cinnamon Raisin (1)	430	56	22	7	280	3-1/2 carb., 4 fat
Muffin, Apple Bran (1)	170	38	0	0	200	2-1/2 carb.
DESSERTS/SHAKES						
Cookies, McDonaldland (1 pkg)	260	41	9	2	270	3 carb., 2 fat
Ice Cream Cone, Vanilla Low-Fat (1)	120	24	0.5	0	115	1-1/2 carb.
Ice Cream Sundae, Strawberry Low-Fat (1)	240	51	1	0.5	170	3-1/2 carb.
Pie, Apple (1)	260	34	13	3.5	200	2 carb., 3 fat
Shake, Vanilla (small)	340	62	5	3	220	4 carb., 1 fat

PIZZA HUT

THIN 'N' CRISPY PIZZA

						Exchanges
Beef (1 medium slice)	229	21	11	5	709	1-1/2 carb., 1 med-fat meat, 1 fat
Cheese (1 medium slice)	205	21	8	4	534	1-1/2 carb., 1 med-fat meat, 1 fat
Ham (1 medium slice)	184	21	7	3	591	1-1/2 carb., 1 med-fat meat
Italian Sausage (1 medium slice)	236	21	12	5	650	1-1/2 carb., 1 med-fat meat, 1 fat
Meat Lover's (1 medium slice)	288	21	13	6	892	1-1/2 carb., 2 med-fat meat, 1 fat
Pepperoni (1 medium slice)	215	21	10	4	627	1-1/2 carb., 1 med-fat meat, 1 fat
Pepperoni Lover's (1 medium slice)	289	22	16	7	862	1-1/2 carb., 2 med-fat meat, 1 fat
Pork Topping (1 medium slice)	237	21	12	5	709	1-1/2 carb., 1 med-fat meat, 1 fat
Supreme (1 medium slice)	257	21	13	5	795	1-1/2 carb., 1 med-fat meat, 2 fat
Veggie Lover's (1 medium slice)	186	22	7	3	545	1-1/2 carb., 1 med-fat meat

HAND-TOSSED PIZZA

						Exchanges
Beef (1 medium slice)	260	29	9	4	797	2 carb., 1 med-fat meat, 1 fat
Cheese (1 medium slice)	235	29	7	4	621	2 carb., 1 med-fat meat
Ham (1 medium slice)	213	29	5	3	657	2 carb., 1 med-fat meat

FAST FOODS

Products	Cal.	Carb. (g)	Fat (g)	Sat. Fat (g)	Sodium (mg)	Exchanges
Italian Sausage (1 medium slice)	267	29	11	5	737	2 carb., 1 med-fat meat, 1 fat
Meat Lover's (1 medium slice)	314	29	11	6	958	2 carb., 2 med-fat meat
Pepperoni (1 medium slice)	238	29	8	4	689	2 carb., 1 med-fat meat, 1 fat
Pepperoni Lover's (1 medium slice)	306	30	14	6	897	2 carb., 1 med-fat meat, 2 fat
Pork Topping (1 medium slice)	268	29	10	5	797	2 carb., 1 med-fat meat, 1 fat
Supreme (1 medium slice)	284	30	12	5	884	2 carb., 1 med-fat meat, 1 fat
Veggie Lover's (1 medium slice)	216	30	6	3	632	2 carb., 1 med-fat meat
PAN PIZZA						
Beef (1 medium slice)	286	28	11	5	501	2 carb., 1 med-fat meat, 2 fat
Cheese (1 medium slice)	261	28	11	5	501	2 carb., 1 med-fat meat, 1 fat
Ham (1 medium slice)	239	28	9	3	537	2 carb., 1 med-fat meat, 1 fat
Italian Sausage (1 medium slice)	293	27	15	5	617	2 carb., 1 med-fat meat, 2 fat
Meat Lover's (1 medium slice)	340	28	18	7	838	2 carb., 1 med-fat meat, 3 fat
Pepperoni (1 medium slice)	265	28	12	4	569	2 carb., 1 med-fat meat, 1 fat

Pepperoni Lover's (1 medium slice)	332	28	17	7	777	2 carb., 1 med-fat meat, 2 fat
Pork Topping (1 medium slice)	294	28	14	5	677	2 carb., 1 med-fat meat, 2 fat
Supreme (1 medium slice)	311	28	15	6	764	2 carb., 1 med-fat meat, 2 fat
Veggie Lover's (1 medium slice)	243	29	10	3	512	2 carb., 1 med-fat meat, 1 fat

PERSONAL PAN PIZZA

Pepperoni (1)	637	69	28	10	1340	4-1/2 carb., 2 med-fat meat, 4 fat
Supreme (1)	722	70	34	12	1760	4-1/2 carb., 3 med-fat meat, 4 fat

SUBWAY

6-INCH COLD SUBS

Classic Italian B.M.T. (1)	434	44	21	7	1586	3 carb., 2 med-fat meat, 2 fat
Club (1)	300	45	6	1	1261	3 carb., 2 lean meat
Cold Cut Trio (1)	347	44	12	3	1222	3 carb., 1 med-fat meat, 1 fat
Ham (1)	273	44	4	1	1291	3 carb., 1 lean meat
Roast Beef (1)	299	44	6	0	837	3 carb., 2 lean meat
Seafood & Crab (1)	415	44	19	3	793	3 carb., 2 med-fat meat, 2 fat
Seafood & Crab w/Light Mayonnaise (1)	333	44	10	2	817	3 carb., 2 med-fat meat,

FAST FOODS

Products	Cal.	Carb. (g)	Fat (g)	Sat. Fat (g)	Sodium (mg)	Exchanges
Tuna (1)	522	44	33	5	824	3 carb., 1 med-fat meat, 6 fat,
Tuna w/Light Mayonnaise (1)	372	45	15	2	877	3 carb., 1 med-fat meat, 2 fat
Turkey Breast (1)	276	45	4	1	1303	3 carb., 1 lean meat
Veggie Delite (1)	223	43	3	0	526	3 carb.
6-INCH HOT SUBS						
Meatball (1)	411	53	15	6	1014	3-1/2 carb., 1 med-fat meat, 2 fat
Melt (1)	361	45	12	5	1680	3 carb., 2 med-fat meat
Roasted Chicken Breast Fillet (1)	321	44	5	1	1065	3 carb., 3 very lean meat
Steak & Cheese (1)	363	47	10	4	1079	3 carb., 2 med-fat meat
SALADS						
Bread Bowl (1)	290	56	4	NA	650	3-1/2 carb.
Club (1)	123	10	3	0	1041	1 lean meat, 2 vegetable
Roasted Chicken Breast Fillet (1)	143	9	3	1	845	2 very lean meat, 2 vegetable
Seafood & Crab (1)	238	9	17	3	573	1 med-fat meat, 2 fat, 2 vegetable

						Exchanges
Seafood & Crab w/Light Mayonnaise (1)	155	10	8	1	597	1 med-fat meat, 1 fat, 2 vegetable
Tuna (1)	345	9	31	5	604	1 med-fat meat, 5 fat, 2 vegetable
Tuna w/Light Mayonnaise (1)	194	10	13	2	657	1 med-fat meat, 2 fat, 2 vegetable
Turkey Breast (1)	99	10	2	1	1083	1 lean meat, 2 vegetable
Veggie Delite (1)	45	8	1	0	306	2 vegetable

OPTIONAL FIXIN'S

Bacon (2 slices)	45	0	4	1	182	1 fat
Cheese (2 triangles)	41	0	3	2	201	1 fat
Mayonnaise (1 tsp)	37	0	4	1	27	1 fat
Mayonnaise, Light (1 tsp)	18	1	2	0	33	free
Mustard (2 tsp)	8	1	0	0	0	free
Olive Oil Blend (1 tsp)	45	0	5	1	0	1 fat
Vinegar (1 tsp)	1	0	0	0	0	free

TACO BELL

TACOS

BLT Soft (1)	340	22	23	8	610	1-1/2 carb., 1 med-fat meat, 4 fat

FAST FOODS

Products	Cal.	Carb. (g)	Fat (g)	Sat. Fat (g)	Sodium (mg)	Exchanges
Double Decker (1)	340	37	15	5	700	2-1/2 carb., 1 med-fat meat, 2 fat
Double Decker Supreme (1)	390	39	18	8	710	2-1/2 carb., 1 med-fat meat, 3 fat
Kid's Soft Roll-Up (1)	290	20	16	8	790	1 carb., 2 med-fat meat, 1 fat
Soft (1)	210	20	10	5	530	1 carb., 1 med-fat meat, 1 fat
Soft Supreme (1)	260	22	14	7	540	1-1/2 carb., 1 med-fat meat, 2 fat
Steak Soft (1)	200	18	7	3	500	1 carb., 2 lean meat
Supreme (1)	220	13	13	6	290	1 carb., 1 med-fat meat, 2 fat
Taco (1)	170	11	10	4	280	1 carb., 1 med-fat meat, 1 fat
BURRITOS						
7-Layer (1)	540	65	24	9	1310	4 carb., 5 fat
Bacon Cheeseburger (1)	560	43	30	12	1360	3 carb., 3 med-fat meat, 3 fat
Bean (1)	380	55	12	4	1140	3-1/2 carb., 2 fat
Chicken Club (1)	540	43	31	10	1290	3 carb., 2 med-fat meat, 4 fat
Chili Cheese (1)	330	37	13	6	880	2-1/2 carb., 1 med-fat meat, 2 fat

						Exchanges
Supreme (1)	440	50	18	8	1220	3 carb., 1 med-fat meat, 3 fat
Supreme, Big Beef (1)	520	52	23	10	1450	3-1/2 carb., 2 med-fat meat, 3 fat

SPECIALTIES

Big Beef MexiMelt (1)	300	21	16	8	860	1-1/2 carb., 2 med-fat meat, 1 fat
Mexican Pizza (1)	570	41	36	11	1050	3 carb., 2 med-fat meat, 5 fat
Taco Salad w/Salsa (1)	840	62	52	15	1670	4 carb., 3 med-fat meat, 7 fat
Taco Salad w/Salsa w/o Shell (1)	840	29	21	11	1420	2 carb., 3 med-fat meat, 1 fat
Tostada (1)	300	31	14	5	700	2 carb., 1 med-fat meat, 2 fat

BORDER FAJITA WRAPS

Chicken (1)	460	49	21	6	1220	3 carb., 1 med-fat meat, 3 fat
Chicken Supreme (1)	500	51	25	8	1230	3-1/2 carb., 1 med-fat meat, 4 fat
Steak (1)	460	48	21	6	1130	3 carb., 2 med-fat meat, 2 fat
Steak Supreme (1)	510	50	25	8	1140	3 carb., 2 med-fat meat, 3 fat
Veggie (1)	420	51	19	5	920	3-1/2 carb., 4 fat
Veggie Supreme (1)	460	53	23	8	930	3-1/2 carb., 5 fat

FAST FOODS

Products	Cal.	Carb. (g)	Fat (g)	Sat. Fat (g)	Sodium (mg)	Exchanges
BORDER LIGHTS						
Burrito, Chicken (1)	310	41	8	2	980	3 carb., 1 med-fat meat, 1 fat
Burrito, Chicken Supreme (1)	430	52	13	3	1410	3-1/2 carb., 2 med-fat meat, 1 fat
Taco, Chicken Soft (1)	180	21	5	2	660	1-1/2 carb., 1 med-fat meat
Taco, Kid's Chicken Soft (1)	180	20	5	2	590	1 carb., 1 med-fat meat
NACHOS AND SIDES						
Cinnamon Twists (1 order)	140	19	6	0	190	1 carb., 1 fat
Mexican Rice (1 order)	190	20	10	4	510	1 carb., 2 fat
Nachos (1 order)	310	34	18	4	540	2 carb., 4 fat
Nachos Bell Grande (1 order)	740	83	39	10	1200	5-1/2 carb., 8 fat
Nachos Supreme, Big Beef (1 order)	430	43	24	7	720	3 carb., 5 fat
Pintos 'N' Cheese (1 order)	190	18	8	4	690	1 carb., 1 med-fat meat, 1 fat

WENDY'S

SANDWICHES

Big Bacon Classic (1)	610	45	33	13	1510	3 carb., 4 med-fat meat, 3 fat
Cheeseburger, Jr. (1)	320	34	13	6	770	2 carb., 2 med-fat meat, 1 fat
Cheeseburger, Jr. Bacon (1)	410	34	21	8	910	2 carb., 2 med-fat meat, 2 fat
Cheeseburger, Jr. Deluxe (1)	360	36	16	6	840	2-1/2 carb., 2 med-fat meat, 1 fat
Cheeseburger, Kid's Meal (1)	320	33	13	6	770	2 carb., 2 med-fat meat, 1 fat
Hamburger, Jr. (1)	270	34	10	3	560	2 carb., 1 med-fat meat, 1 fat
Hamburger, Kid's Meal (1)	270	33	10	3	560	2 carb., 2 med-fat meat
Hamburger, Single, Plain (1)	360	31	16	6	460	2 carb., 3 med-fat meat
Hamburger, Single w/Everything (1)	420	37	20	7	810	2-1/2 carb., 3 med-fat meat, 1 fat
Sandwich, Breaded Chicken (1)	440	44	18	3	840	3 carb., 3 med-fat meat, 1 fat
Sandwich, Chicken Club (1)	500	44	23	5	1090	3 carb., 3 med-fat meat, 2 fat
Sandwich, Grilled Chicken (1)	290	35	7	1.5	720	2 carb., 3 lean meat
Sandwich, Spicy Chicken (1)	440	45	20	4	1220	3 carb., 2 med-fat meat, 2 fat

FAST FOODS

Products	Cal.	Carb. (g)	Fat (g)	Sat. Fat (g)	Sodium (mg)	Exchanges
BAKED POTATOES AND FRENCH FRIES						
Baked Potato, Plain (1)	310	71	0	0	25	5 carb.
Baked Potato w/Bacon & Cheese (1)	540	78	18	4	1430	5 carb., 4 fat
Baked Potato w/Broccoli & Cheese (1)	470	80	14	3	470	5 carb., 3 fat
Baked Potato w/Cheese (1)	570	78	23	9	640	5 carb., 1 med-fat meat, 4 fat
Baked Potato w/Chili & Cheese (1)	620	83	24	9	780	5-1/2 carb., 1 med-fat meat, 4 fat
Baked Potato w/Sour Cream & Chives (1)	380	74	6	4	40	5 carb., 1 fat
French Fries (1 medium order)	380	47	19	4	120	3 carb., 4 fat
Sour Cream (1 pkt)	60	1	6	4	15	1 fat
CHILI AND CHICKEN NUGGETS						
Chicken Nuggets (5-piece)	230	10	16	4	500	1/2 carb., 1 med-fat meat, 2 fat
Chili (1)	210	21	7	2.5	800	1-1/2 carb., 1 med-fat meat
Sauce, Barbeque (1 pkt)	50	11	0	0	100	1 carb.
Sauce, Honey Mustard (1 pkt)	130	6	12	2	220	1/2 carb., 2 fat

Sauce, Spicy Buffalo Wing (1 pkt)	30	4	2	0	210	free
Sauce, Sweet & Sour (1 pkt)	50	12	0	0	120	1 carb.
FRESH SALADS TO GO						
Salad, Caesar Side w/o dressing (1)	110	8	5	2	660	1 med-fat meat, 1 vegetable
Salad, Deluxe Garden (1)	110	10	6	1	320	2 vegetable, 1 med-fat meat
Salad, Grilled Chicken w/o dressing (1)	200	10	8	1.5	690	3 med-fat meat, 2 vegetables
Salad, Side w/o dressing (1)	60	5	3	.5	160	1 vegetable, 1 fat
Salad, Taco (1)	590	53	30	11	1230	3-1/2 carb., 3 med-fat meat, 3 fat
Soft Breadstick (1)	130	24	3	.5	250	1-1/2 carb., 1 fat
SALAD DRESSINGS						
Blue Cheese (2 Tbsp)	170	0	19	3	190	4 fat
French (2 Tbsp)	120	6	10	1.5	330	1/2 carb., 2 fat
French, Fat-Free (2 Tbsp)	30	8	0	0	150	1/2 carb.
Hidden Valley Ranch (2 Tbsp)	90	1	10	1.5	240	2 fat
Hidden Valley Ranch, Reduced-Fat/Calorie (2 Tbsp)	60	2	5	1	240	1 fat

FAST FOODS

Products	Cal.	Carb. (g)	Fat (g)	Sat. Fat (g)	Sodium (mg)	Exchanges
Italian Caesar (2 Tbsp)	150	1	16	2.5	250	3 fat
Italian, Reduced-Fat/Calorie (2 Tbsp)	40	2	3	0	340	1 fat
Salad Oil (1 Tbsp)	130	0	14	2	0	3 fat
Sweet Red French (2 Tbsp)	130	9	10	1.5	230	1/2 carb., 2 fat
Thousand Island (2 Tbsp)	130	3	13	2	170	3 fat
DESSERTS						
Cookies, Chocolate Chip (1)	270	38	11	8	150	2-1/2 carb., 2 fat
Frosty Dairy Dessert (1 medium)	460	76	13	7	260	5 carb., 3 fat

FATS, OILS, AND SALAD DRESSINGS

Products	Cal.	Carb. (g)	Fat (g)	Sat. Fat (g)	Sodium (mg)	Exchanges
Butter, Reduced-Fat (1 Tbsp)	50	0	6	4	70	1 fat
Butter, Stick (1 tsp)	36	0	4	3	41	1 fat
Butter, Whipped (2 tsp)	40	0	5	3	50	1 fat
Chitterlings, Boiled (2 Tbsp)	42	0	4	1	6	1 fat
Cream Cheese, Fat-Free (1 Tbsp)	15	1	0	0	2	free
Creamer, Nondairy, Liquid, Regular (1 Tbsp)	18	2	1	1	0	free
Creamer, Nondairy, Powder, Regular (1 tsp)	22	2	1	1	0	free
Dressing, Oil & Vinegar (2 Tbsp)	144	<1	16	3	<1	3 fat
Dressing, Yogurt (1 Tbsp)	11	1	<1	<1	59	free
Lard (1 tsp)	36	0	4	2	0	1 fat
Margarine, Fat-Free/Nonfat (4 Tbsp)	20	0	0	0	0	free
Margarine, Lower Fat (1 Tbsp)	50	0	6	1	60	1 fat

FATS, OILS, AND SALAD DRESSINGS

Products	Cal.	Carb. (g)	Fat (g)	Sat. Fat (g)	Sodium (mg)	Exchanges
Margarine, Reduced-Calorie (1 Tbsp)	50	0	6	1	90	1 fat
Margarine, Squeeze (1 tsp)	30	0	3	<1	37	1 fat
Margarine, Stick (1 tsp)	34	0	4	<1	44	1 fat
Margarine, Tub (1 tsp)	30	0	4	<1	33	1 fat
Mayonnaise (1 tsp)	33	0	4	<1	26	1 fat
Mayonnaise, Fat-Free (1 Tbsp)	10	2	0	0	NA	free
Mayonnaise, Light/Reduced-Calorie (1 Tbsp)	40	3	3	<1	120	1 fat
Oil, Canola (1 tsp)	41	0	5	<1	0	1 fat
Oil, Cocoa Butter (1 tsp)	40	0	5	3	0	1 fat
Oil, Coconut (1 tsp)	39	0	5	4	0	1 fat
Oil, Cod Liver/Fish (1 tsp)	41	0	5	1	0	1 fat
Oil, Corn (1 tsp)	44	0	5	<1	0	1 fat
Oil, Cottonseed (1 tsp)	40	0	5	1	0	1 fat
Oil, Olive (1 tsp)	40	0	5	<1	0	1 fat

Oil, Palm Kernel (1 tsp)	39	0	5	4	0	1 fat
Oil, Palm (1 tsp)	40	0	5	2	0	1 fat
Oil, Peanut (1 tsp)	40	0	5	<1	0	1 fat
Oil, Safflower (1 tsp)	44	0	5	<1	0	1 fat
Oil, Sardine/Fish (1 tsp)	41	0	5	1	0	1 fat
Oil, Sesame (1 tsp)	40	0	5	<1	0	1 fat
Oil, Soybean (1 tsp)	44	0	5	<1	0	1 fat
Salad Dressing, Fat-Free (1 Tbsp)	20	5	0	0	0	free
Salad Dressing, Light/Reduced-Calorie/Reduced-Fat (2 Tbsp)	80	5	6	1	307	1 fat
Salad Dressing, Regular (1 Tbsp)	64	2	6	NA	150	1 fat
Salt Pork, Raw, Cured (1/2 oz)	52	0	6	2	100	1 fat
Shortening (1 tsp)	35	0	4	1	0	1 fat
Sour Cream, Fat-Free (1 Tbsp)	15	3	0	0	0	free
Sour Cream, Light (1 Tbsp)	18	2	1	<1	5	free
Sour Cream, Reduced-Fat (3 Tbsp)	45	2	4	3	20	1 fat

FATS, OILS, AND SALAD DRESSINGS

Products	Cal.	Carb. (g)	Fat (g)	Sat. Fat (g)	Sodium (mg)	Exchanges
Sour Cream, Regular (2 Tbsp)	52	1	5	3	12	1 fat
BLUE BONNET						
Margarine (1 Tbsp)	100	0	11	2	110	2 fat
Margarine, Liquid (1 Tbsp)	100	0	11	2	125	2 fat
Margarine, Stick (1 Tbsp)	90	<1	11	2	110	2 fat
Margarine Spread, Tub (1 Tbsp)	62	<1	7	1	110	1 fat
BREAKSTONE						
Sour Cream (2 Tbsp)	60	1	5	4	15	1 fat
BUTTER BUDS						
Butter Replacement, Dry (1 Tbsp)	19	5	<1	<1	60	free
CARNATION						
Lite Creamer, Coffee-Mate (1 Tbsp)	10	1	<1	0	0	free
Nondairy Creamer, Coffee-Mate (1 Tbsp)	73	10	5	5	0	1/2 carb., 1 fat

CREMORA

Nondairy Creamer (1 Tbsp)	10	1	<1	<1	5	free
Nondairy Creamer, Powder, Lite (1 Tbsp)	8	2	<1	0	3	free

CRISCO

Vegetable Shortening (1 Tbsp)	113	0	13	3	0	3 fat

ESTEE

Dressing, Blue Cheese (2 Tbsp)	15	1	<1	0	80	free
Dressing, Creamy French-Style (2 Tbsp)	10	2	0	0	80	free
Dressing, Creamy Garlic (2 Tbsp)	10	2	0	0	80	free
Dressing, Creamy Italian (2 Tbsp)	15	2	<1	0	80	free
Dressing, Italian (2 Tbsp)	5	1	0	0	80	free
Dressing, Thousand Island (2 Tbsp)	10	2	0	0	80	free

FLEISCHMANN'S

Fat-Free 5-Calorie Spread, Buttery Original (1 Tbsp)	5	5	1	0	130	free
Fat-Free 10-Calorie Spread, Cheddar (1 Tbsp)	10	1	0	0	120	free
Margarine, Corn Oil (1 Tbsp)	102	<1	11	2	96	2 fat

FATS, OILS, AND SALAD DRESSINGS

Products	Cal.	Carb. (g)	Fat (g)	Sat. Fat (g)	Sodium (mg)	Exchanges
Margarine, Corn Oil, White (1 Tbsp)	100	0	11	2	115	2 fat
Margarine, Diet, Tub (1 Tbsp)	49	<1	6	<1	50	1 fat
Margarine, Light, Stick (1 Tbsp)	65	<1	7	1	70	1 fat
Margarine, Tub (1 Tbsp)	102	<1	11	2	96	2 fat
Margarine "90" (1 Tbsp)	110	0	13	3	110	3 fat
Margarine Spread, Light, Tub (1 Tbsp)	65	<1	8	1	70	2 fat
Oil, Harvest Blend (1 Tbsp)	122	0	14	1	0	3 fat
IMPERIAL						
Margarine, Diet, Tub (1 Tbsp)	49	<1	6	<1	140	1 fat
Margarine, Light, Tub (1 Tbsp)	56	<1	6	1	110	1 fat
Margarine, Tub (1 Tbsp)	102	<1	11	2	105	2 fat
KNUDSEN						
Sour Cream, Light (2 Tbsp)	40	2	3	2	20	1 fat
Sour Cream, Nonfat (2 Tbsp)	35	6	0	0	25	1/2 carb.

KRAFT

Dressing, Bacon & Tomato (2 Tbsp)	140	2	14	3	260	3 fat
Dressing, Buttermilk (2 Tbsp)	150	2	16	3	230	3 fat
Dressing, Caesar (2 Tbsp)	130	2	13	3	370	3 fat
Dressing, Caesar Ranch (2 Tbsp)	140	1	15	3	300	3 fat
Dressing, Catalina French (2 Tbsp)	140	8	11	2	390	1/2 carb., 2 fat
Dressing, Catalina w/Honey (2 Tbsp)	140	8	12	2	310	1/2 carb., 2 fat
Dressing, Coleslaw (2 Tbsp)	150	8	12	2	420	1/2 carb., 2 fat
Dressing, Creamy Garlic (2 Tbsp)	110	2	11	2	350	2 fat
Dressing, Creamy Italian (2 Tbsp)	110	3	11	4	230	2 fat
Dressing, Cucumber Ranch (2 Tbsp)	150	2	15	3	220	3 fat
Dressing, Deliciously Right 1000 Island (2 Tbsp)	70	8	4	1	320	1/2 carb., 1 fat
Dressing, Deliciously Right Bacon & Tomato (2 Tbsp)	60	3	5	1	300	1 fat
Dressing, Deliciously Right Caesar (2 Tbsp)	60	2	5	1	560	1 fat
Dressing, Deliciously Right Catalina French (2 Tbsp)	80	9	4	<1	400	1/2 carb., 1 fat
Dressing, Deliciously Right Creamy Italian (2 Tbsp)	50	3	5	1	250	1 fat

FATS, OILS, AND SALAD DRESSINGS

Products	Cal.	Carb. (g)	Fat (g)	Sat. Fat (g)	Sodium (mg)	Exchanges
Dressing, Deliciously Right Cucumber (2 Tbsp)	60	2	5	1	450	1 fat
Dressing, Deliciously Right French (2 Tbsp)	50	6	3	<1	260	1 fat
Dressing, Deliciously Right Italian (2 Tbsp)	70	3	7	1	240	1 fat
Dressing, Deliciously Right Ranch (2 Tbsp)	100	5	9	2	320	2 fat
Dressing, Fat-Free Blue Cheese (2 Tbsp)	50	12	0	0	340	1 carb.
Dressing, Fat-Free Catalina (2 Tbsp)	45	11	0	0	360	1 carb.
Dressing, Fat-Free French (2 Tbsp)	40	12	0	0	300	1 carb.
Dressing, Fat-Free Honey Dijon (2 Tbsp)	50	11	0	0	330	1/2 carb.
Dressing, Fat-Free Italian (2 Tbsp)	10	2	0	0	290	free
Dressing, Fat-Free Peppercorn Ranch (2 Tbsp)	50	11	0	0	360	1 carb.
Dressing, Fat-Free Ranch (2 Tbsp)	50	11	0	0	310	1 carb.
Dressing, Fat-Free Red Wine Vinegar (2 Tbsp)	15	3	0	0	400	free
Dressing, Fat-Free Thousand Island (2 Tbsp)	45	11	0	0	300	1 carb.
Dressing, Fat-Free, Oil-Free, Italian (2 Tbsp)	5	2	0	0	450	free

Dressing, French (2 Tbsp)	120	4	12	2	260	3 fat
Dressing, Honey Dijon (2 Tbsp)	150	4	15	2	200	3 fat
Dressing, House Italian (2 Tbsp)	120	3	12	2	240	2 fat
Dressing, Light Mayonnaise (1 Tbsp)	50	1	5	1	110	1 fat
Dressing, Peppercorn Ranch (2 Tbsp)	170	1	18	3	340	4 fat
Dressing, Presto Italian (2 Tbsp)	140	2	15	3	290	3 fat
Dressing, Ranch (2 Tbsp)	170	2	18	3	270	4 fat
Dressing, Roka Brand Blue Cheese (2 Tbsp)	90	5	7	4	470	2 fat
Dressing, Russian (2 Tbsp)	130	10	10	2	280	1/2 carb., 2 fat
Dressing, Salsa Ranch (2 Tbsp)	130	1	13	2	320	3 fat
Dressing, Salsa Zesty Garden (2 Tbsp)	70	3	6	1	280	1 fat
Dressing, Seven Seas Viva Italian (2 Tbsp)	110	2	11	2	580	2 fat
Dressing, Sour Cream & Onion Ranch (2 Tbsp)	170	1	18	3	240	4 fat
Dressing, Thousand Island & Bacon (2 Tbsp)	120	5	12	2	190	3 fat
Dressing, Thousand Island (2 Tbsp)	110	5	10	2	310	2 fat
Dressing, Zesty Italian (2 Tbsp)	110	2	11	2	530	2 fat

FATS, OILS, AND SALAD DRESSINGS

Products	Cal.	Carb. (g)	Fat (g)	Sat. Fat (g)	Sodium (mg)	Exchanges
Margarine, Chiffon Soft (1 Tbsp)	100	0	11	2	105	2 fat
Margarine, Chiffon Whipped (1 Tbsp)	70	0	7	2	70	1 fat
Margarine, Parkay (1 Tbsp)	60	0	7	2	110	1 fat
Margarine, Parkay, Squeeze (1 Tbsp)	80	<1	9	2	120	2 fat
Margarine, Parkay, Stick (1 Tbsp)	90	0	10	2	110	2 fat
Margarine, Parkay, Tub (1 Tbsp)	70	0	7	2	120	1 fat
Margarine, Parkay Light, Tub (1 Tbsp)	50	0	6	1	120	1 fat
Margarine, Parkay Soft, Tub (1 Tbsp)	100	0	11	2	105	2 fat
Margarine, Parkay Soft, Diet (1 Tbsp)	50	0	6	1	110	1 fat
Margarine, Parkay Whipped (1 Tbsp)	70	0	7	2	70	1 fat
Margarine, Touch-Of-Butter (1 Tbsp)	60	0	7	2	110	1 fat
Margarine, Touch-Of-Butter, Squeeze (1 Tbsp)	80	0	9	2	115	2 fat
Mayonnaise, Fat-Free (1 Tbsp)	10	2	0	0	105	free
Mayonnaise, Real (1 Tbsp)	100	0	11	2	75	2 fat

Miracle Whip Dressing (1 Tbsp)	70	2	7	1	85	1 fat
Miracle Whip Free Nonfat Dressing (1 Tbsp)	15	3	0	0	120	free
Miracle Whip Free Nonfat Mayonnaise (1 Tbsp)	15	3	0	0	120	free
Miracle Whip Light Dressing (1 Tbsp)	40	3	3	0	120	1 fat
LIPTON						
Dressing, Fat-Free Blue Cheese (2 Tbsp)	35	7	0	0	310	1/2 carb.
Dressing, Fat-Free Creamy Italian (2 Tbsp)	35	8	0	0	170	1/2 carb.
Dressing, Fat-Free Creamy Roasted Garlic (2 Tbsp)	40	9	0	0	280	1/2 carb.
Dressing, Fat-Free Honey Dijon (2 Tbsp)	45	10	0	0	270	1/2 carb.
Dressing, Fat-Free Italian (2 Tbsp)	15	2	0	0	280	free
Dressing, Fat-Free Ranch (2 Tbsp)	40	9	0	0	270	1/2 carb.
Dressing, Fat-Free Sweet Spicy French (2 Tbsp)	30	7	0	0	220	1/2 carb.
Dressing, Fat-Free Thousand Island (2 Tbsp)	35	8	0	0	290	1/2 carb.
Dressing, Lite Italian (2 Tbsp)	15	2	<1	0	380	free
Dressing, Lite Thousand Island (2 Tbsp)	80	7	5	1	250	1/2 carb., 1 fat

FATS, OILS, AND SALAD DRESSINGS

Products	Cal.	Carb. (g)	Fat (g)	Sat. Fat (g)	Sodium (mg)	Exchanges
MARIE'S						
Dressing, Coleslaw (2 Tbsp)	150	6	13	2	210	1/2 carb., 3 fat
Dressing, Low-Fat Creamy Blue Cheese (2 Tbsp)	45	7	2	0	270	1/2 carb.
Dressing, Low-Fat Creamy Italian Herb (2 Tbsp)	40	6	2	0	290	1/2 carb.
Dressing, Low-Fat Creamy Parmesan (2 Tbsp)	45	7	2	0	270	1/2 carb.
Dressing, Low-Fat Zesty Ranch (2 Tbsp)	45	7	2	0	330	1/2 carb.
Dressing/Dip, Buttermilk Ranch (2 Tbsp)	180	4	18	3	230	3 fat
Dressing/Dip, Chunky Blue Cheese (2 Tbsp)	180	3	19	4	170	4 fat
Dressing/Dip, Creamy Ranch (2 Tbsp)	190	3	20	3	170	4 fat
Dressing/Dip, Honey Mustard (2 Tbsp)	160	8	15	2	160	1/2 carb., 3 fat
Dressing/Dip, Low-Calorie Blue Cheese (2 Tbsp)	100	7	7	1	250	1/2 carb., 1 fat
Dressing/Dip, Low-Calorie Creamy Ranch (2 Tbsp)	100	7	7	<1	240	1/2 carb., 1 fat
Dressing/Dip, Parmesan Ranch (2 Tbsp)	180	3	19	3	160	4 fat
Dressing/Dip, Poppyseed (2 Tbsp)	150	8	12	2	200	1/2 carb., 2 fat

Food						Exchanges
Dressing/Dip. Sour Cream & Dill (2 Tbsp)	190	3	20	3	160	4 fat
Dressing/Dip, Tangy French (2 Tbsp)	130	8	11	2	260	1/2 carb., 2 fat
Dressing/Dip, Thousand Island (2 Tbsp)	240	7	23	4	320	1/2 carb., 5 fat
Vinaigrette, Fat-Free Honey Dijon (2 Tbsp)	50	11	0	0	125	1 carb.
Vinaigrette, Fat-Free Red Wine (2 Tbsp)	40	10	0	0	300	1/2 carb.
Vinaigrette, Fat-Free White Wine (2 Tbsp)	40	10	0	0	310	1/2 carb.
Vinaigrette, Zesty Fat-Free Herb (2 Tbsp)	30	7	0	0	250	1/2 carb.
Vinaigrette, Zesty Fat-Free Italian (2 Tbsp)	35	8	0	0	280	1/2 carb.
Vinaigrette, Zesty Fat-Free Raspberry (2 Tbsp)	35	8	0	0	35	1/2 carb.
NABISCO						
Margarine, Tastex Colored (1 Tbsp)	100	0	11	3	170	2 fat
Margarine, Tastex White (1 Tbsp)	100	0	11	3	170	2 fat
NUCOA						
Margarine, Stick (1 Tbsp)	102	<1	12	2	160	2 fat
PARKAY						
Margarine, Soft, Tub (1 Tbsp)	102	<1	11	2	105	2 fat

FATS, OILS, AND SALAD DRESSINGS

Products	Cal.	Carb. (g)	Fat (g)	Sat. Fat (g)	Sodium (mg)	Exchanges
Margarine, Squeeze Liquid (1 Tbsp)	102	0	11	2	110	2 fat
PROMISE						
Margarine Spread, Extra Light, Tub (1 Tbsp)	50	<1	6	<1	50	1 fat
Margarine Spread, Tub (1 Tbsp)	90	<1	10	2	90	2 fat
SAFFOLA						
Margarine, Stick (1 Tbsp)	102	<1	11	2	95	2 fat
Margarine, Tub (1 Tbsp)	100	<1	11	1	95	2 fat
Margarine, Unsalted, Stick (1 Tbsp)	102	<1	11	2	0	2 fat
SEALTEST						
Sour Cream (2 Tbsp)	60	1	5	4	15	1 fat
Sour Cream, Free Fat-Free (2 Tbsp)	35	6	0	0	25	free
Sour Cream, Light (2 Tbsp)	40	2	3	2	20	1 fat
SEVEN SEAS						
Dressing, Chunky Blue Cheese (2 Tbsp)	90	5	7	4	470	2 fat

Dressing, Creamy Caesar (2 Tbsp)	140	1	15	3	300	3 fat
Dressing, Creamy Italian (2 Tbsp)	110	2	12	2	510	3 fat
Dressing, Creamy Italian, Low-Calorie (2 Tbsp)	60	2	5	1	490	1 fat
Dressing, Fat-Free Italian (2 Tbsp)	10	2	0	0	480	free
Dressing, Fat-Free Ranch (2 Tbsp)	50	12	0	0	330	1 carb.
Dressing, Fat-Free Red Wine Vinegar (2 Tbsp)	15	3	0	0	400	free
Dressing, Green Goddess (2 Tbsp)	120	1	13	2	260	3 fat
Dressing, Herbs & Spices (2 Tbsp)	120	1	12	2	320	3 fat
Dressing, Italian (1 Tbsp)	70	2	8	1	118	2 fat
Dressing, Italian & Olive Oil, Low-Calorie (2 Tbsp)	50	2	5	1	450	1 fat
Dressing, Ranch (2 Tbsp)	150	2	16	3	250	3 fat
Dressing, Red Wine Vinegar & Oil (2 Tbsp)	110	2	11	2	510	2 fat
Dressing, Two-Cheese Italian (2 Tbsp)	70	3	7	1	240	1 fat
Dressing, Vinegar & Oil, Low-Calorie (2 Tbsp)	60	2	5	1	310	1 fat
Dressing, Viva Caesar (2 Tbsp)	120	2	12	2	500	3 fat
Dressing, Viva Italian (2 Tbsp)	110	2	11	2	580	2 fat

FATS, OILS, AND SALAD DRESSINGS

Products	Cal.	Carb. (g)	Fat (g)	Sat. Fat (g)	Sodium (mg)	Exchanges
Dressing, Viva Italian, Low-Calorie (2 Tbsp)	45	2	4	1	390	1 fat
Dressing, Viva Russian (2 Tbsp)	150	3	16	3	230	3 fat
SHEDD'S SPREAD						
Margarine Spread, Tub (1 Tbsp)	60	<1	6	<1	110	1 fat
WEIGHT WATCHERS						
Dressing, Salad Celebrations 3-Chez Caesar (2 Tbsp)	40	5	2	0	190	1 fat
Dressing, Salad Celebrations Fat-Free Caesar (2 Tbsp)	10	1	0	0	390	free
Dressing, Salad Celebrations Fat-Free French (2 Tbsp)	40	9	0	0	200	1/2 carb.
Dressing, Salad Celebrations Fat-Free Honey Dijon (2 Tbsp)	45	11	0	0	150	1 carb.
Dressing, Salad Celebrations Fat-Free Italian (2 Tbsp)	30	7	0	0	360	1/2 carb.
Dressing, Salad Celebrations Russian (2 Tbsp)	45	8	2	0	190	1/2 carb.
Extra Light Spread (1 Tbsp)	49	<1	6	1	136	1 fat
Margarine, Light (1 Tbsp)	45	2	4	1	70	1 fat

Margarine, Reduced-Fat, Stick (1 Tbsp)	60	0	7	2	130	1 fat
Margarine, Sodium-Free Light (1 Tbsp)	45	2	4	1	0	1 fat
Mayonnaise, Fat-Free (1 Tbsp)	10	3	0	0	105	free
Mayonnaise, Low-Sodium Light (1 Tbsp)	25	1	2	1	40	1/2 fat
Salad Dressing, Fat-Free Whipped (1 Tbsp)	15	3	0	0	95	free
WESSON						
Best Blend (1 Tbsp)	122	0	14	1	0	3 fat
Oil, Soybean (1 tsp)	40	0	5	<1	0	1 fat
Oil, Stir-Fry (1 Tbsp)	122	0	14	1	0	3 fat
Oil, Sunlite Sunflower (1 tsp)	40	0	5	<1	0	1 fat
WISH-BONE						
Dressing, Caesar w/Olive Oil (2 Tbsp)	100	2	10	2	400	2 fat
Dressing, Chunky Blue Cheese (2 Tbsp)	170	2	17	3	280	3 fat
Dressing, Classic House Italian (2 Tbsp)	140	2	14	2	360	3 fat
Dressing, Creamy Italian (2 Tbsp)	100	3	10	2	310	2 fat
Dressing, Creamy Roasted Garlic (2 Tbsp)	140	3	13	2	240	3 fat

FATS, OILS, AND SALAD DRESSINGS

Products	Cal.	Carb. (g)	Fat (g)	Sat. Fat (g)	Sodium (mg)	Exchanges
Dressing, Deluxe French (2 Tbsp)	120	5	11	2	170	2 fat
Dressing, Honey Dijon (2 Tbsp)	130	9	10	2	390	1/2 carb., 2 fat
Dressing, Italian (2 Tbsp)	100	3	9	2	590	2 fat
Dressing, Lite Chunky Blue Cheese (2 Tbsp)	80	2	7	2	380	2 fat
Dressing, Lite Ranch (2 Tbsp)	100	5	8	2	240	2 fat
Dressing, Olive Oil Italian (2 Tbsp)	70	4	6	1	400	1 fat
Dressing, Olive Oil Vinaigrette (2 Tbsp)	60	4	5	<1	250	1 fat
Dressing, Ranch (2 Tbsp)	160	1	17	3	210	3 fat
Dressing, Robusto Italian (2 Tbsp)	100	4	10	2	610	2 fat
Dressing, Russian (2 Tbsp)	110	15	6	1	350	1 carb., 1 fat
Dressing, Sante Fe (2 Tbsp)	150	3	15	3	220	3 fat
Dressing, Sierra (2 Tbsp)	150	2	16	3	260	3 fat
Dressing, Sweet & Sour Spicy French (2 Tbsp)	130	6	12	2	330	1/2 carb., 2 fat

FRUITS AND FRUIT JUICES

FRUITS

Products	Cal.	Carb. (g)	Fat (g)	Sat. Fat (g)	Sodium (mg)	Exchanges
Apple, Unpeeled (1 large)	125	32	<1	<1	0	2 fruit
Apple, Unpeeled (1 small)	63	16	<1	<1	0	1 fruit
Apples, Dried (4 rings)	63	17	<1	0	23	1 fruit
Applesauce, Unsweetened (1/2 cup)	52	14	<1	0	2	1 fruit
Apricots, Canned, Extra Light Syrup (1/2 cup)	60	15	<1	0	2	1 fruit
Apricots, Canned, Juice Pack (1/2 cup)	60	15	0	0	5	1 fruit
Apricots, Dried (8 halves)	66	17	<1	0	2	1 fruit
Apricots, Fresh (4)	68	16	1	0	1	1 fruit
Banana (1 small)	64	16	<1	<1	1	1 fruit
Banana Chips (1/2 cup)	120	14	8	7	1	1 fruit, 2 fat
Blackberries, Fresh (1/2 cup)	56	14	<1	0	0	1 fruit

FRUITS AND FRUIT JUICES

Products	Cal.	Carb. (g)	Fat (g)	Sat. Fat (g)	Sodium (mg)	Exchanges
Blackberries, Frozen, Unsweetened (1/2 cup)	73	18	<1	NA	2	1 fruit
Blueberries, Fresh (1/2 cup)	61	15	<1	0	7	1 fruit
Blueberries, Frozen, Unsweetened (1/2 cup)	58	14	<1	NA	1	1 fruit
Cantaloupe, Fresh (1 cup)	56	13	<1	0	14	1 fruit
Cherries, Sweet, Canned, Juice Pack (1/2 cup)	68	17	0	0	4	1 fruit
Cherries, Sweet, Fresh (12)	59	14	<1	<1	0	1 fruit
Cranberries (1 cup)	47	12	<1	<1	<1	1 fruit
Cranberry Sauce, Canned (1/2 cup)	105	27	<1	<1	20	1-1/2 fruit
Dates (3)	68	18	<1	0	0	1 fruit
Figs, Dried (1-1/2)	71	18	<1	<1	3	1 fruit
Figs, Fresh (1-1/2 large)	71	18	<1	<1	1	1 fruit
Fruit Cocktail, Canned, Extra Light Syrup (1/2 cup)	55	14	<1	0	5	1 fruit
Fruit Cocktail, Canned, Juice Pack (1/2 cup)	57	15	0	0	5	1 fruit
Fruit Salad, Fresh (1/2 cup)	50	13	<1	<1	<1	1 fruit

Grapefruit, Canned (1/2 cup)	69	17	<1	0	13	1 fruit
Grapefruit, Fresh (1/2 cup)	51	13	<1	0	0	1 fruit
Grapes, Fresh, Seedless (17)	60	15	<1	<1	2	1 fruit
Honeydew Melon, Fresh (1 cup)	59	16	<1	0	15	1 fruit
Kiwi, Fresh (1)	56	14	<1	0	5	1 fruit
Mango, Fresh (1/2)	68	18	<1	<1	2	1 fruit
Melon Balls, Mixed, Frozen (1 cup)	57	14	<1	<1	54	1 fruit
Mixed Fruit, Dried (1/2 cup)	83	22	<1	<1	6	1-1/2 fruit
Nectarine, Fresh (1)	67	16	<1	0	0	1 fruit
Orange, Fresh (1)	62	15	<1	0	0	1 fruit
Oranges, Mandarin, Canned, Juice Pack (1/2 cup)	69	18	<1	0	9	1 fruit
Papaya, Fresh (1/2 medium)	59	15	<1	<1	4	1 fruit
Peach, Fresh (1 medium)	57	15	<1	0	0	1 fruit
Peaches, Canned, Extra Light Syrup (1/2 cup)	52	14	<1	0	6	1 fruit
Peaches, Canned, Juice Pack (1/2 cup)	55	14	0	0	5	1 fruit
Pear, Fresh (1/2 large)	59	15	<1	0	0	1 fruit

FRUITS AND FRUIT JUICES

Products	Cal.	Carb. (g)	Fat (g)	Sat. Fat (g)	Sodium (mg)	Exchanges
Pears, Canned (1/2 cup)	62	16	<1	0	5	1 fruit
Pears, Canned, Light Syrup (1/2 cup)	58	15	<1	0	3	1 fruit
Pineapple, Canned, Juice Pack (1/2 cup)	74	20	0	0	1	1 fruit
Pineapple, Fresh (1/2 cup)	57	14	<1	0	1	1 fruit
Plums, Canned, Juice Pack (1/2 cup)	73	19	0	0	2	1 fruit
Plums, Fresh (2 small)	73	17	<1	<1	0	1 fruit
Prunes, Dried, Uncooked (3)	60	16	<1	0	1	1 fruit
Raisins, Dark, Seedless (2 Tbsp)	54	14	<1	0	2	1 fruit
Raspberries, Black, Fresh (1 cup)	60	14	<1	0	0	1 fruit
Rhubarb, Diced (2 cups)	52	12	<1	<1	10	1 fruit
Strawberries, Fresh (1-1/2 cups)	56	13	<1	0	2	1 fruit
Strawberries, Frozen, Unsweetened (1-1/2 cups)	65	17	<1	0	4	1 fruit
Tangerines, Fresh (2 small)	74	19	<1	0	2	1 fruit
Watermelon, Fresh (1-1/2 cups)	64	15	<1	NA	4	1 fruit

JUICES

Apple Juice/Cider, Canned/Bottled (1/2 cup)	58	15	<1	0	4	1 fruit
Apricot Nectar, Canned (1/2 cup)	71	18	<1	<1	4	1 fruit
Cranberry Juice Cocktail, Bottled (1/3 cup)	48	12	<1	0	2	1 fruit
Cranberry Juice Cocktail, Reduced-Calorie (1 cup)	50	11	0	0	7	1 fruit
Fruit Juice Blends, 100% Juice (1/3 cup)	50	12	<1	0	10	1 fruit
Grape Juice, Bottled (1/3 cup)	51	13	<1	0	3	1 fruit
Grapefruit Juice, Canned (1/2 cup)	47	11	<1	0	1	1 fruit
Orange Juice, Canned (1/2 cup)	52	12	<1	<1	3	1 fruit
Orange Juice, Fresh (1/2 cup)	56	13	<1	0	1	1 fruit
Orange Juice, Frozen, Reconstituted (1/2 cup)	56	13	<1	0	1	1 fruit
Pineapple Juice, Canned (1/2 cup)	70	17	<1	0	1	1 fruit
Prune Juice, Bottled (1/3 cup)	60	15	0	0	3	1 fruit

GRAINS, NOODLES, AND RICE

GRAINS, NOODLES, AND RICE

Products	Cal.	Carb. (g)	Fat (g)	Sat. Fat (g)	Sodium (mg)	Exchanges
Barley, Cooked (1/2 cup)	135	30	1	<1	<1	2 strch
Barley, Pearled, Cooked (1/2 cup)	97	22	<1	<1	3	1-1/2 strch
Brown Rice, Long-Grain, Cooked (1/2 cup)	108	23	1	<1	5	1-1/2 strch
Brown Rice, Medium-Grain, Cooked (1/2 cup)	110	23	<1	<1	<1	1-1/2 strch
Bulgur Wheat, Cooked (1/2 cup)	76	17	<1	<1	5	1 strch
Couscous, Cooked (1/2 cup)	100	21	<1	<1	5	1-1/2 strch
Noodles, Egg, Cooked (1/2 cup)	107	20	1	<1	6	1 strch
Fried Rice, Meatless (1 cup)	264	34	12	2	286	2 strch, 2 fat
Grits, Yellow Corn, Cooked (1/2 cup)	73	16	<1	<1	0	1 strch
Lasagna, Cut, Cooked (1/2 cup)	99	20	<1	<1	<1	1 strch
Linguine, Cooked (1/2 cup)	99	20	<1	<1	<1	1 strch
Macaroni, Cooked (1/2 cup)	99	20	<1	<1	<1	1 strch
Macaroni, Vegetable, Cooked (1/2 cup)	86	18	<1	<1	4	1 strch

Macaroni, Whole-Wheat, Cooked (1/2 cup)	87	19	<1	<1	2	1 strch
Millet, Cooked (1/2 cup)	143	28	1	<1	2	2 strch
Noodles, Chow Mein (1/2 cup)	116	13	7	1	97	1 strch, 1 fat
Noodles, Ramen, Cooked (1 cup)	156	29	2	<1	1349	2 strch
Noodles, Rice, Cooked (1/2 cup)	62	15	<1	<1	4	1 strch
Noodles, Spinach Egg, Cooked (1/2 cup)	106	20	1	<1	10	1 strch
Pasta, Homemade w/o Egg, Cooked (2 oz)	70	14	<1	<1	42	1 strch
Pasta/Noodles, Egg, Homemade, Cooked (2 oz)	74	13	<1	<1	47	1 strch
Pasta/Noodles, Fresh, Cooked (2 oz)	74	14	<1	<1	3	1 strch
Pasta/Noodles, Spinach, Fresh, Cooked (2 oz)	74	14	<1	<1	3	1 strch
Rice Pilaf (1 cup)	268	46	7	1	754	3 strch, 1 fat
Rotini, Cooked (1/2 cup)	99	20	<1	<1	<1	2 strch
Shells, Jumbo, Cooked (2)	65	13	<1	<1	<1	1 strch
Shells, Small, Cooked (1/2 cup)	81	17	<1	<1	<1	1 strch
Shells, Whole-Wheat, Cooked (1/2 cup)	87	19	<1	<1	2	1 strch
Spaghetti, Cooked (1/2 cup)	99	20	<1	<1	<1	1 strch

GRAINS, NOODLES, AND RICE

Products	Cal.	Carb. (g)	Fat (g)	Sat. Fat (g)	Sodium (mg)	Exchanges
Spaghetti, Spinach, Cooked (1/2 cup)	91	19	<1	<1	10	1 strch
Spaghetti, Whole-Wheat, Cooked (1/2 cup)	87	19	<1	<1	2	1 strch
Spirals, Cooked (1/2 cup)	95	19	<1	<1	<1	1 strch
Vermicelli, Cooked (1/2 cup)	99	20	<1	<1	<1	1 strch
Wagon Wheels, Cooked (1/2 cup)	99	20	<1	<1	<1	1 strch
Wheat Bran (1/2 cup)	65	19	1	<1	<1	1 strch
Wheat Germ, Toasted (1 Tbsp)	27	4	<1	<1	<1	free
White Flour, All-Purpose (1 Tbsp)	28	6	<1	<1	<1	1/2 strch
White Hominy, Canned (1/2 cup)	58	12	<1	<1	168	1 strch
White Rice, Long-Grain, Cooked (1/2 cup)	134	29	<1	<1	1	2 strch
White Rice, Long-Grain, Instant, Cooked (1/2 cup)	81	18	<1	<1	3	1 strch
White Rice, Long-Grain, Parboiled, Cooked (1/2 cup)	100	22	<1	<1	3	1/2 strch
White Rice, Medium-Grain, Cooked (1/2 cup)	134	29	<1	<1	0	2 strch
White Rice, Short-Grain, Cooked (1/2 cup)	134	29	<1	<1	0	2 strch

Food	Cal	Carb	Fat	Sod	Exchanges
Wild Rice, Cooked (1/2 cup)	83	18	<1	3	1 strch
ALBER'S					
Cornmeal, Yellow (1 Tbsp)	37	8	0	0	1/2 strch
Grits, Hominy Quick (1/2 cup)	140	31	<1	0	2 strch
DI GIORNO					
Angel Hair Pasta (2 oz)	160	31	1	190	2 strch
KRAFT					
Macaroni & Cheese (1 cup)	390	48	17	730	3 strch, 3 fat
Macaroni & Cheese, Deluxe Original (1 cup)	320	44	10	730	3 strch, 1 med-fat meat, 1 fat
Macaroni & Cheese, Shaped Pastas (1 cup)	390	48	17	770	3 strch, 3 fat
Macaroni & Cheese, Thick'n Creamy (1 cup)	320	50	10	730	3 strch, 2 fat
Macaroni & Cheese, White Cheddar (1 cup)	390	48	17	730	3 strch, 3 fat
Velveeta Rotini & Cheese w/Broccoli (1 cup)	400	46	16	1240	3 strch, 1 med-fat meat, 2 fat
Velveeta Shells & Cheese, Bacon (1 cup)	360	43	14	1140	3 strch, 1 med-fat meat, 2 fat
Velveeta Shells & Cheese, Original (1 cup)	360	44	13	1030	3 strch, 1 med-fat meat, 2 fat
Velveeta Shells & Cheese, Salsa (1 cup)	380	47	14	1180	3 strch, 1 med-fat meat, 2 fat

GRAINS, NOODLES, AND RICE

Products	Cal.	Carb. (g)	Fat (g)	Sat. Fat (g)	Sodium (mg)	Exchanges
LA CHOY						
Fried Rice (1 cup)	236	53	1	<1	1024	3-1/2 strch
Noodles, Chow Mein (1/2 cup)	137	19	6	1	217	1 strch, 1 fat
Noodles, Crispy Wide (1/2 cup)	148	16	8	2	289	1 strch, 2 fat
Noodles, Rice (1/2 cup)	121	21	3	<1	378	1-1/2 strch, 1 fat
LIPTON						
Noodles & Sauce, Alfredo Broccoli, Dry (2/3 cup)	260	39	7	4	940	2-1/2 strch, 1 fat
Noodles & Sauce, Butter Herb, Dry (2/3 cup)	250	41	7	3	860	3 strch, 1 fat
Pasta & Sauce, Cheddar Broccoli, Dry (1/2 cup)	260	46	4	2	870	3 strch, 1 fat
Pasta & Sauce, Creamy Garlic, Dry (2/3 cup)	260	45	6	3	840	3 strch, 1 fat
Pasta & Sauce, Herb Tomato, Dry (2/3 cup)	240	48	2	<1	690	3 strch
Pasta & Sauce, Three-Cheese, Dry (1/2 cup)	240	41	5	3	870	3 strch, 1 fat
Pasta Saute, Angel Hair Chicken, Dry (1/3 cup)	210	44	2	<1	850	3 strch
Pasta Saute, Chicken Herb Primavera, Dry (1/2 cup)	230	45	3	2	830	3 strch, 1 fat

Pasta Saute, Rotini w/Garlic & Butter, Dry (1/3 cup)	210	41	3	1	790	3 strch, 1 fat
Pasta Saute, Spirals, Garlic & Butter, Dry (1/2 cup)	230	43	3	2	790	3 strch, 1 fat
Pasta Saute, Stir-Fry, Chicken, Dry (1/2 cup)	220	45	2	0	850	3 strch
Rice & Beans, Cajun, Dry (1/2 cup)	260	53	1	0	540	3-1/2 strch
Rice & Sauce, Alfredo Broccoli, Dry (1/2 cup)	250	44	5	2	860	3 strch, 1 fat
Rice & Sauce, Beef Broccoli, Dry (1/2 cup)	230	46	1	0	940	3 strch
Rice & Sauce, Beef Flavor, Dry (1/2 cup)	230	47	1	0	940	3 strch
Rice & Sauce, Cajun, Dry (1/2 cup)	230	49	1	0	930	3 strch
Rice & Sauce, Cheddar Broccoli, Dry (1/2 cup)	250	48	3	1	940	3 strch, 1 fat
Rice & Sauce, Chicken Broccoli, Dry (1/2 cup)	250	48	2	1	940	3 strch
Rice & Sauce, Chicken Flavor, Dry (1/2 cup)	240	48	2	<1	900	3 strch
Rice & Sauce, Chicken Risotto, Dry (1/2 cup)	230	44	2	<1	740	3 strch
Rice & Sauce, Creamy Chicken, Dry (1/2 cup)	260	46	5	1	770	3 strch, 1 fat
Rice & Sauce, Herb & Butter, Dry (1/2 cup)	240	43	4	2	920	3 strch, 1 fat
Rice & Sauce, Medley, Dry (1/2 cup)	240	46	2	<1	810	3 strch
Rice & Sauce, Oriental, Dry (1/2 cup)	230	46	1	0	750	3 strch

GRAINS, NOODLES, AND RICE

Products	Cal.	Carb. (g)	Fat (g)	Sat. Fat (g)	Sodium (mg)	Exchanges
Rice & Sauce, Original Long-Grain, Dry (1/2 cup)	250	51	1	0	890	3-1/2 strch
Rice & Sauce, Pilaf, Dry (1/2 cup)	230	46	1	0	850	3 strch
Rice, Golden Saute, Fried Rice, Dry (1/2 cup)	240	47	1	0	900	3 strch
Rice, Golden Saute, Onion Mushroom, Dry (1/2 cup)	240	45	4	2	850	3 strch, 1 fat
Rice, Golden Saute, Oriental, Dry (1/2 cup)	240	43	5	2	910	3 strch, 1 fat
Rice, Golden Saute, Spanish, Dry (1/2 cup)	250	46	5	2	910	3 strch, 1 fat
MINUTE RICE						
Brown Rice, Whole-Grain, Instant, Cooked (2/3 cup)	170	34	2	0	10	2 strch
Rice, Boil-In-Bag, Cooked (1 cup)	190	42	0	0	10	3 strch
White Rice, Instant, Cooked (1/2 cup)	170	37	0	0	5	2-1/2 strch
PILLSBURY						
Shake & Blend Flour (2 Tbsp)	95	20	<1	<1	<1	1 strch
RICE-A-RONI						
Beef, As Prepared (1 cup)	310	52	9	9	1160	3-1/2 strch, 2 fat

Chicken, As Prepared (1 cup)	310	52	9	2	980	3-1/2 strch, 2 fat
Red Beans & Rice, As Prepared (1 cup)	290	51	7	2	1190	3-1/2 strch, 1 fat
STOVE TOP						
Stuffing Mix, Long-Grain & Wild Rice (1/2 cup)	110	22	1	0	490	1-1/2 strch
Stuffing Mix, Mushroom & Onion (1/2 cup)	110	20	2	0	410	1 strch
UNCLE BEN'S						
Brown Rice, Fast-Cook Whole-Grain (1 cup)	190	42	2	0	20	3 strch
Brown Rice, Lightly Milled (1 cup)	170	35	2	0	0	2 strch
Brown Rice, Original (1 cup)	170	37	2	0	0	2-1/2 strch
Brown Rice & Wild Mushroom Flavor (2/3 cup)	140	31	1	0	460	2 strch
Converted Rice (1 cup)	170	38	0	0	0	2-1/2 strch
Converted Rice, Boil-In-Bag (1 cup)	170	40	<1	0	15	2-1/2 strch
Converted Rice, Fast-Cook (1 cup)	190	43	<1	0	15	3 strch
Long-Grain & Wild Rice, Fast-Cook (1 cup)	200	42	0	0	850	3 strch
Long-Grain & Wild Rice, Original Natural (1 cup)	190	42	<1	0	630	3 strch

GRAINS, NOODLES, AND RICE

Products	Cal.	Carb. (g)	Fat (g)	Sat. Fat (g)	Sodium (mg)	Exchanges
Long-Grain Rice & Wild Chicken Stock Sauce (1/2 cup)	200	40	2	0	410	2-1/2 strch
Long-Grain Rice & Wild Garden Vegetable Blend (1/2 cup)	200	41	2	0	750	3 strch
Multi-Grain Blend, Specialty Blends (1 cup)	160	35	1	0	0	2 strch
Pilaf, Specialty Blends (1 cup)	170	36	<1	0	0	2-1/2 strch
Wild Rice, Specialty Blends (1 cup)	160	36	<1	0	0	2-1/2 strch

Products	Cal.	Carb. (g)	Fat (g)	Sat. Fat (g)	Sodium (mg)	Exchanges
LEGUMES						
Baby Lima Beans, Cooked (1/2 cup)	115	21	<1	<1	3	1-1/2 strch
Baked Beans w/Beef, Canned (1/2 cup)	161	23	5	2	632	1-1/2 strch, 1 med-fat meat
Baked Beans, Homemade (1/2 cup)	190	27	7	3	532	2 strch, 1 fat
Baked Beans, Vegetarian, Canned (1/2 cup)	118	26	<1	<1	504	2 strch
Black Beans, Cooked (1/2 cup)	114	21	<1	<1	<1	1-1/2 strch
Black Turtle Soup Beans, Cooked (1/2 cup)	120	22	<1	<1	3	1-1/2 strch
Black-Eyed Cowpeas w/Pork (1/2 cup)	100	20	2	<1	420	1 strch
Fava/Broadbeans, Canned (1/2 cup)	91	16	<1	<1	580	1 strch, 1 very lean meat
French Beans, Cooked (1/2 cup)	111	21	<1	<1	5	1-1/2 strch
Garbanzo Beans/Chickpeas, Cooked (1/2 cup)	135	23	2	<1	6	1-1/2 strch, 1 very lean meat
Great Northern Beans, Cooked (1/2 cup)	105	19	<1	<1	2	1 strch, 1 very lean meat
Hummus (1/2 cup)	210	25	11	2	300	1-1/2 strch, 2 fat

LEGUMES

Products	Cal.	Carb. (g)	Fat (g)	Sat. Fat (g)	Sodium (mg)	Exchanges
Kidney Beans, California Red, Cooked (1/2 cup)	109	20	<1	<1	4	1 strch, 1 very lean meat
Kidney Beans, Canned, Not Drained (1/2 cup)	104	19	<1	<1	444	1 strch, 1 very lean meat
Kidney Beans, Red, Cooked (1/2 cup)	112	20	<1	<1	2	1 strch, 1 very lean meat
Kidney Beans, Royal Red, Cooked (1/2 cup)	108	19	<1	<1	4	1 strch, 1 very lean meat
Lentils, Cooked (1/2 cup)	115	20	<1	<1	2	1 strch, 1 very lean meat
Navy Beans, Cooked (1/2 cup)	129	24	<1	<1	1	1-1/2 strch, 1 very lean meat
Pink Beans, Cooked (1/2 cup)	125	23	<1	<1	2	1-1/2 strch
Pinto Beans, Cooked (1/2 cup)	117	22	<1	<1	2	1-1/2 strch
Pork & Beans in Sweet Sauce, Canned (1/2 cup)	140	27	2	<1	425	2 strch
Pork & Beans in Tomato Sauce, Canned (1/2 cup)	124	25	1	<1	557	1-1/2 strch
Refried Beans/Frijoles, Canned (1/2 cup)	136	24	1	<1	536	1-1/2 strch
Split Peas, Cooked (1/2 cup)	115	21	<1	<1	2	1-1/2 strch, 1 very lean meat
White Beans, Cooked (1/2 cup)	125	23	<1	<1	5	1-1/2 strch
White Beans, Small, Cooked (1/2 cup)	127	23	<1	<1	2	1-1/2 strch

Yellow Beans, Cooked (1/2 cup)	127	22	<1	<1	4	1-1/2 strch

B & M

Baked Beans, 99% Fat-Free (1/2 cup)	160	31	1	0	220	2 strch
Baked Beans, Barbeque (1/2 cup)	170	32	2	<1	360	2 strch
Baked Beans, Brick-Oven (1/2 cup)	180	32	2	<1	390	2 strch
Baked Beans, Extra Hearty (1/2 cup)	190	32	2	<1	450	2 strch
Baked Beans, Red Kidney (1/2 cup)	170	32	2	<1	440	2 strch
Baked Beans, Yellow Eye (1/2 cup)	170	28	2	<1	460	2 strch
Baked Beans w/Honey (1/2 cup)	170	30	2	0	450	2 strch

CAMPBELL'S

Brown Sugar Bacon-Flavor Beans (1/2 cup)	170	29	3	1	490	2 strch, 1 fat
Chili Beans in Zesty Sauce (1/2 cup)	130	21	3	1	490	1-1/2 strch, 1 fat
Homestyle Beans (1/2 cup)	150	27	2	<1	490	1 strch
New England-Style Baked Beans (1/2 cup)	180	32	3	1	460	2 strch, 1 fat
Old-Fashioned Barbecue Beans (1/2 cup)	170	29	3	<1	460	2 strch, 1 fat
Pork & Beans in Tomato Sauce (1/2 cup)	130	24	2	<1	420	1-1/2 strch

LEGUMES

Products	Cal.	Carb. (g)	Fat (g)	Sat. Fat (g)	Sodium (mg)	Exchanges
Vegetarian Beans w/Tomato Sauce (1/2 cup)	130	24	2	1	460	1-1/2 strch
FRIENDS						
Baked Beans, Original (1/2 cup)	160	32	1	0	390	2 strch
Baked Beans, Red Kidney (1/2 cup)	160	32	1	0	510	2 strch
GEBHARDT						
Chili Beans (1/2 cup)	134	31	1	<1	630	2 strch
Pinto Beans (1/2 cup)	92	18	1	0	505	1 strch, 1 very lean meat
Refried Beans, Jalapeño (1/2 cup)	105	19	3	1	380	1 strch, 1 fat
Refried Beans, No-Fat (1/2 cup)	92	20	<1	0	480	1 strch, 1 very lean meat
Refried Beans, Traditional (1/2 cup)	109	20	3	1	497	1 strch, 1 fat
Refried Beans, Vegetarian (1/2 cup)	118	21	2	<1	550	1-1/2 strch
GREEN GIANT						
Baked Beans in Sauce (1/2 cup)	152	30	1	<1	554	2 strch
Black Beans (1/2 cup)	110	20	<1	<1	575	1 strch

	Cal	Carb	Fat		Sod	Exchanges
Black-Eyed Peas (1/2 cup)	103	19	<1	0	276	1 strch
Butter Beans (1/2 cup)	89	16	<1	0	448	1 strch
Chili Beans in Sauce (1/2 cup)	84	19	1	0	551	1 strch
Garbanzo Beans (1/2 cup)	107	18	2	<1	363	1 strch
Great Northern Beans (1/2 cup)	100	18	<1	<1	288	1 strch
Joan Of Arc Baked Beans w/Onion (1/2 cup)	143	28	1	<1	622	2 strch
Joan Of Arc Barbecue Beans (1/2 cup)	138	28	<1	<1	459	2 strch
Joan Of Arc Honey-Baked Beans (1/2 cup)	186	34	<1	<1	488	2 strch
Joan Of Arc Italian Beans (1/2 cup)	122	24	<1	<1	476	1-1/2 strch
Joan Of Arc Mexican Beans (1/2 cup)	115	21	1	<1	526	1-1/2 strch
Kidney Beans, Dark Red (1/2 cup)	112	19	<1	<1	339	1 strch
Kidney Beans, Light Red (1/2 cup)	112	19	<1	<1	339	1 strch, 1 very lean meat
Pinto Beans (1/2 cup)	107	20	<1	<1	280	1 strch
Red Beans (1/2 cup)	105	19	<1	<1	342	1 strch
HEALTH VALLEY						
Honey-Baked Beans, Fat-Free, Salted (1/2 cup)	110	24	0	0	135	1-1/2 strch

LEGUMES

Products	Cal.	Carb. (g)	Fat (g)	Sat. Fat (g)	Sodium (mg)	Exchanges
HEARTLAND						
Iron Kettle Baked Beans (1/2 cup)	150	29	1	0	400	2 strch
HUNT'S						
Big John's Beans & Fixin's (1/2 cup)	127	23	4	1	590	1-1/2 strch, 1 fat
Chili Beans (1/2 cup)	87	17	<1	0	597	1 strch
Kidney Beans (1/2 cup)	94	20	<1	0	484	1 strch
Pork & Beans (1/2 cup)	130	28	1	<1	516	2 strch
Red Beans, Small (1/2 cup)	89	19	<1	0	713	1 strch
OLD EL PASO						
Black Beans (1/2 cup)	100	17	1	0	400	1 strch, 1 very lean meat
Garbanzo Beans (1/2 cup)	120	20	3	0	280	1 strch, 1 lean meat
Mexe Beans (1/2 cup)	110	19	<1	0	630	1 strch, 1 very lean meat
Pinto Beans (1/2 cup)	110	19	<1	0	420	1 strch, 1 very lean meat
Refried Beans (1/2 cup)	110	17	2	1	500	1 strch, 1 lean meat

Refried Beans, Fat-Free (1/2 cup)	110	20	0	0	480	1 strch, 1 very lean meat
Refried Beans, Spicy (1/2 cup)	140	22	3	2	560	1-1/2 strch, 1 fat
Refried Beans, Vegetarian (1/2 cup)	100	16	1	0	490	1 strch
Refried Beans & Cheese (1/2 cup)	130	18	4	2	500	1 strch, 1 med-fat meat
Refried Beans w/Green Chili (1/2 cup)	110	19	<1	0	720	1 strch, 1 very lean meat
Refried Beans w/Sausage (1/2 cup)	200	14	13	5	360	1 strch, 1 med-fat meat, 2 fat
Refried Black Beans (1/2 cup)	120	18	2	0	340	1 strch, 1 lean meat
ORTEGA						
Refried Beans/Frijoles (1/2 cup)	140	23	3	<1	480	1-1/2 strch, 1 fat
ORVAL KENT						
Barbeque Beans (1/2 cup)	160	34	<1	0	700	1 strch
Four-Bean Salad (1/2 cup)	100	19	<1	0	300	1 strch
PROGRESSO						
Black Beans (1/2 cup)	100	17	1	0	400	1 strch, 1 very lean meat
Cannellini Beans (1/2 cup)	100	18	<1	0	270	1 strch
Chickpeas (1/2 cup)	120	20	3	0	280	1 strch, 1 fat

LEGUMES

Products	Cal.	Carb. (g)	Fat (g)	Sat. Fat (g)	Sodium (mg)	Exchanges
Fava Beans (1/2 cup)	110	20	<1	0	250	1 strch
Kidney Beans, Red (1/2 cup)	110	20	<1	0	280	1 strch, 1 very lean meat
Pinto Beans (1/2 cup)	110	18	1	0	250	1 strch, 1 very lean meat
ROSARITA						
Refried Beans, Bacon (1/2 cup)	116	19	3	1	489	1 strch, 1 med-fat meat
Refried Beans, Green Chili (1/2 cup)	110	20	3	2	495	1 strch, 1 fat
Refried Beans, Nacho Cheese (1/2 cup)	137	24	3	2	703	1-1/2 strch, 1 fat
Refried Beans, No-Fat (1/2 cup)	123	28	<1	0	574	2 strch
Refried Beans, Onion (1/2 cup)	114	21	3	1	508	1-1/2 strch, 1 fat
Refried Beans, Spicy (1/2 cup)	118	22	3	1	574	1-1/2 strch, 1 fat
Refried Beans, Traditional (1/2 cup)	125	22	3	1	585	1-1/2 strch, 1 fat
Refried Beans, Vegetarian (1/2 cup)	121	23	2	<1	562	1-1/2 strch
Refried Beans w/Green Chiles & Lime, No-Fat (1/2 cup)	101	22	<1	0	565	1-1/2 strch

Refried Beans w/Zesty Salsa, No-Fat (1/2 cup)	99	22	<1	0	554	1-1/2 strch
Refried Black Beans, Low-Fat (1/2 cup)	107	23	<1	0	569	1-1/2 strch

MEATS, FISH, AND POULTRY

MEATS, FISH, AND POULTRY

Products	Cal.	Carb. (g)	Fat (g)	Sat. Fat (g)	Sodium (mg)	Exchanges
Anchovies in Oil, Canned, Drained (5)	42	0	2	<1	734	1 lean meat
Bacon (3 slices)	105	0	9	3	288	1 high-fat meat
Beef, Chipped, Dried (1 oz)	47	0	1	<1	948	1 very lean meat
Beef, Chuck/Blade Pot Roast (1 oz)	62	0	2	<1	19	1 lean meat
Beef, Corned Brisket (1 oz)	72	<1	5	2	323	1 med-fat meat
Beef, Cubed Steak (1 oz)	58	0	2	<1	15	1 lean meat
Beef, Flank Steak, Lean (1 oz)	59	0	3	1	24	1 lean meat
Beef, Ground, Extra Lean (1 oz)	73	0	5	2	20	1 med-fat meat
Beef, Ground, Lean (1 oz)	78	0	5	2	22	1 med-fat meat
Beef, Ground, Regular (1 oz)	82	0	6	2	24	1 med-fat meat
Beef, Ground Round (1 oz)	56	0	1	<1	13	1 lean meat
Beef, Heart (1 oz)	50	<1	2	<1	18	1 lean meat
Beef, Liver (1 oz)	46	1	1	<1	20	1 lean meat

Food						Exchange
Beef, Prime Rib (1 oz)	83	0	6	2	21	1 med-fat meat
Beef, Rib Roast, Lean (1 oz)	65	0	4	1	21	1 lean meat
Beef, Round Steak, Lean (1 oz)	55	0	2	<1	18	1 lean meat
Beef, Rump Roast, Lean (1 oz)	60	0	2	<1	15	1 lean meat
Beef, Shortribs (1 oz)	83	0	5	2	16	1 med-fat meat
Beef, Sirloin (1 oz)	54	0	2	<1	19	1 lean meat
Beef, Jerky (1 oz)	94	4	4	2	796	1 med-fat meat
Beef Kidney (1 oz)	41	<1	1	<1	38	1 very lean meat
Beef Tenderloin, Lean (1 oz)	67	0	4	1	18	1 lean meat
Beef Tongue (1 oz)	80	<1	6	3	17	1 med-fat meat
Bologna, Beef & Pork (1 oz)	89	<1	8	3	289	1 high-fat meat
Bratwurst, Pork (1 oz)	85	<1	7	3	158	1 high-fat meat
Buffalo (1 oz)	40	0	<1	<1	16	1 very lean meat
Canadian Bacon (1 oz)	53	<1	2	<1	441	1 lean meat
Catfish Fillet (1 oz)	43	0	2	<1	23	1 lean meat
Caviar, Black/Red, Granular (2 Tbsp)	81	1	6	1	480	1 med-fat meat

MEATS, FISH, AND POULTRY

Products	Cal.	Carb. (g)	Fat (g)	Sat. Fat (g)	Sodium (mg)	Exchanges
Chicken, Dark Meat, w/o Skin (1 oz)	58	0	3	<1	26	1 lean meat
Chicken, Dark Meat, w/Skin (1 oz)	72	0	5	1	25	1 med-fat meat
Chicken, Fried, Flour-Coated (1 oz)	76	<1	4	1	24	1 med-fat meat
Chicken, Light Meat, w/Skin (1 oz)	63	0	3	<1	21	1 lean meat
Chicken, Liver (1 oz)	45	<1	2	<1	15	1 lean meat
Chicken, White Meat, w/o Skin (1 oz)	49	0	1	<1	22	1 very lean meat
Chicken Patty, Breaded (1 = 2.7 oz)	213	11	13	4	399	1 strch, 1 med-fat meat, 2 fat
Clams, Canned, Drained Solids (1 oz)	42	1	<1	<1	32	1 very lean meat
Clams, Fresh, Steamed (1 oz)	42	1	<1	<1	32	1 very lean meat
Cod (1 oz)	30	0	<1	0	22	1 very lean meat
Cornish Hen, w/o Skin (1 oz)	38	0	1	<1	18	1 very lean meat
Crab (1 oz)	38	<1	2	<1	151	1 lean meat
Crab, Canned, Drained Solids (1 oz)	28	0	<1	<1	95	1 very lean meat
Duck, Domestic (1 oz)	57	0	3	1	19	1 lean meat

Escargot or Snails (1 oz)	32	1	<1	<1	33	1 very lean meat
Fish, Fried, Cornmeal-Coated (1 oz)	65	2	<1	1	79	1 med-fat meat
Fish Sticks, Frozen, Heated (2)	155	14	7	2	332	1 strch, 1 med-fat meat
Flounder (1 oz)	33	0	<1	<1	29	1 very lean meat
Goose (1 oz)	68	0	4	1	22	1 lean meat
Haddock (1 oz)	32	0	<1	0	20	1 very lean meat
Halibut (1 oz)	40	0	<1	<1	20	1 very lean meat
Ham, Boiled, Lean, Sandwich-Type (1 oz)	46	<1	2	<1	362	1 lean meat
Ham, Canned (1 oz)	48	<1	2	<1	304	1 lean meat
Ham, Cured (1 oz)	45	0	2	<1	378	1 lean meat
Ham, Fresh, Baked (1 oz)	60	0	3	<1	18	1 lean meat
Ham Salad Spread (1/2 cup)	130	6	9	3	547	1 high-fat meat
Herring, Smoked (1 oz)	62	0	4	<1	262	1 lean meat
Hot Dog, Beef & Pork (1)	144	1	13	5	504	1 high-fat meat, 1 fat
Hot Dog, Chicken (1)	116	3	9	3	617	1 high-fat meat
Hot Dog, Fat-Free (1)	30	3	<1	<1	286	1 very lean meat

MEATS, FISH, AND POULTRY

Products	Cal.	Carb. (g)	Fat (g)	Sat. Fat (g)	Sodium (mg)	Exchanges
Hot Dog, Low-Fat (1)	50	<1	2	<1	450	1 lean meat
Hot Dog, Turkey (1)	102	<1	8	2	642	1 high-fat meat
Imitation Shellfish, From Surimi (1 oz)	29	3	<1	<1	238	1 very lean meat
Knockwurst (1 oz)	87	<1	8	3	286	1 high-fat meat
Lamb, Ground (1 oz)	80	<1	6	2	23	1 med-fat meat
Lamb, Rib Roast (1 oz)	67	0	4	1	24	1 med-fat meat
Lamb Leg, Sirloin, Lean (1 oz)	58	0	3	<1	20	1 lean meat
Lamb Loin, Roast/Chop (1 oz)	57	0	3	1	19	1 lean meat
Liver Pate, Canned (2 Tbsp)	52	2	3	1	100	1 lean meat
Liverwurst (1/2 cup)	160	3	14	5	380	1 high-fat meat, 1 fat
Lobster, Fresh, Steamed (1 oz)	28	<1	<1	<1	108	1 very lean meat
Mackerel (1 oz)	57	0	3	<1	31	1 lean meat
Meat Loaf (1 oz)	57	<1	4	3	186	1 med-fat meat
Meat Sticks, Smoked (1 oz)	153	15	14	6	410	1 strch, 1 high-fat meat, 1 fat

Food						Exchange
Meatball, Beef or Pork (1 oz)	55	2	3	1	104	1 lean meat
Octopus (1 oz)	46	1	<1	<1	130	1 very lean meat
Orange Roughy (1 oz)	25	0	<1	<1	23	1 very lean meat
Oyster, Medium (6)	58	3	2	<1	177	1 lean meat
Peanut Butter, Smooth, Salted (2 Tbsp)	188	7	16	3	153	1 high-fat meat, 1 fat
Pepperoni Sausage, Beef & Pork (1 oz)	139	<1	12	5	571	1 high-fat meat, 1 fat
Pheasant, w/o Skin (1 oz)	38	0	1	<1	10	1 very lean meat
Pickle & Pimento Loaf (1 oz)	74	2	6	2	394	1 high-fat meat
Pickled Beef Tripe (1 oz)	18	0	<1	<1	13	1 very lean meat
Pork, Boston Blade (1 oz)	66	0	4	2	25	1 med-fat meat
Pork, Ground (1 oz)	84	0	6	2	21	1 high-fat meat
Pork, Spareribs (1 oz)	113	0	9	3	27	1 high-fat meat
Pork Cutlet (1 oz)	50	0	2	<1	13	1 med-fat meat
Pork Loin, Roast/Chop, Center Cut (1 oz)	60	0	3	1	16	1 lean meat
Pork Sausage, Fresh, Pattie/Link (1 oz)	105	<1	9	3	369	1 high-fat meat
Pork Tenderloin (1 oz)	47	0	1	<1	16	1 lean meat

MEATS, FISH, AND POULTRY

Products	Cal.	Carb. (g)	Fat (g)	Sat. Fat (g)	Sodium (mg)	Exchanges
Rabbit (1 oz)	58	0	2	<1	10	1 lean meat
Rainbow Trout Fillet (1 oz)	42	0	2	<1	16	1 lean meat
Salami, Beef & Pork (1 oz)	71	<1	6	2	302	1 high-fat meat
Salmon, Canned in Water (1 oz)	40	0	2	<1	139	1 lean meat
Salmon Fillet (1 oz)	61	0	3	<1	19	1 lean meat
Sardines, Oil-Packed, Drained (2)	50	0	3	<1	121	1 lean meat
Sausage, Hard, Fat-Free (1 oz)	35	3	<1	<1	290	1 very lean meat
Sausage, Italian, Pork (1 oz)	92	<1	7	3	263	1 high-fat meat
Sausage, Polish (1 oz)	92	<1	8	3	248	1 high-fat meat
Sausage, Smoked (1 oz)	96	<1	9	3	269	1 high-fat meat
Sausage, Vienna, Canned (1 oz)	78	<1	7	3	266	1 high-fat meat
Scallops, Fresh, Steamed (1 oz)	32	0	<1	<1	78	1 very lean meat
Sea Bass (1 oz)	35	0	<1	<1	25	1 very lean meat
Shrimp, Canned, Drained Solids (1 oz)	34	<1	<1	<1	48	1 very lean meat

Food					Exchange
Shrimp, Fresh, Cooked in Water (1 oz)	28	0	<1	<1	64	1 very lean meat
Smoked Clams in Oil, Canned, Small (5)	88	1	6	1	161	1 med-fat meat
Squid, Pickled (1 oz)	26	1	<1	<1	397	1 very lean meat
Steak, Porterhouse (1 oz)	62	0	3	1	19	1 lean meat
Steak, T-Bone (1 oz)	61	0	3	1	19	1 lean meat
Swordfish (1 oz)	43	0	1	<1	32	1 very lean meat
Tempeh (1/2 cup)	83	7	3	<1	2	1 med-fat meat
Tofu (1/2 cup)	88	2	6	<1	8	1 med-fat meat
Trout (1 oz)	54	0	2	<1	19	1 very lean meat
Tuna, Canned in Oil, Drained (1 oz)	56	0	2	<1	100	1 lean meat
Tuna, Canned, Water-Packed, Solids Only (1 oz)	33	0	<1	<1	96	1 very lean meat
Turkey, Dark Meat, w/o Skin (1 oz)	53	0	2	<1	22	1 lean meat
Turkey, Ground (1 oz)	67	0	4	1	30	1 med-fat meat
Turkey, White Meat, w/o Skin (1 oz)	44	0	<1	<1	18	1 very lean meat
Turkey Ham (1 oz)	36	<1	1	<1	282	1 very lean meat
Turkey Kielbasa, Low-Fat (1 oz)	45	2	3	1	300	1 lean meat

MEATS, FISH, AND POULTRY

Products	Cal.	Carb. (g)	Fat (g)	Sat. Fat (g)	Sodium (mg)	Exchanges
Turkey Pastrami, Low-Fat (1 oz)	40	<1	2	<1	296	1 lean meat
Veal Cutlet, Lean (1 oz)	58	0	6	>1	19	1 med-fat meat
Veal Loin, Chop (1 oz)	50	0	2	<1	27	1 lean meat
Veal Parmigiana (7.25 oz)	430	27	21	8	1463	2 strch, 4 med-fat meat
Veal Brisket, Lean (1 oz)	47	0	2	<1	26	1 lean meat
Venison (1 oz)	45	0	<1	<1	15	1 very lean meat
BANQUET						
Chicken, Country-Fried (3 oz)	270	13	18	5	620	1 strch, 2 med-fat meat, 2 fat
Chicken, Hot'n Spicy Fried (1)	260	13	18	5	590	1 strch, 2 med-fat meat, 2 fat
Chicken, Original Fried (3 oz)	270	13	18	5	620	1 strch, 2 med-fat meat, 2 fat
Chicken, Skinless Fried (3 oz)	210	7	13	3	480	1/2 strch, 2 med-fat meat, 1 fat
Chicken, Southern Fried (1)	270	13	18	5	590	1 strch, 2 med-fat meat, 2 fat
Chicken Breasts, Fried (1)	410	18	26	13	600	1 strch, 3 med-fat meat, 2 fat

Chicken Breasts, Fried Original (1)	410	18	26	13	600	1 strch, 3 med-fat meat, 2 fat
Chicken Nuggets, Southern Fried (9)	230	14	15	3	500	1 strch, 1 med-fat meat, 2 fat
Chicken Patties, Boneless (1)	200	11	12	25	400	1 strch, 1 med-fat meat, 1 fat
Chicken Patties, Southern Fried (1)	190	12	12	3	480	1 strch, 1 med-fat meat, 1 fat
Chicken Tenders (3)	210	13	10	2	470	1 strch, 2 med-fat meat
Chicken Tenders, Southern Fried (3)	210	14	10	2	490	1 strch, 2 med-fat meat
Chicken Wings, Hot'n Spicy Breaded (4)	230	5	16	5	280	2 med-fat meat, 1 fat
Snack Chicken, Hot'n Spicy (4)	240	11	16	4	480	1 strch, 1 med-fat meat, 2 fat
BRYAN FOODS						
Beef in Broth, Cubed (1 oz)	60	0	1	NA	234	1 lean meat
Bologna, Beef & Pork (1 oz)	91	<1	9	3	298	1 high-fat meat
Chicken w/Broth, Boned (1 oz)	74	0	3	NA	153	1 med-fat meat
Chicken w/Skin & Broth, Boned (1 oz)	82	0	4	NA	156	1 med-fat meat
Ham, Smoked, 95% Fat-Free (1 oz)	31	<1	1	<1	357	1 very lean meat
Pepperoni (1 oz)	162	1	13	5	581	1 high-fat meat, 1 fat
Salami (2 oz)	71	<1	6	2	284	1 med-fat meat

MEATS, FISH, AND POULTRY

Products	Cal.	Carb. (g)	Fat (g)	Sat. Fat (g)	Sodium (mg)	Exchanges
Turkey Breast, Deli Classics (1 oz)	54	0	2	<1	17	1 lean meat
COUNTRY SKILLET						
Chicken, Fried (3 oz)	270	13	18	5	620	1 strch, 2 med-fat meat, 2 fat
Chicken Chunks (5)	270	18	17	3	720	1 strch, 2 med-fat meat, 2 fat
Chicken Chunks, Southern Fried (5)	250	16	15	3	550	1 strch, 1 med-fat meat, 2 fat
Chicken Nuggets (10)	280	16	18	4	620	1 strch, 2 med-fat meat, 2 fat
Chicken Patties (1)	190	12	12	3	500	1 strch, 1 med-fat meeat, 1 fat
Chicken Patties, Southern Fried (1)	190	12	12	3	450	1 strch, 1 med-fat meat, 1 fat
HEALTHY CHOICE						
Franks, Low-Fat (1)	60	6	2	<1	430	1 lean meat
Ham, Deli Thin Cooked (6 slices)	60	1	2	<1	470	1 lean meat
Turkey Breast, Deli Thin (6 slices)	60	2	2	2	470	1 lean meat

LIBBY'S

Chicken Vienna Sausage (3)	100	0	8	3	450	1 high-fat meat
Corned Beef (2 oz)	120	0	7	3	490	2 lean meat
Potted Meat (1/2 cup)	110	0	7	2	440	1 high-fat meat
Vienna Sausage (3)	130	0	12	3	300	1 high-fat meat, 1 fat
Vienna Sausage in BBQ Sauce (3)	140	2	12	3	310	1 high-fat meat, 1 fat

LOUIS RICH

Chicken, White, Oven-Roasted, Cold Cut (1 slice)	40	<1	2	<1	350	1 lean meat
Chicken Breast, Deluxe Roasted, Cold Cut (1 slice)	29	<1	<1	<1	333	1 very lean meat
Chicken Breast, Hickory-Smoked, Cold Cut (1 slice)	30	1	1	0	360	1 very lean meat
Chicken Breast, Roasted, Deli Thin (4 slices)	60	1	2	<1	620	1 lean meat
Franks, Turkey & Chicken (1)	80	1	6	2	480	1 med-fat meat
Franks, Turkey & Chicken, Bun-Length (1)	110	2	8	3	630	1 high-fat meat
Franks, Turkey & Cheese (1)	91	2	7	2	463	1 high-fat meat
Ham, Baked in Juices (2 slices)	45	1	1	0	510	1 very lean meat
Ham, Dinner Slice, Baked (1 slice)	84	0	2	<1	1133	2 very lean meat

MEATS, FISH, AND POULTRY

Products	Cal.	Carb. (g)	Fat (g)	Sat. Fat (g)	Sodium (mg)	Exchanges
Ham, Honey, Thin-Cut (6 slices)	70	2	2	1	760	1 lean meat
Ham, Honey, Traditional (2 slices)	50	1	2	<1	530	1 lean meat
Ham, Smoked (2 slices)	46	<1	1	<1	566	1 very lean meat
Turkey, Ground (3 oz)	141	0	9	3	114	3 lean meat
Turkey, White, Smoked (1 slice)	30	<1	<1	<1	284	1 very lean meat
Turkey & Cheddar Smoked Sausage (2 oz)	94	2	6	2	547	2 lean meat
Turkey Bacon (1 slice)	34	<1	3	<1	184	1 fat
Turkey Bologna (1 slice)	58	<1	5	2	242	1 med-fat meat
Turkey Bologna, Chunk (2 oz)	101	3	7	2	549	2 med-fat meat
Turkey Breast, Carving Board (2 slices)	40	0	<1	0	560	1 very lean meat
Turkey Breast, Hickory-Smoked, Dinner Slice (1 slice)	80	2	1	0	1060	2 very lean meat
Turkey Breast, Hickory-Smoked, Fat-Free (1 slice)	23	1	<1	<1	300	1 very lean meat
Turkey Breast, Hickory-Smoked, Skinless (2 oz)	53	1	<1	<1	746	1 very lean meat
Turkey Breast, Honey-Roasted, Cold Cut (1 slice)	30	1	<1	<1	320	1 very lean meat

Turkey Breast, Honey-Roasted, Dinner Slice (1 slice)	80	3	1	<1	940	2 very lean meat
Turkey Breast, Oven-Roasted (2 oz)	52	<1	<1	<1	666	2 very lean meat
Turkey Breast, Oven-Roasted, Cold Cut (1 slice)	28	1	<1	<1	311	1 very lean meat
Turkey Breast, Oven-Roasted, Dinner Slice (1 slice)	70	NA	1	0	910	2 very lean meat
Turkey Breast, Roasted, Chunk (2 oz)	60	2	2	<1	640	2 very lean meat
Turkey Breast, Roasted, Deli Thin (4 slices)	50	2	1	0	580	1 very lean meat
Turkey Breast, Roasted, Fat-Free (1 slice)	22	1	<1	<1	387	1 very lean meat
Turkey Breast, Smoked, Carving Board (2 slices)	41	<1	<1	<1	540	1 very lean meat
Turkey Breast, Smoked, Cold Cut (1 slice)	28	<1	<1	<1	259	1 very lean meat
Turkey Breast, Smoked, Deli Thin (4 slices)	50	1	1	0	490	1 very lean meat
Turkey Cotto Salami (1 slice)	42	<1	3	<1	285	1 lean meat
Turkey Ham (1 slice)	30	<1	<1	<1	302	1 very lean meat
Turkey Ham, Chopped (1 slice)	42	<1	3	<1	297	1 lean meat
Turkey Ham, Chunk (2 oz)	65	<1	2	<1	616	1 lean meat
Turkey Ham, Deli Thin (4 slices)	60	0	2	<1	580	1 lean meat
Turkey Ham, Honey-Cured (3 slices)	70	2	2	<1	652	1 lean meat

MEATS, FISH, AND POULTRY

Products	Cal.	Carb. (g)	Fat (g)	Sat. Fat (g)	Sodium (mg)	Exchanges
Turkey Nuggets, Breaded (4)	254	14	16	3	625	1 strch, 1 med-fat meat, 2 fat
Turkey Pastrami, Chunk (2 oz)	68	<1	3	<1	584	2 very lean meat
Turkey Patties (1)	115	0	6	2	338	2 lean meat
Turkey Polska Kielbasa Sausage (2 oz)	82	1	5	2	506	2 lean meat
Turkey Roast, Honey-Roasted, Skinless (2 oz)	58	3	<1	<1	669	2 very lean meat
Turkey Salami (1 slice)	41	<1	3	<1	281	1 lean meat
Turkey Salami, Chunk (2 oz)	106	<1	8	3	508	2 med-fat meat
Turkey Sausage Links (2)	93	0	6	2	472	1 med-fat meat
Turkey Sausage, Ground (2-1/2 oz)	124	<1	8	3	437	2 med-fat meat
Turkey Sausage, Smoked (2 oz)	87	2	5	2	507	2 lean meat
Turkey Sticks, Breaded (3)	230	12	15	3	580	1 strch, 1 med-fat meat, 2 fat
MRS. PAUL'S						
Fish Fillet, Healthy Treasure Breaded (1)	130	16	3	1	220	1 strch, 1 lean meat
Fish Portions, Battered (2)	250	20	16	5	430	1 strch, 1 med-fat meat, 2 fat

Food	Cal					Exchanges
Fish Portions, Breaded (2)	190	16	10	3	280	1 strch, 1 med-fat meat, 1 fat
Fish Sandwich w/Cheese (4.3 oz)	330	38	15	4	630	2-1/2 strch, 1 med-fat meat, 2 fat
Fish Shapes, Sea Pals Breaded (5)	190	18	9	3	320	1 strch, 1 med-fat meat, 1 fat
Fish Sticks, Breaded (6)	210	19	11	2	370	1 strch, 1 med-fat meat, 1 fat
Fish Sticks, Breaded Minis (12)	220	20	11	3	330	1 strch, 1 med-fat meat, 1 fat
Fish Sticks, Healthy Treasure Breaded (4)	170	20	3	2	350	1 strch, 1 lean meat
Premium Fillets, Haddock (1)	230	18	11	3	450	1 strch, 2 med-fat meat
Premium Fillets, Sole (1)	250	22	13	4	510	1-1/2 strch, 2 med-fat meat, 1 fat
Shrimp, Breaded, Garlic & Herb (1)	340	33	15	3	910	2 strch, 2 med-fat meat, 1 fat
Shrimp, Breaded, Special Recipe (1)	350	32	16	3	720	2 strch, 2 med-fat meat, 1 fat

OSCAR MAYER

Food	Cal					Exchanges
Bacon (2 slices)	60	0	5	2	250	1 med-fat meat
Bacon, 1/8-inch Thick Cut (1 slice)	60	0	5	2	250	1 med-fat meat
Bacon, Canadian-Style (2 slices)	50	0	2	1	620	1 lean meat

MEATS, FISH, AND POULTRY

Products	Cal.	Carb. (g)	Fat (g)	Sat. Fat (g)	Sodium (mg)	Exchanges
Bacon, Lower Sodium (2 slices)	60	0	4	2	170	1 med-fat meat
Bacon Bits, Real (1 Tbsp)	25	0	2	<1	220	1 fat
Bologna (1 slice)	90	1	8	3	290	1 high-fat meat
Bologna, Beef (1 slice)	90	1	8	4	310	1 high-fat meat
Bologna, Beef, Light (1 slice)	60	2	4	2	310	1 med-fat meat
Bologna, Fat-Free (1 slice)	20	1	0	0	280	1 very lean meat
Bologna, Garlic (1 slice)	130	1	12	5	420	1 high-fat meat, 1 fat
Bologna, Light (1 slice)	60	2	4	2	310	1 med-fat meat
Bologna, Wisconsin-Made Ring (2 oz)	180	2	16	6	460	1 high-fat meat, 2 fat
Chicken Breast, Honey-Glazed, Deli Thin (4 slices)	60	2	<1	0	730	1 very lean meat
Chicken Breast, Oven-Roasted, Fat-Free (4 slices)	45	1	0	0	650	1 very lean meat
Franks, Beef (1)	140	1	13	6	460	1 high-fat meat, 1 fat
Franks, Beef, Bun-Length (1)	180	2	17	7	580	1 high-fat meat, 2 fat
Franks, Beef, Fat-Free (1)	35	2	0	0	480	1 very lean meat

Franks, Beef, Light (1)	110	2	8	4	620	1 high-fat meat
Franks, Big & Juicy Deli-Style (1)	230	1	22	10	680	2 high-fat meat, 1 fat
Franks, Big & Juicy Original Beef (1)	240	1	22	9	700	2 high-fat meat, 1 fat
Franks, Big & Juicy Quarter Pound Beef (1)	350	2	33	13	1050	2 high-fat meat, 3 fat
Ham, Baked (3 slices)	70	2	3	1	790	1 lean meat
Ham, Baked, Fat-Free (3 slices)	35	1	0	0	520	1 very lean meat
Ham, Boiled (3 slices)	60	0	3	1	820	1 lean meat
Ham, Boiled, Deli Thin (4 slices)	50	1	2	<1	700	1 lean meat
Ham, Chopped w/Natural Juices (1 slice)	50	1	3	1	320	1 lean meat
Ham, Honey (3 slices)	70	2	3	1	760	1 lean meat
Ham, Honey, Deli Thin (4 slices)	60	2	2	<1	650	1 lean meat
Ham, Honey, Fat-Free (3 slices)	35	2	0	0	580	1 very lean meat
Ham, Lower Sodium (3 slices)	70	2	3	1	520	1 lean meat
Ham, Smoked (3 slices)	60	0	3	1	750	1 lean meat
Ham, Smoked, Cooked, Deli Thin (4 slices)	50	0	2	1	630	1 lean meat
Ham, Smoked, Fat-Free (3 slices)	35	1	0	0	550	1 very lean meat

MEATS, FISH, AND POULTRY

Products	Cal.	Carb. (g)	Fat (g)	Sat. Fat (g)	Sodium (mg)	Exchanges
Ham & Cheese Loaf (1 slice)	70	1	5	3	350	1 med-fat meat
Head Cheese (1 slice)	50	0	4	2	360	1 med-fat meat
Honey Loaf (1 slice)	35	1	1	0	380	1 very lean meat
Hot Dogs, Cheese (1)	140	1	13	5	530	1 high-fat meat, 1 fat
Hot Dogs, Fat-Free (1)	40	2	0	0	490	1 very lean meat
Liver Cheese (1 slice)	120	1	10	4	420	1 high-fat meat
Luncheon Loaf, Spiced (1 slice)	70	2	5	2	340	1 med-fat meat
Old-Fashioned Loaf (1 slice)	70	1	5	2	330	1 med-fat meat
Olive Loaf (1 slice)	70	2	6	2	370	1 med-fat meat
Pepperoni (15 slices)	140	0	13	5	550	1 high-fat meat, 1 fat
Pickle & Pimento Loaf (1 slice)	80	3	6	2	360	1 med-fat meat
Roast Beef, Deli Thin (4 slices)	60	1	2	<1	530	1 lean meat
Salami for Beer (2 slices)	110	1	9	3	580	1 high-fat meat
Salami, Hard (3 slices)	100	0	9	3	510	1 high-fat meat

Item						Exchanges
Salami, Cotto (2 slices)	110	0	9	4	500	1 high-fat meat
Salami, Cotto, Beef (2 slices)	90	1	7	3	590	1 high-fat meat
Salami, Genoa (3 slices)	100	0	9	3	490	1 high-fat meat
Sandwich Spread (2 oz)	130	8	10	4	460	1/2 strch, 1 high-fat meat
Sausage, Liver, B'raunschweiger (1 slice)	100	1	9	3	320	1 high-fat meat
Sausage, Liver, Braunschweiger Spread (2 oz)	190	1	17	6	630	1 high-fat meat, 2 fat
Sausage, New England Brand (2 slices)	60	1	3	1	570	1 lean meat
Sausage, Pork Links (2)	180	1	16	6	450	2 high-fat meat
Sausage, Smokie Links (1)	130	1	12	4	430	1 high-fat meat, 1 fat
Sausage, Smokies Little (6)	170	1	16	6	580	1 high-fat meat, 2 fat
Sausage, Smokies Little Cheese (6)	180	1	16	6	590	1 high-fat meat, 2 fat
Sausage, Summer (2 slices)	140	0	13	5	650	1 high-fat meat, 1 fat
Sausage, Summer, Beef (2 slices)	140	1	12	5	640	1 high-fat meat, 1 fat
Turkey, White, Oven-Roasted (1 slice)	30	2	1	0	320	1 very lean meat
Turkey, White, Smoked (1 slice)	30	1	1	0	330	1 very lean meat
Turkey Breast, Oven-Roasted (4 slices)	40	2	0	0	670	1 very lean meat

MEATS, FISH, AND POULTRY

Products	Cal.	Carb. (g)	Fat (g)	Sat. Fat (g)	Sodium (mg)	Exchanges
Turkey Breast, Smoked, Fat-Free (4 slices)	40	2	0	0	570	1 very lean meat
Turkey Breast/White Turkey, Roasted, Deli Thin (4 slices)	50	2	1	0	610	1 very lean meat
Turkey Breast/White Turkey, Smoked/Honey-Roasted, Deli Thin (4 slices)	50	2	1	0	500	1 very lean meat
Wieners (1)	150	1	13	5	460	1 high-fat meat, 1 fat
Wieners, Big & Juicy Hot 'N Spicy (1)	220	1	20	8	750	2 high-fat meat, 1 fat
Wieners, Big & Juicy Original (1)	240	1	22	9	690	2 high-fat meat, 1 fat
Wieners, Big & Juicy Smokie Links (1)	220	1	19	7	770	2 high-fat meat, 1 fat
Wieners, Bun-Length (1)	190	2	17	6	570	1 high-fat meat, 2 fat
Wieners, Light (1)	110	2	9	3	590	1 high-fat meat
Wieners, Little (6)	180	2	17	6	570	1 high-fat meat, 2 fat
Wieners, Little, Hot & Spicy (6)	170	1	16	6	580	1 high-fat meat, 2 fat

PROGRESSO

Food						Exchanges
Clams, Minced (1/2 cup)	50	4	0	0	500	1 very lean meat

RED DEVIL

Food						Exchanges
Snackers, Chunky Chicken (1/2 cup)	169	13	10	2	450	1 strch, 1 high-fat meat
Snackers, Deviled Ham (1 pkg)	310	11	18	6	680	1 strch, 2 high-fat meat
Snackers, Honey Ham (1 pkg)	320	19	22	6	560	1 strch, 2 high-fat meat, 1 fat

SWANSON

Food						Exchanges
Chicken, Chunk (1/2 cup)	90	2	3	<1	200	2 lean meat
Chicken, Chunk White, in Water (1/2 cup)	80	<1	<1	<1	240	2 very lean meat
Chicken, Grilled, in Garlic Sauce (1)	270	35	7	3	640	2 strch, 2 lean meat
Chicken, Premium Chunk, in Water (1/2 cup)	90	<1	3	<1	240	2 lean meat
Turkey, Chunk White, in Water (1/2 cup)	90	4	2	<1	220	2 very lean meat
Turkey, Premium Chunk, in Water (1/2 cup)	100	2	4	<1	230	2 lean meat

TOMBSTONE

Food						Exchanges
Beef Jerky (1)	35	1	0	0	310	1 very lean meat
Beef Sticks (1)	110	0	10	5	270	1 med-fat meat, 1 fat

MEATS, FISH, AND POULTRY

Products	Cal.	Carb. (g)	Fat (g)	Sat. Fat (g)	Sodium (mg)	Exchanges
Beef Sticks, Snappy (1)	110	1	10	5	260	1 high-fat meat, 1 fat
TYSON						
Chicken Breast Fillet, Marinated (3 oz)	88	<1	2	<1	204	3 very lean meat
Chicken Nuggets (3 oz)	207	9	14	4	383	1/2 strch, 1 med-fat meat, 2 fat
Pork Chop, Marinated (3 oz)	130	<1	7	3	261	2 lean meat
UNDERWOOD						
Chicken Spread, Chunky (1/2 cup)	120	2	8	3	470	1 high-fat meat
Ham Spread, Deviled (1/2 cup)	160	0	14	5	440	1 high-fat meat, 1 fat
Ham Spread, Honey (1/2 cup)	170	1	15	5	330	1 high-fat meat, 1 fat
VAN DE KAMP'S						
Fish Fillet, Battered (1)	180	12	11	2	340	1 strch, 1 med-fat meat, 1 fat
Fish Fillets, Breaded (2)	280	17	19	3	270	1 strch, 1 med-fat meat, 3 fat
Fish Nuggets, Battered (8)	280	20	18	3	600	1 strch, 1 med-fat meat, 3 fat

Fish Sticks, Battered (6)	260	18	16	3	540	1 strch, 1 med-fat meat, 2 fat
Fish Sticks, Breaded (6)	260	21	14	3	350	1-1/2 strch, 1 med-fat meat, 2 fat
Fish Sticks Snack Pack (6)	260	21	14	3	350	1-1/2 strch, 1 med-fat meat, 2 fat
Flounder Natural Fillet (1)	110	0	2	0	105	3 very lean meat
Haddock Fillets, Battered (2)	260	18	16	3	530	1 strch, 1 med-fat meat, 2 fat
Haddock Fillets, Breaded (2)	280	19	17	3	310	1 strch, 1 med-fat meat, 2 fat
Halibut Fillets, Battered (3)	330	22	21	3	520	1-1/2 strch, 1 med-fat meat, 3 fat
Ocean Perch, Today's Catch (4 oz)	110	0	2	NA	70	3 very lean meat
Perch Fillets, Battered (2)	300	19	20	3	480	1 strch, 1 med-fat meat, 3 fat
Shrimp, Butterfly, Breaded (7)	280	28	14	3	580	2 strch, 1 med-fat meat, 2 fat
Shrimp, Popcorn, Breaded (20)	270	28	13	2	610	2 strch, 1 med-fat meat, 2 fat
Shrimp, Whole, Breaded (7)	240	26	10	2	520	2 strch, 1 med-fat meat, 1 fat
Sole Natural Fillet (1)	110	0	2	0	125	3 very lean meat

MILK AND YOGURT

MILK AND YOGURT

Products	Cal.	Carb. (g)	Fat (g)	Sat. Fat (g)	Sodium (mg)	Exchanges
Buttermilk, Skim, Cultured (1 cup)	99	12	2	1	257	1 skim milk
Carob Flavor Beverage Mix w/Milk (1 cup)	195	23	8	5	133	1 whole milk, 1 carb.
Carob Flavor Beverage Mix, Powder (3 Tbsp)	45	11	<1	<1	12	1 carb.
Chocolate Drink, Syrup w/Reduced-Fat Milk (1 cup)	181	30	5	3	140	1 reduced-fat milk, 1 carb.
Chocolate Malted Milk Drink (1 cup)	228	30	9	6	172	1 whole milk, 1 carb.
Cocoa, Sugar-Free, Mix w/Water, (1 pkt)	49	9	<1	<1	177	1/2 skim milk
Cocoa/Hot Chocolate Mix w/Water (1 pkt)	102	22	1	<1	143	1/2 skim milk, 1 carb.
Cocoa/Hot Chocolate Mix w/Whole Milk (1 cup)	218	26	9	6	123	1 whole milk, 1 carb.
Cocoa Mix, Sugar-Free, w/Reduced-Fat Milk (1 cup)	136	15	6	3	160	1 reduced-fat milk
Cocoa Mix, Sugar-Free w/Water (1 cup)	63	11	<1	<1	225	1 skim milk
Eggnog (1 cup)	343	34	19	11	138	1 whole milk, 1-1/2 carb., 2 fat
Eggnog, 2% Reduced-Fat (1 cup)	189	17	8	4	155	1 whole milk

Food					Exchange
Instant Breakfast Powder (1 pkt)	131	25	<1	142	1 skim milk, 1 carb.
Milk, 1%, Reduced-Fat (1 cup)	102	12	3	123	1 skim milk
Milk, 1%, Reduced-Fat, Acidophilus (1 cup)	101	12	3	122	1 skim milk
Milk, 1%, Reduced-Fat, Chocolate (1 cup)	158	26	3	152	1 skim milk, 1 carb.
Milk, 1%, Reduced-Fat, Protein-Fortified (1 cup)	119	14	3	143	1 skim milk
Milk, 2%, Reduced-Fat (1 cup)	121	12	5	122	1 reduced-fat milk
Milk, 2%, Reduced-Fat, Chocolate (1 cup)	179	26	5	151	1 reduced-fat milk, 1 carb.
Milk, 2%, Reduced-Fat, Protein-Fortified (1 cup)	137	14	5	145	1 reduced-fat milk
Milk, Evaporated Skim Canned (1 cup)	199	29	<1	293	2 skim milk
Milk, Evaporated Whole (1 cup)	338	25	19	267	2 whole milk
Milk, Goat (1 cup)	168	11	10	122	1 whole milk
Milk, Nonfat Chocolate (1 cup)	144	27	1	121	1 skim milk, 1 carb.
Milk, Nonfat Powder w/Water (1 cup)	82	12	<1	131	1 skim milk
Milk, Nonfat Skim (1 cup)	86	12	<1	126	1 skim milk
Milk, Nonfat Skim, Lactose-Reduced (1 cup)	86	12	<1	126	1 skim milk
Milk, Nonfat Skim, Protein-Fortified (1 cup)	100	14	<1	144	1 skim milk

MILK AND YOGURT

Products	Cal.	Carb. (g)	Fat (g)	Sat. Fat (g)	Sodium (mg)	Exchanges
Milk, Soy (1 cup)	79	4	5	<1	29	1 reduced-fat milk
Milk, Sweetened Condensed, Canned (1 cup)	982	166	27	17	389	3 whole milk, 9 carb.
Milk, Whole (1 cup)	150	11	8	5	120	1 whole milk
Milk, Whole, Chocolate (1 cup)	209	26	9	5	149	1 whole milk, 1 carb.
Yogurt, Low-Fat, Custard-Style, Fruit (1 cup)	250	47	3	2	143	1-1/2 skim milk, 2 carb.
Yogurt, Low-Fat, Fruit & Nuts (1 cup)	290	47	7	2	139	1-1/2 low-fat milk, 2 carb.
Yogurt, Low-Fat, Fruit (1 cup)	250	47	3	2	143	1-1/2 skim milk, 2 carb.
Yogurt, Low-Fat, Plain (1 cup)	155	17	4	3	172	1 reduced-fat milk
Yogurt, Nonfat, Fruit w/LoCal Sweetener (1 cup)	122	19	<1	<1	139	1 skim milk, 1/2 carb.
Yogurt, Nonfat, Plain (1 cup)	137	19	<1	<1	187	1-1/2 skim milk
Yogurt, Whole-Milk, Plain (1 cup)	150	11	8	5	114	1 whole milk
A L B A						
Shake Mix, Chocolate, w/Water (1 pkt)	65	11	<1	<1	177	1 skim milk
Shake Mix, Diet Vanilla, w/Water (1 cup)	105	17	<1	<1	257	1 skim milk

Shake Mix, Low-Calorie Chocolate, w/Water (1 cup)	86	15	<1	<1	233	1 skim milk

CARNATION

Cocoa Mix w/Marshmallow (1 pkt)	110	25	1	<1	95	1-1/2 carb.
Cocoa Mix, Rich & Creamy (3 Tbsp)	110	24	2	0	130	1-1/2 carb.
Cocoa Mix, Rich Chocolate (1 pkt)	110	24	1	0	100	1-1/2 carb.
Instant Breakfast, Cafe Mocha (10-oz can)	220	35	3	<1	210	1 skim milk, 1-1/2 carb.
Instant Breakfast, Chocolate (10-oz can)	220	37	3	1	230	1 skim milk, 1-1/2 carb.
Instant Breakfast, Chocolate Malt (1 pkt)	130	26	1	<1	130	1/2 skim milk, 1 carb.
Instant Breakfast, Chocolate Malt, No Sugar Added (1 pkg)	70	11	2	<1	120	1 skim milk
Instant Breakfast, Chocolate Malt, No Sugar Added (1 pkt)	160	24	2	<1	240	1-1/2 skim milk
Instant Breakfast, French Vanilla (10-oz can)	200	31	3	<1	180	1 skim milk, 1 carb.
Instant Breakfast, French Vanilla (1 pkt)	130	27	0	0	110	2 carb.
Instant Breakfast, Milk Chocolate (1 pkt)	130	28	1	<1	100	2 carb.

MILK AND YOGURT

Products	Cal.	Carb. (g)	Fat (g)	Sat. Fat (g)	Sodium (mg)	Exchanges
Instant Breakfast, Milk Chocolate, No Sugar Added (1 pkt)	120	21	2	<1	154	1 skim milk, 1/2 carb.
Instant Breakfast, Strawberry Cream (10-oz can)	220	35	3	<1	210	1 skim milk, 1-1/2 carb.
Instant Breakfast, Strawberry Cream (1 pkt)	130	28	0	0	160	2 carb.
Instant Breakfast, Vanilla, No Sugar Added (1 pkt)	70	12	0	0	90	1/2 skim milk, 1/2 carb.
Milk, Evaporated Reduced-Fat (2 Tbsp)	25	3	<1	<1	35	free
Milk, Evaporated (1 cup)	320	24	16	12	267	2 whole milk
Milk, Sweetened Condensed (2 Tbsp)	130	22	3	2	45	1-1/2 carb., 1 fat
Quik Strawberry Beverage Mix (1 Tbsp)	84	21	<1	<1	8	1-1/2 carb.
Sweet Success Creamy Milk Chocolate Powder (1 scoop)	90	24	1	<1	125	1-1/2 carb.
Sweet Success Creamy Milk Chocolate Shake (10 oz)	200	36	3	<1	230	1 skim milk, 1-1/2 carb.
Sweet Success Creamy Vanilla Delight (10 oz)	200	37	3	<1	220	1 skim milk, 1-1/2 carb.

DANNON

Double Delights, Chocolate Eclair (6 oz)	220	45	1	<1	150	1 skim milk, 2 carb.
Double Delights, Peach/Apricot 'N Cream (6 oz)	170	33	1	<1	100	1 skim milk, 1 carb.
Double Delights, Strawberry Banana Split (6 oz)	160	32	1	<1	100	1 skim milk, 1 carb.
Double Delights, Strawberry Cheesecake (6 oz)	170	33	1	<1	100	1 skim milk, 1 carb.
Duets, Strawberry Cheesecake (6 oz)	90	18	0	0	70	1 skim milk
Duets, Strawberry Sundae (6 oz)	90	18	0	0	70	1 skim milk
Yogurt, Fat-Free Blended, Raspberry (4.4 oz)	120	24	0	0	75	1 skim milk, 1 carb.
Yogurt, Fat-Free Blended, Strawberry Banana (4.4 oz)	110	23	0	0	80	1 skim milk, 1 carb.
Yogurt, Fat-Free Chunky Fruit, Peach (6 oz)	160	34	0	0	110	1 skim milk, 1 carb.
Yogurt, Fat-Free Chunky Fruit, Strawberry (6 oz)	160	32	0	0	105	1 skim milk, 1 carb.
Yogurt, Fat-Free Light, Non-Fat, w/Aspartame, Peach (4.4 oz)	50	9	0	0	65	1/2 skim milk
Yogurt, Fruit-On-The-Bottom, Fresh Lemon (8 oz)	210	36	3	2	160	1 skim milk, 1-1/2 carb.
Yogurt, Fruit-On-The-Bottom, Peach (8 oz)	240	45	3	2	140	1 skim milk, 2 carb.
Yogurt, Fruit-On-The-Bottom, Strawberry (8 oz)	240	46	3	2	135	1 skim milk, 2 carb.

MILK AND YOGURT

Products	Cal.	Carb. (g)	Fat (g)	Sat. Fat (g)	Sodium (mg)	Exchanges
Yogurt, Light, Banana Creme Pie (8 oz)	100	15	0	0	120	1 skim milk
Yogurt, Light, Blueberry (8 oz)	100	18	0	0	115	1 skim milk
Yogurt, Light, Cherry Vanilla (8 oz)	100	18	0	0	115	1 skim milk
Yogurt, Light, Strawberry (8 oz)	100	17	0	0	115	1 skim milk
Yogurt, Light 'N Crunchy, Mint Chocolate Chip (8 oz)	140	27	0	0	150	1 skim milk, 1 carb.
Yogurt, Sprinkl'ins (4.1 oz)	130	24	2	<1	85	1 skim milk, 1 carb.
KRAFT						
Instant Malted Milk w/2%, Chocolate (1 cup)	200	29	6	3	160	1 reduced-fat milk, 1 carb.
Yogurt, Kid Pack Low-Fat Banana Berry, 1% (4.4 oz)	130	24	1	1	65	1 skim milk, 1 carb.
Yogurt, Kid Pack Low-Fat Berry Blue, 1% (4.4 oz)	150	30	1	<1	65	1 skim milk, 1 carb.
Yogurt, Kid Pack Low-Fat Cherry, 1% (4.4 oz)	140	27	1	<1	65	1 skim milk, 1 carb.
Yogurt, Kid Pack Low-Fat Grape, 1% (4.4 oz)	130	24	1	1	65	1 skim milk, 1 carb.
Yogurt, Kid Pack Low-Fat Orange, 1% (4.4 oz)	150	29	1	<1	65	1 skim milk, 1 carb.
Yogurt, Kid Pack Low-Fat Tropical Punch (4.4 oz)	140	27	1	<1	65	1 skim milk, 1 carb.

Product	Cal	Carb	Fat	Cal	Exchanges
Yogurt, Kid Pack Low-Fat Wild Berry (4.4 oz)	140	27	1	<1	65	1 skim milk, 1 carb.
Yogurt, Kid Pack Low-Fat Wild Strawberry (4.4 oz)	140	28	1	<1	65	1 skim milk, 1 carb.
Yogurt, Light N' Lively Free Nonfat Berry (6 oz)	170	34	0	0	105	1 skim milk, 1-1/2 carb.
Yogurt, Light N' Lively Free Nonfat Lemon (6 oz)	170	35	0	0	105	1 skim milk, 1-1/2 carb.
Yogurt, Light N' Lively Free Nonfat Peach (6 oz)	170	35	0	0	105	1 skim milk, 1-1/2 carb.
Yogurt, Light N' Lively Free Nonfat Raspberry (6 oz)	180	36	0	0	105	1 skim, 1-1/2 carb.
Yogurt, Light N' Lively Free Nonfat Strawberry (6 oz)	170	35	0	0	105	1 skim milk, 1-1/2 carb.
Yogurt, Light N' Lively Low-Fat Blueberry (4.4 oz)	140	27	1	<1	65	1 skim milk, 1 carb.
Yogurt, Light N' Lively Low-Fat Peach (4.4 oz)	140	27	1	<1	65	1 skim milk, 1 carb.
Yogurt, Light N' Lively Low-Fat Pineapple (4.4 oz)	140	27	1	<1	60	1 skim milk, 1 carb.
Yogurt, Light N' Lively Low-Fat Red Raspberry (4.4 oz)	130	24	1	1	65	1 skim milk, 1 carb.
Yogurt, Light N' Lively Low-Fat Strawberry (4.4 oz)	140	26	1	1	65	1 skim milk, 1 carb.
Yogurt, Light N' Lively Nonfat Blueberry (6 oz)	190	38	0	0	105	1 skim milk, 1-1/2 carb.
Yogurt, Light N' Lively Nonfat Vanilla (6 oz)	160	32	0	0	105	1 skim milk, 1 carb.
Yogurt, Low-Fat Strawberry Banana (4.4 oz)	140	28	1	<1	60	1 skim milk, 1 carb.

MILK AND YOGURT

Products	Cal.	Carb. (g)	Fat (g)	Sat. Fat (g)	Sodium (mg)	Exchanges
Yogurt, Low-Fat Strawberry Fruit Cup (4.4 oz)	140	27	1	<1	60	1 skim milk, 1 carb.
LACTAID						
Milk, Lactaid 100, Reduced-Fat (1 cup)	80	13	0	0	125	1 skim milk
Milk, Lactaid 70, 2% Low-Fat (1 cup)	130	12	5	3	125	1 reduced-fat milk
Milk, Lactaid 70, Non-Fat (1 cup)	80	13	0	0	125	1 skim milk
OVALTINE						
Cocoa Mix & Water, Sugar-Free (1 cup)	49	9	<1	<1	107	1 skim milk
Malted Milk Drink, Fortified (1 cup)	231	28	9	5	204	1 whole milk, 1 carb.
Malted Milk Drink, Fortified Chocolate (1 cup)	225	29	9	6	244	1 whole milk, 1 carb.
PET						
Milk, Regular Evaporated (2 Tbsp)	40	3	2	1	30	1 fat
Milk, Skimmed Evaporated (2 Tbsp)	25	3	0	0	35	free
PILLSBURY						
Instant Breakfast, Chocolate (1 envelope)	134	28	1	<1	189	2 carb.

Instant Breakfast, Variety Pack (1 envelope)	134	28	1	<1	189	2 carb.
SWISS MISS						
Cocoa Mix w/Milk, Sugar-Free (1 cup)	136	15	6	3	160	1 reduced-fat milk
ULTRA SLIM FAST						
Chocolate (11 oz can)	230	42	3	NA	200	1-1/2 slim milk, 1-1/2 carb.
Chocolate Malt (1 scoop)	120	24	1	<1	100	1 skim milk, 1 carb.
French Vanilla (1 scoop)	110	22	<1	0	130	1 skim milk, 1 carb.
Orange Pineapple (11.5 oz can)	220	48	2	<1	260	1 skim milk, 2 carb.
Powder w/Skim Milk, Chocolate (1 cup)	200	36	1	NA	230	1-1/2 skim milk, 1 carb.
Powder w/Skim Milk, Strawberry (1 cup)	190	32	1	<1	220	1-1/2 skim milk, 1 carb.
Vanilla (11 oz can)	220	38	3	1	460	1-1/2 skim milk, 1 carb.
WEIGHT WATCHERS						
Hot Cocoa Mix (1 pkt)	70	10	0	0	160	1 skim milk
Milk, Nonfat Skim (1 cup)	90	13	0	0	130	1 skim milk
Sweet Success Drink, Chocolate Chip (8 oz)	180	30	3	2	288	1 skim milk, 1 carb.
Sweet Success Drink, Chocolate Fudge (8 oz)	180	30	2	NA	336	1 skim milk, 1 carb.

MILK AND YOGURT

Products	Cal.	Carb. (g)	Fat (g)	Sat. Fat (g)	Sodium (mg)	Exchanges
Sweet Success Drink, Chocolate Mocha (8 oz)	180	30	1	1	336	1 skim milk, 1 carb.
Sweet Success Drink, Milk Chocolate (8 oz)	180	30	2	1	336	1 skim milk, 1 carb.
Sweet Success Drink, Vanilla (8 oz)	180	33	1	<1	312	1 skim milk, 1-1/2 carb.
Sweet Success Shake, Chocolate Almond (10 oz)	197	38	3	0	238	1 skim milk, 2 carb.
Sweet Success Shake, Chocolate Fudge (10 oz)	197	38	3	0	219	1 skim milk, 2 carb.
Sweet Success Shake, Chocolate Mocha (10 oz)	197	38	3	0	219	1 skim milk, 2 carb.
Sweet Success Shake, Chocolate Raspberry Truffle (10 oz)	197	38	3	0	219	1 skim milk, 2 carb.
Sweet Success Shake, Milk Chocolate (10 oz)	197	38	3	0	238	1 skim milk, 2 carb.
Sweet Success Shake, Vanilla Creme (10 oz)	197	38	3	0	219	1 skim milk, 2 carb.
YOPLAIT						
Yogurt, Crunchy Light, Vanilla (7 oz)	140	22	2	0	150	1 skim milk, 1/2 carb.
Yogurt, Custard-Style, Strawberry (6 oz)	190	32	3	2	100	1 skim milk, 1 carb.
Yogurt, Custard-Style, Strawberry Banana (6 oz)	190	32	3	2	100	1 skim milk, 1 carb.

Food						Exchanges
Yogurt, Custard-Style, Thick & Creamy Vanilla (6 oz)	190	32	3	2	95	1 skim milk, 1 carb.
Yogurt, Light Fat-Free, Blueberry Patch (6 oz)	90	16	0	0	75	1 skim milk
Yogurt, Light Fat-Free, Carmel Apple (6 oz)	90	16	0	0	75	1 skim milk
Yogurt, Light Fat-Free, Harvest Peach (6 oz)	90	16	0	0	75	1 skim milk
Yogurt, Light Fat-Free, Strawberries 'N Bananas (6 oz)	90	16	0	0	75	1 skim milk
Yogurt, Original 99% Fat-Free, Cafe Au Lait (6 oz)	170	31	2	1	90	1 skim milk, 1 carb.
Yogurt, Original 99% Fat-Free, Lemon Burst (6 oz)	180	33	2	1	125	1 skim milk, 1 carb.
Yogurt, Original 99% Fat-Free, Strawberry Banana (6 oz)	180	33	2	1	125	1 skim milk, 1 carb.
Yogurt, Original 99% Fat-Free, Tropical Peach (6 oz)	180	33	2	1	125	1 skim milk, 1 carb.

NUTS, SEEDS, AND NUT/SEED PRODUCTS

NUTS, SEEDS, AND NUT/SEED PRODUCTS

Products	Cal.	Carb. (g)	Fat (g)	Sat. Fat (g)	Sodium (mg)	Exchanges
Almond Butter, Plain (1 Tbsp)	101	3	10	<1	2	2 fat
Almond Butter, Salted (1 Tbsp)	98	3	9	<1	70	2 fat
Almonds, Dried, Whole (1 oz)	165	6	15	1	3	1 med-fat meat, 2 fat
Almonds, Dry-Roasted (1 oz)	164	7	14	1	218	1 med-fat meat, 2 fat
Almonds, Dry-Roasted, Whole, Unsalted (1 oz)	164	7	14	1	3	1 med-fat meat, 2 fat
Almonds, Oil-Roasted (1 oz)	173	5	16	2	218	1 med-fat meat, 2 fat
Almonds, Toasted (1 oz)	167	7	14	1	3	1 med-fat meat, 2 fat
Beechnuts, Dried (1 oz)	164	10	14	2	11	1/2 strch, 3 fat
Brazil Nuts, Dried (1 oz)	186	4	19	5	<1	1 med-fat meat, 3 fat
Cashew Butter, Unsalted (1 Tbsp)	94	4	8	2	2	2 fat
Cashews, Dry-Roasted (1 oz)	161	9	13	3	179	1/2 strch, 3 fat
Cashews, Oil-Roasted (1 oz)	161	8	14	3	175	1/2 strch, 3 fat
Chinese Chestnuts, Dried (1 oz)	103	23	<1	<1	1	1-1/2 strch

Chinese Chestnuts, Roasted (1 oz)	68	15	<1	<1	1	1 strch
Coconut, Dried, Shredded, Sweetened (1/4 cup)	233	11	8	7	61	1 strch, 2 fat
Coconut, Fresh (2.5 x 2-inch piece)	159	7	15	13	9	1/2 strch, 3 fat
Coconut, Toasted (1 oz)	168	13	13	12	11	1 strch, 3 fat
Coconut Milk, Raw (1 cup)	552	13	57	51	36	1 strch, 11 fat
English Walnut Halves, Dried (1 oz)	180	5	17	2	3	1 med-fat meat, 2 fat
European Chestnuts, Roasted (1 oz)	69	15	<1	<1	<1	1 strch
Filberts/Hazelnuts, Dried, Whole (1 oz)	177	4	18	1	<1	1 med-fat meat, 3 fat
Filberts/Hazelnuts, Dry Roasted, Salted (1 oz)	188	5	18	1	221	3 fat
Filberts/Hazelnuts, Oil Roasted, Salted (1 oz)	187	6	18	1	223	1/2 strch, 3 fat
Hickory Nuts, Dried (1 oz)	186	5	18	2	<1	4 fat
Japanese Chestnuts, Dried (1 oz)	101	23	<1	<1	10	1-1/2 strch
Japanese Chestnuts, Roasted (1 oz)	57	13	<1	<1	5	1 strch
Macadamia Nuts (1 oz)	196	4	21	3	1	4 fat
Macadamia Nuts, Oil Roasted (1 oz)	201	4	20	3	73	4 fat
Mixed Nuts, Dry Roasted (1 oz)	166	7	14	2	187	1/2 strch, 3 fat

NUTS, SEEDS, AND NUT/SEED PRODUCTS

Products	Cal.	Carb. (g)	Fat (g)	Sat. Fat (g)	Sodium (mg)	Exchanges
Mixed Nuts, Oil Roasted (1 oz)	172	6	16	3	183	1/2 strch, 3 fat
Mixed Nuts, Oil Roasted, No Peanuts (1 oz)	172	6	16	3	196	1/2 strch, 3 fat
Mixed Nuts, Oil Roasted, Unsalted (1 oz)	173	6	16	2	3	1 med-fat meat, 2 fat
Peanut Butter, Chunky (1 Tbsp)	94	4	8	2	78	1 med-fat meat, 1 fat
Peanut Butter, Natural, Salted (1 Tbsp)	94	3	8	1	40	1 med-fat meat, 1 fat
Peanut Butter, Natural, Unsalted (1 Tbsp)	94	3	8	1	<1	1 med-fat meat, 1 fat
Peanut Butter, Smooth (1 Tbsp)	94	3	8	2	77	1 med-fat meat, 1 fat
Peanuts, Dry-Roasted, Unsalted (1 oz)	164	6	14	2	2	1 med-fat meat, 2 fat
Peanuts, Oil-Roasted (1 oz)	163	5	14	2	121	1 med-fat meat, 2 fat
Peanuts, Spanish, Raw (1 oz)	160	4	14	2	6	1 med-fat meat, 2 fat
Pecans, Dried Halves (1 oz)	187	5	19	2	<1	4 fat
Pecans, Dry-Roasted (1 oz)	187	6	18	2	222	3 fat
Pecans, Oil-Roasted (1 oz)	192	5	20	2	212	4 fat
Pine (Pignolia) Nuts, Dried (1 oz)	146	4	14	2	1	1 med-fat meat, 2 fat

Pistachio Nuts, Dry-Roasted (1 oz)	170	8	15	2	218	1/2 strch, 3 fat
Pumpkin Kernels, Roasted (1 oz)	146	3	12	2	161	1 med-fat meat, 1 fat
Pumpkin Seeds, Roasted (1 oz)	125	15	5	1	161	1 strch, 1 fat
Sesame Seeds, Dried, Whole (1 Tbsp)	52	2	5	1	1	1 fat
Sunflower Seeds, Dry (1 oz)	159	5	14	2	<1	1 med-fat meat, 2 fat
Sunflower Seeds, Dry-Roasted (1 oz)	163	7	14	2	<1	1 med-fat meat, 2 fat
Sunflower Seeds, Oil-Roasted (1 oz)	172	4	16	2	169	1 med-fat meat, 2 fat
Tahini or Sesame Butter (1 Tbsp)	91	3	9	1	<1	2 fat
BAKER'S						
Coconut, Angel Flake (2 Tbsp)	70	7	5	4	45	1/2 strch, 1 fat
Coconut, Premium Shredded (2 Tbsp)	60	6	4	4	35	1/2 strch, 1 fat
BEER NUTS						
Cashew Halves (1 oz)	170	8	13	3	80	1 med-fat meat, 2 fat
Peanuts (1 oz)	170	7	14	3	80	1 med-fat meat, 2 fat
BLUE DIAMOND						
Almonds, Whole, Dry Roasted (1 oz)	168	4	16	1	0	1 med-fat meat, 2 fat

NUTS, SEEDS, AND NUT/SEED PRODUCTS

Products	Cal.	Carb. (g)	Fat (g)	Sat. Fat (g)	Sodium (mg)	Exchanges
CORNUTS						
Barbeque (1 oz)	130	20	4	1	280	1 strch, 1 fat
Chili Picante (1 oz)	130	20	4	1	260	1 strch, 1 fat
Original (1 oz)	130	20	4	4	170	1 strch, 1 fat
Pepperoni Pizza (1 oz)	130	20	4	1	190	1 strch, 1 fat
Ranch (1 oz)	130	20	4	1	190	1 strch, 1 fat
ESTEE						
Peanut Butter, Creamy/Chunky (2 Tbsp)	190	7	15	3	0	1 high-fat meat, 1 fat
FISHER						
Mixed Nuts (1 oz)	180	5	16	3	110	1 med-fat meat, 2 fat
Peanuts, Golden-Roasted, Lightly Salted (1 oz)	170	6	14	3	95	1 med-fat meat, 2 fat
JIFF						
Peanut Butter, Creamy (2 Tbsp)	190	7	16	3	150	1 high-fat meat, 2 fat
Peanut Butter, Extra Crunchy (2 Tbsp)	190	7	16	3	130	1 high-fat meat, 2 fat

Peanut Butter, Reduced-Fat, Creamy (2 Tbsp)	190	15	12	3	250	1 carb., 1 high-fat meat, 1 fat
Peanut Butter, Reduced-Fat, Crunchy (2 Tbsp)	190	15	12	3	220	1 carb., 1 high-fat meat
Peanut Butter, Simply Jiff, Creamy (2 Tbsp)	190	6	16	3	65	1 high-fat meat, 2 fat
LAURA SCUDDER'S						
Peanut Butter, Nutty (2 Tbsp)	200	6	16	3	110	1 high-fat meat, 2 fat
Peanut Butter, Smooth (2 Tbsp)	200	6	16	3	110	1 high-fat meat, 2 fat
Peanut Butter, Smooth, Reduced-Fat (2 Tbsp)	200	12	12	2	120	1 carb., 1 high-fat meat, 1 fat
PETER PAN						
Peanut Butter, Creamy (2 Tbsp)	190	7	16	3	150	1 high-fat meat, 2 fat
Peanut Butter, Extra Crunchy (2 Tbsp)	190	7	16	3	120	1 high-fat meat, 2 fat
Peanut Butter Spread, Smart Choice (2 Tbsp)	180	14	11	2	150	1 carb., 1 high-fat meat, 1 fat
PLANTERS						
Cashews, Honey-Roasted (1 oz)	155	12	12	2	120	1 carb., 2 fat
Nut Topping (2 Tbsp)	100	3	9	9	0	2 fat
Peanuts, Honey-Roasted (1 oz)	160	8	13	2	90	1/2 carb., 1 med-fat meat, 2 fat

NUTS, SEEDS, AND NUT/SEED PRODUCTS

Products	Cal.	Carb. (g)	Fat (g)	Sat. Fat (g)	Sodium (mg)	Exchanges
Peanuts, Reduced-Fat Honey-Roasted (1 oz)	130	12	7	1	150	1 carb, 1 high-fat meat
Select Mix, Cashews, Almonds, & Macadamias (1 oz)	170	6	16	3	90	1 med-fat meat, 2 fat
REESE'S						
Peanut Butter, Creamy (2 Tbsp)	200	6	16	3	115	1 high-fat meat, 2 fat
Peanut Butter, Extra Crunchy (2 Tbsp)	200	6	16	3	80	1 high-fat meat, 2 fat
SKIPPY						
Peanut Butter, Creamy (2 Tbsp)	190	7	16	4	150	1 high-fat meat, 2 fat
Peanut Butter, Creamy, Roasted Honey Nut (2 Tbsp)	190	6	17	4	125	1 high-fat meat, 2 fat
Peanut Butter, Reduced-Fat Creamy (2 Tbsp)	190	14	12	3	190	1 carb., 1 high-fat meat, 1 fat
Peanut Butter, Reduced-Fat Super Chunk (2 Tbsp)	180	13	12	3	170	1 carb., 1 high-fat meat, 1 fat
Peanut Butter, Super Chunk (2 Tbsp)	190	6	17	4	140	1 high-fat meat, 2 fat
Peanut Butter, Super Chunk, Roasted Honey Nut (2 Tbsp)	190	7	17	4	120	1 high-fat meat, 2 fat

SAUCES, CONDIMENTS, AND GRAVIES

Products	Cal.	Carb. (g)	Fat (g)	Sat. Fat (g)	Sodium (mg)	Exchanges
Apple Butter (2 Tbsp)	65	17	<1	<1	0	1 carb.
Catsup/Ketchup (1 Tbsp)	16	4	<1	<1	182	free
Catsup/Ketchup, Low-Sodium (1 Tbsp)	16	4	<1	<1	3	free
Chutney (1 Tbsp)	26	7	<1	<1	38	1/2 carb.
Gravy, Au Jus, Canned (1/2 cup)	19	3	<1	<1	60	free
Gravy, Beef, Canned (1/2 cup)	62	6	3	1	652	1/2 carb., 1 fat
Gravy, Beef, Homemade (1/2 cup)	89	7	5	2	767	1/2 carb., 1 fat
Gravy, Brown, Dry Mix w/Water (1/2 cup)	38	7	<1	<1	538	1/2 carb.
Gravy, Chicken, Canned (1/2 cup)	94	7	7	2	687	1/2 carb., 1 fat
Gravy, Chicken Giblet, Homemade (1/2 cup)	97	6	5	1	683	1/2 carb., 1 fat
Gravy, Mushroom, Canned (1/2 cup)	60	7	6	<1	678	1/2 carb., 1 fat
Gravy, Sausage (1/2 cup)	206	8	16	6	408	1/2 carb., 3 fat

SAUCES, CONDIMENTS, AND GRAVIES

Products	Cal.	Carb. (g)	Fat (g)	Sat. Fat (g)	Sodium (mg)	Exchanges
Gravy, Turkey, Canned (1/2 cup)	61	6	3	<1	687	1/2 strch, 1 fat
Guacamole w/Tomatoes (1 Tbsp)	17	1	2	<1	27	free
Honey (1 Tbsp)	64	17	0	0	<1	1 carb.
Horseradish, Prepared (1 Tbsp)	6	1	<1	<1	14	free
Jam, Cherry/Strawberry (1 Tbsp)	54	14	<1	0	2	1 carb.
Jam, Not Cherry or Strawberry (1 Tbsp)	54	14	<1	0	2	1 carb.
Jam/Marmalade, Artificially Sweetened (1 Tbsp)	2	11	<1	<1	0	free
Jam/Marmalade/Preserves, Reduced-Sugar (1 Tbsp)	36	9	<1	<1	5	1/2 carb.
Jam/Preserves (1 Tbsp)	48	13	<1	<1	8	1 carb.
Jelly (1 Tbsp)	49	13	<1	<1	7	1 carb.
Jelly, Blackberry (1 Tbsp)	50	13	0	0	10	1 carb.
Jelly, Dietetic (1 Tbsp)	6	11	0	0	<1	free
Jelly, Reduced-Sugar (1 Tbsp)	34	9	<1	<1	<1	1/2 carb.
Marmalade, Orange (1 Tbsp)	49	13	0	0	11	1 carb.

Mustard, Dijon (1 Tbsp)	19	2	1	<1	379	free
Mustard, Prepared (1 Tbsp)	12	1	<1	<1	196	free
Olives, Green, Pitted (10)	45	<1	5	<1	936	1 fat
Olives, Small Ripe, Canned (10)	37	2	3	<1	279	1 fat
Olives, Stuffed Green (10)	41	<1	5	<1	827	1 fat
Peppers, Pickled Hot Jalapeño (2)	8	2	<1	<1	121	free
Pickle, Dill (1)	12	3	<1	<1	833	free
Pickle, Dill, Low-Sodium (1)	7	2	<1	<1	12	free
Pickle, Sour (1)	4	<1	<1	<1	423	free
Pickle, Sweet (1 medium)	41	11	<1	<1	329	1/2 carb.
Pickle Slices, Dill (10)	11	3	<1	<1	769	free
Pickle Slices, Dill, Low-Sodium (10)	11	3	<1	<1	11	free
Pickle Slices, Fresh Pack (4)	22	5	<1	0	202	free
Pickle Slices, Sour (10)	8	2	<1	<1	846	free
Relish, Hot Dog (1 Tbsp)	18	4	<1	<1	81	free
Relish, Sweet Pickle (1 Tbsp)	21	5	<1	<1	109	free

SAUCES, CONDIMENTS, AND GRAVIES

Products	Cal.	Carb. (g)	Fat (g)	Sat. Fat (g)	Sodium (mg)	Exchanges
Sauce, Bearnaise, Homemade (1/2 cup)	317	1	33	20	436	7 fat
Sauce, Black Bean (1/2 cup)	129	14	6	1	1322	1 strch, 1 fat
Sauce, Cheese (1/2 cup)	216	6	17	8	539	1/2 carb., 1 med-fat meat, 2 fat
Sauce, Curry (1/2 cup)	74	3	6	1	392	1 fat
Sauce, Hollandaise (1/2 cup)	171	1	36	20	312	7 fat
Sauce, Hot Chili/Red Pepper (2 Tbsp)	7	1	<1	<1	8	free
Sauce, Hot Green Chili (1 Tbsp)	3	<1	<1	0	4	free
Sauce, Marinara Tomato (1/2 cup)	85	13	4	<1	786	1 carb., 1 fat
Sauce, Salsa/Mexican, Homemade (1/2 cup)	24	5	<1	<1	468	1 vegetable
Sauce, Soy (1 Tbsp)	10	2	<1	<1	1028	free
Sauce, Spanish-Style Tomato (1/2 cup)	40	9	<1	<1	576	1/2 carb.
Sauce, Tartar (1 Tbsp)	74	<1	8	2	99	2 fat
Sauce, Teriyaki (1 Tbsp)	15	3	0	0	690	free

Sauce, White, Homemade (1/2 cup)	178	10	14	4	185	1/2 strch, 3 fat
Sauce, Worcestershire (1 Tbsp)	11	3	0	0	167	free
Spaghetti Sauce, Meat, Canned (1/2 cup)	150	19	7	1	590	1 carb., 2 fat
Spaghetti Sauce, Meat, Homemade (1/2 cup)	145	11	8	2	565	2 carb., 1 med-fat meat, 1 fat
Spaghetti Sauce, Canned (1/2 cup)	136	20	6	<1	618	1 carb., 1 fat
Syrup, Maple (1 Tbsp)	52	13	<1	0	2	1 carb.
Syrup, Pancake (1 Tbsp)	56	15	0	0	16	1 carb.
CAMPBELL'S						
Spaghetti Sauce, Italian-Style (1/2 cup)	120	25	2	0	550	1-1/2 carb.
Spaghetti Sauce, Marinara, Homestyle (1/2 cup)	90	18	1	0	510	1 carb.
Spaghetti Sauce, Mushroom Garlic (1/2 cup)	90	19	1	0	540	1 carb.
Spaghetti Sauce, Mushroom (1/2 cup)	100	22	1	0	530	1-1/2 carb.
Spaghetti Sauce w/Ground Beef Flavor (1/2 cup)	100	19	2	0	600	1 carb.
Spaghetti Sauce, Traditional (1/2 cup)	120	25	2	0	550	1-1/2 carb.
Spaghetti Sauce, Xtra Garlic Onion (1/2 cup)	60	12	1	0	370	1 carb.

SAUCES, CONDIMENTS, AND GRAVIES

Products	Cal.	Carb. (g)	Fat (g)	Sat. Fat (g)	Sodium (mg)	Exchanges
CARY'S						
Syrup, Sugar-Free (1/4 cup)	35	9	0	0	135	1/2 carb.
CHEF MATE						
Gravy, Country Sausage (1/4 cup)	103	4	8	2	248	2 fat
Sauce, Basic Cheese (1/2 cup)	134	13	8	3	788	1 carb., 2 fat
Sauce, Coney Island-Style (1/4 cup)	33	3	3	<1	208	1 fat
Sauce, Golden Cheese (1/2 cup)	231	3	18	10	824	1 med-fat meat, 3 fat
Sauce, Hot Dog Chili (1/4 cup)	38	5	1	<1	216	1/2 carb.
Sauce, Sharp Cheddar Cheese (1/2 cup)	216	6	16	8	776	1/2 carb., 1 med-fat meat, 2 fat
Sauce, Sloppy Joe Barbecue (1/3 cup)	111	9	6	3	539	1/2 carb., 1 fat
CLAUSSEN						
Pickle Relish, Sweet (1 Tbsp)	13	3	<1	<1	85	free
Pickles, Bread'n Butter Chips (4)	19	4	<1	<1	173	free

Food	Cal.	Carb. (g)	Fat (g)	Sat. Fat (g)	Sod. (mg)	Exchanges/Choices
Pickles, Hamburger Dill Chips (10)	4	<1	<1		421	free
Pickles, Kosher Dill Halves (1)	4	<1	<1		325	free
Pickles, Kosher Dill Slices (4)	3	<1	<1		320	free
Pickles, Kosher Dill Spears (1)	4	<1	<1		312	free
Pickles, Kosher Mini Dills (1)	4	<1	<1		300	free
CONTADINA						
Pasta Ready Tomatoes & 3-Cheeses (1/2 cup)	70	8	4	0	650	1/2 carb., 1 fat
Pasta Ready Tomatoes & Mushrooms (1/2 cup)	50	9	1	0	641	1/2 carb.
Pasta Ready Tomatoes & Olives (1/2 cup)	60	8	2	0	641	1/2 carb.
Pasta Ready Tomatoes & Red Pepper (1/2 cup)	60	8	2	0	691	1/2 carb.
Pasta Ready Tomatoes Primavera (1/2 cup)	50	8	1	0	600	1/2 carb.
Pizza Sauce, All-Purpose (1/4 cup)	25	6	0	0	20	1/2 carb.
Pizza Sauce, Chunky, Basic (1/4 cup)	30	6	0	0	280	1/2 carb.
Pizza Sauce, Deluxe (1/4 cup)	30	5	1	0	120	1/2 carb.
Pizza Sauce, Fully Prepared (1/4 cup)	25	6	0	0	270	1/2 carb.
Pizza Sauce & 3-Cheeses, Chunky (1/4 cup)	35	5	<1	0	190	1/2 carb.

SAUCES, CONDIMENTS, AND GRAVIES

Products	Cal.	Carb. (g)	Fat (g)	Sat. Fat (g)	Sodium (mg)	Exchanges
Pizza Sauce & Mushrooms, Chunky (1/4 cup)	30	5	0	0	290	1/2 carb.
Pizza Sauce w/Basil (1/4 cup)	25	6	0	0	20	1/2 carb.
Pizza Sauce w/Cheese (1/4 cup)	30	4	1	0	350	1/2 carb.
Pizza Sauce w/Pepperoni (1/4 cup)	30	4	1	0	359	1/2 carb.
Pizza Sauce, Original (1/4 cup)	24	4	<1	0	288	1/2 carb.
Pizza Sauce, Squeeze (1/4 cup)	34	6	1	0	337	1/2 carb.
Pizza Sauce, Squeeze, Italian Cheese (1/4 cup)	40	6	1	0	420	1/2 carb.
Spaghetti Sauce (1/2 cup)	70	14	2	0	560	1 carb.
Spaghetti Sauce, Deluxe (1/2 cup)	80	14	2	0	600	1 carb.
Sauce, Marinara, Deluxe (1/2 cup)	80	12	4	<1	470	1 carb., 1 fat
Sauce, Multi-Purpose Tomato (1/2 cup)	35	8	0	0	20	1/2 carb.
Sauce, Sweet 'n Sour (1/2 cup)	165	33	4	0	473	2 carb., 1 fat
DEL MONTE						
Spaghetti Sauce, Traditional (1/2 cup)	60	14	1	0	500	1 carb.

Food						Exchanges
Spaghetti Sauce w/Garlic & Onion (1/2 cup)	60	13	1	0	460	1 carb.
Spaghetti Sauce w/Green Peppers & Mushrooms (1/2 cup)	60	12	1	0	390	1 carb.
Spaghetti Sauce w/Meat (1/2 cup)	70	13	2	0	510	1 carb.
Spaghetti Sauce w/Mushrooms (1/2 cup)	70	15	1	0	520	1 carb.
DI GIORNO						
Sauce, Alfredo (1/4 cup)	230	2	22	10	550	1 med-fat meat, 3 fat
Sauce, Alfredo, Reduced-Fat (1/4 cup)	170	16	10	6	600	1 carb., 1 med-fat meat, 1 fat
Sauce, Four-Cheese (1/4 cup)	200	2	19	11	410	1 med-fat meat, 3 fat
Sauce, Lite Chunky Tomato & Basil (1/2 cup)	70	16	0	0	290	1 carb.
Sauce, Marinara (1/2 cup)	100	12	5	1	530	1 carb., 1 fat
Sauce, Olive Oil & Garlic & Cheeses (1/4 cup)	370	3	36	8	540	1 med-fat meat, 6 fat
Sauce, Pesto (1/4 cup)	320	3	31	7	500	1 med-fat meat, 5 fat
Sauce, Plum Tomato & Mushroom (1/2 cup)	70	15	0	0	310	1 carb.
Sauce, Traditional Meat (1/2 cup)	120	12	6	2	610	1 carb., 1 med-fat meat

SAUCES, CONDIMENTS, AND GRAVIES

Products	Cal.	Carb. (g)	Fat (g)	Sat. Fat (g)	Sodium (mg)	Exchanges
ESTEE						
Syrup, Blueberry Breakfast (1/4 cup)	80	20	0	0	70	1 carb.
Syrup, Maple Breakfast (1/4 cup)	80	20	0	0	125	1 carb.
FEATHERWEIGHT						
Syrup, Lite Pancake (1/4 cup)	80	20	0	0	125	1 carb.
FRANCO-AMERICAN						
Gravy, Au Jus (1/4 cup)	10	2	<1	0	310	free
Gravy, Beef (1/4 cup)	30	4	2	.997	300	1 fat
Gravy, Brown, w/Onions (1/2 cup)	50	8	2	0	680	1/2 carb.
Gravy, Chicken (1/4 cup)	45	3	4	<1	270	1 fat
Gravy, Chicken Giblet (1/4 cup)	30	3	2	0	310	1 fat
Gravy, Creamy Mushroom (1/4 cup)	20	4	<1	0	310	free
Gravy, Golden Pork (1/4 cup)	45	3	4	2	340	1 fat
Gravy, Mushroom (1/4 cup)	20	3	<1	0	300	free

Gravy, Turkey (1/4 cup)	25	3	<1	0	290	free
GENERAL MILLS						
Bac-O-Bits, Salad Topping (1 Tbsp)	25	2	<1	NA	103	free
Spaghetti Sauce (1/2 cup)	79	10	3	<1	699	1/2 carb., 1 fat
GREEN GIANT						
Relish, Corn, Canned (1 Tbsp)	20	5	<1	0	42	free
Sauce, Sloppy Joe Sandwich (1/4 cup)	51	11	<1	<1	423	1 carb.
GREY POUPON						
Country Dijon Mustard (1 Tbsp)	15	<1	0	0	360	free
HEALTHY CHOICE						
BBQ Sauce, Hickory (2 Tbsp)	26	6	<1	0	226	1/2 carb.
BBQ Sauce, Hot & Spicy (2 Tbsp)	25	6	<1	0	229	1/2 carb.
BBQ Sauce, Original (2 Tbsp)	25	6	<1	0	229	1/2 carb.
Ketchup (1 Tbsp)	9	2	<1	0	97	free
Pasta Sauce, Extra Chunky Garlic & Onion (1/2 cup)	43	8	<1	0	368	1/2 carb.
Pasta Sauce, Extra Chunky Italian Vegetable (1/2 cup)	39	8	<1	0	380	1/2 carb.

SAUCES, CONDIMENTS, AND GRAVIES

Products	Cal.	Carb. (g)	Fat (g)	Sat. Fat (g)	Sodium (mg)	Exchanges
Pasta Sauce, Extra Chunky Mushroom (1/2 cup)	41	8	<1	0	352	1/2 carb.
Pasta Sauce, Traditional (1/2 cup)	47	10	<1	0	391	1/2 carb.
Pasta Sauce, Super Chunky Mushroom & Sweet Peppers (1/2 cup)	44	9	<1	0	366	1/2 carb.
Pasta Sauce, Super Chunky Vegetable Primavera (1/2 cup)	45	9	<1	0	358	1/2 carb.
Pasta Sauce, Super Tomato, Mushroom, & Garlic (1/2 cup)	46	9	<1	0	411	1/2 carb.
Pasta Sauce Flavored w/Meat (1/2 cup)	47	8	1	0	384	1/2 carb.
Pasta Sauce w/Garlic & Herbs (1/2 cup)	47	10	<1	NA	391	1/2 carb.
Pasta Sauce w/Mushrooms (1/2 cup)	47	10	<1	NA	391	1/2 carb.
HUNGRY JACK						
Syrup, Maple, Butter (1 Tbsp)	52	13	0	0	23	1 carb.
Syrup, Maple, Butter, Lite (1 Tbsp)	28	7	0	0	52	1/2 carb.

Syrup, Pancake, Regular (1 Tbsp)	52	13	0	0	23	1 carb.
Syrup, Pancake, Regular Lite (1 Tbsp)	28	7	0	0	52	1/2 carb.
HUNT'S						
BBQ Sauce, Bold Original (2 Tbsp)	46	11	<1	0	315	1 carb.
BBQ Sauce, Hickory (2 Tbsp)	38	9	<1	0	410	1/2 carb.
BBQ Sauce, Hickory & Brown Sugar (2 Tbsp)	75	18	<1	0	382	1 carb.
BBQ Sauce, Honey Mustard (2 Tbsp)	48	12	<1	0	450	1 carb.
BBQ Sauce, Hot & Spicy (2 Tbsp)	48	12	<1	0	450	1 carb.
BBQ Sauce, Light (2 Tbsp)	23	6	<1	0	169	1/2 carb.
BBQ Sauce, Mesquite (2 Tbsp)	40	9	<1	0	361	1/2 carb.
BBQ Sauce, Mild Dijon (2 Tbsp)	39	9	<1	0	400	1/2 carb.
BBQ Sauce, Original (2 Tbsp)	39	9	<1	0	399	1/2 carb.
BBQ Sauce, Teriyaki (2 Tbsp)	46	11	<1	0	351	1 carb.
Chicken Sensations, BBQ Flavor (1 Tbsp)	35	3	3	<1	308	1 fat
Chicken Sensations, Italian Garlic (1 Tbsp)	30	1	3	<1	326	1 fat
Chicken Sensations, Lemon Herb (1 Tbsp)	31	2	3	<1	378	1 fat

SAUCES, CONDIMENTS, AND GRAVIES

Products	Cal.	Carb. (g)	Fat (g)	Sat. Fat (g)	Sodium (mg)	Exchanges
Chicken Sensations, Southwestern (1 Tbsp)	27	1	3	<1	281	1 fat
Salsa, Alfresco, Medium (2 Tbsp)	10	2	0	0	199	free
Salsa, Homestyle, Medium (2 Tbsp)	27	6	<1	0	236	1 vegetable
Sauce, Pepper, Original & Hot (1 tsp)	0	<1	0	0	205	free
Sauce, Picante, Medium (2 Tbsp)	11	2	<1	0	256	free
Sauce, Steak (1 Tbsp)	10	2	<1	0	256	free
Spaghetti Sauce, Chunky Italian-Style Vegetable (1/2 cup)	63	13	1	<1	528	1 carb.
Spaghetti Sauce, Chunky Marinara (1/2 cup)	60	12	2	<1	526	1 carb.
Spaghetti Sauce, Home Style Traditional (1/2 cup)	56	7	3	<1	596	1/2 carb., 1/2 fat
Spaghetti Sauce, Italian Sausage (1/2 cup)	77	12	3	<1	596	1 carb., 1/2 fat
Spaghetti Sauce, Italian-Style Cheese & Garlic (1/2 cup)	65	9	2	<1	690	1/2 carb., 1/2 fat
Spaghetti Sauce, Old Country Traditional (1/2 cup)	53	7	3	<1	542	1/2 carb., 1/2 fat

Spaghetti Sauce, Original Traditional (1/2 cup)	65	11	2	<1	621	1 carb.
Spaghetti Sauce Flavored w/Meat, Home Style (1/2 cup)	56	7	3	1	596	1/2 carb., 1/2 fat
Spaghetti Sauce Flavored w/Meat, Original (1/2 cup)	65	11	2	<1	604	1 carb.
Spaghetti Sauce w/Garlic & Herbs, Old Country (1/2 cup)	63	9	3	<1	522	1/2 carb., 1/2 fat
Spaghetti Sauce w/Mushrooms, Old Country (1/2 cup)	53	7	3	<1	542	1/2 carb., 1/2 fat
Spaghetti Sauce w/Mushrooms, Original (1/2 cup)	65	11	2	<1	604	1 carb.
Spaghetti Sauce w/Parmesan, Classic Italian (1/2 cup)	50	8	2	<1	634	1/2 carb.
Spaghetti Sauce w/Tomato & Basil, Classic Italian (1/2 cup)	48	8	2	<1	613	1/2 carb.
KRAFT						
BBQ Sauce, Charcoal Grill (2 Tbsp)	60	12	1	0	440	1 carb.
BBQ Sauce, Garlic (2 Tbsp)	40	9	0	0	420	1/2 carb.
BBQ Sauce, Hickory Smoke (2 Tbsp)	40	10	0	0	440	1/2 carb.
BBQ Sauce, Hickory Smoke Onion Bits (2 Tbsp)	50	11	0	0	340	1 carb.

SAUCES, CONDIMENTS, AND GRAVIES

Products	Cal.	Carb. (g)	Fat (g)	Sat. Fat (g)	Sodium (mg)	Exchanges
BBQ Sauce, Honey (2 Tbsp)	50	13	0	0	320	1 carb.
BBQ Sauce, Hot (2 Tbsp)	40	9	0	0	540	1/2 carb.
BBQ Sauce, Hot Hickory Smoke (2 Tbsp)	40	9	0	0	360	1/2 carb.
BBQ Sauce, Italian Seasonings (2 Tbsp)	45	10	<1	0	280	1/2 carb.
BBQ Sauce, Kansas City-Style (2 Tbsp)	45	11	0	0	280	1 carb.
BBQ Sauce, Mesquite Smoke (2 Tbsp)	40	9	0	0	210	1/2 carb.
BBQ Sauce, Onion Bits (2 Tbsp)	50	11	0	0	340	1 carb.
BBQ Sauce, Original (2 Tbsp)	40	10	0	0	460	1/2 carb.
BBQ Sauce, Salsa-Style (2 Tbsp)	40	9	0	0	420	1/2 carb.
BBQ Sauce, Teriyaki (2 Tbsp)	60	12	1	0	430	1 carb.
BBQ Sauce, Thick'n Spicy Hickory Smoke (2 Tbsp)	50	12	0	0	440	1 carb.
BBQ Sauce, Thick'n Spicy Honey (2 Tbsp)	60	13	0	0	350	1 carb.
BBQ Sauce, Thick'n Spicy Mesquite (2 Tbsp)	50	12	0	0	440	1 carb.
BBQ Sauce, Thick'n Spicy Original (2 Tbsp)	50	12	0	0	440	1 carb.

BBQ Sauce, Xtra Rich Original (2 Tbsp)	50	12	0	0	360	1 carb.
Fruit Spread, Reduced-Calorie, Grape (1 Tbsp)	20	5	0	0	20	free
Fruit Spread, Reduced-Calorie, Strawberry (1 Tbsp)	20	5	0	0	20	free
Jam, Grape (1 Tbsp)	60	14	0	0	10	1 carb.
Jam, Red Plum (1 Tbsp)	60	13	0	0	10	1 carb.
Jam, Strawberry (1 Tbsp)	50	13	0	0	10	1 carb.
Jelly, Apple (1 Tbsp)	60	14	0	0	10	1 carb.
Jelly, Apple Strawberry (1 Tbsp)	50	13	0	0	10	1 carb.
Jelly, Grape (1 Tbsp)	50	14	0	0	10	1 carb.
Jelly, Guava (1 Tbsp)	50	13	0	0	10	1 carb.
Jelly, Red Current (1 Tbsp)	50	13	0	0	10	1 carb.
Jelly, Strawberry (1 Tbsp)	60	14	0	0	10	1 carb.
Preserves, Apricot (1 Tbsp)	50	13	0	0	10	1 carb.
Preserves, Blackberry (1 Tbsp)	50	13	0	0	10	1 carb.
Preserves, Orange Marmalade (1 Tbsp)	50	14	0	0	10	1 carb.
Preserves, Peach (1 Tbsp)	50	14	0	0	10	1 carb.

SAUCES, CONDIMENTS, AND GRAVIES

Products	Cal.	Carb. (g)	Fat (g)	Sat. Fat (g)	Sodium (mg)	Exchanges
Preserves, Pineapple (1 Tbsp)	50	14	0	0	10	1 carb.
Preserves, Red Raspberry (1 Tbsp)	50	13	0	0	10	1 carb.
Preserves, Strawberry (1 Tbsp)	50	13	0	0	10	1 carb.
Sandwich Spread & Burger Sauce (1 Tbsp)	50	5	3	<1	100	1 fat
Sauce, Horseradish, Cream-Style (1 Tbsp)	0	0	0	0	50	free
Sauce, Horseradish, Mustard (1 Tbsp)	0	0	0	0	55	free
Sauce, Nonfat Tartar (2 Tbsp)	23	5	0	0	197	free
Sauce, Pure Prepared Horseradish (1 Tbsp)	0	0	0	0	60	free
Sauce, Sauceworks Cocktail (1 Tbsp)	15	3	<1	0	200	free
Sauce, Sauceworks Horseradish (1 Tbsp)	20	1	2	0	35	free
Sauce, Sauceworks Lemon Herb Tartar (2 Tbsp)	150	1	16	3	170	3 fat
Sauce, Sauceworks Sweet & Sour (2 Tbsp)	60	14	0	0	125	1 carb.
Sauce, Sauceworks Tartar (2 Tbsp)	100	4	10	4	180	2 fat
Sauce, Steak (2 Tbsp)	19	5	<1	<1	455	free

LA CHOY

Sauce, Brown Gravy (1/4 cup)	275	66	0	0	320	4 carb.
Sauce, Chun King Hot Teriyaki (1 Tbsp)	17	3	0	0	994	free
Sauce, Plum (1 Tbsp)	25	6	<1	0	4	1/2 carb.
Sauce, Soy (1 Tbsp)	11	1	<1	0	1315	free
Sauce, Soy, Lite (1 Tbsp)	15	2	<1	0	505	free
Sauce, Stir-Fry Mandarin Soy (1/2 cup)	71	16	<1	0	852	1 carb.
Sauce, Stir-Fry Sweet & Sour (1/2 cup)	137	36	0	0	754	2 carb.
Sauce, Stir-Fry Szechwan (1/2 cup)	84	19	<1	0	624	1 carb.
Sauce, Stir-Fry Teriyaki (1/2 cup)	95	22	<1	0	1154	1-1/2 carb.
Sauce, Sweet & Sour (2 Tbsp)	58	14	<1	0	104	1 carb.
Sauce, Teriyaki (1 Tbsp)	17	3	<1	0	917	free
Sauce, Teriyaki, Light (1 Tbsp)	18	4	<1	0	439	free

LIBBY'S

Gravy, Country Chicken (1/2 cup)	120	6	8	1	660	1/2 carb., 2 fat
Gravy, Country Sausage (1/2 cup)	180	6	14	3	560	1/2 carb., 3 fat

SAUCES, CONDIMENTS, AND GRAVIES

Products	Cal.	Carb. (g)	Fat (g)	Sat. Fat (g)	Sodium (mg)	Exchanges
Sauce, Sloppy Joe (1/3 cup)	45	10	0	0	430	1/2 carb.
Sauce, Tomato (1/4 cup)	20	4	0	0	280	free
MRS. BUTTERWORTH'S						
Syrup, Pancake, Buttery (1 Tbsp)	58	15	<1	<1	19	1 carb.
Syrup, Pancake, Buttery, LoCal (1 Tbsp)	29	8	0	0	37	1/2 carb.
NESTLE						
Sauce, All-Purpose Stir-Fry (1 Tbsp)	15	2	1	0	260	free
Sauce, Creole (1/4 cup)	25	4	1	0	340	free
Sauce, Hoisin (1 Tbsp)	35	7	<1	0	250	1/2 carb.
Sauce, Italian (1/4 cup)	30	4	2	0	300	1 fat
Sauce, Lemon (2 Tbsp)	40	10	<1	0	15	1/2 carb.
Sauce, Sweet & Sour Glaze (2 Tbsp)	50	12	0	0	260	1 carb.
Sauce, Sweet 'n Sour (2 Tbsp)	40	8	1	0	110	1/2 carb.
Sauce, Szechuan (1 Tbsp)	20	3	1	0	255	free

Sauce, Teriyaki (1 Tbsp)	20	4	<1	0	210	free
OLD EL PASO						
Enchilada Sauce, Green Chili (1/4 cup)	30	3	2	NA	330	1/2 fat
Enchilada Sauce, Mild (1/4 cup)	25	4	1	NA	160	free
Relish, Jalapeño (1 Tbsp)	5	1	0	0	110	free
Salsa, Green Chili, Medium (2 Tbsp)	10	2	0	0	110	free
Salsa, Homestyle, Mild (2 Tbsp)	5	1	0	0	110	free
Salsa, Picante, Hot (2 Tbsp)	10	2	0	0	230	free
Salsa, Picante, Medium (2 Tbsp)	10	2	0	0	230	free
Salsa, Picante, Mild (2 Tbsp)	10	2	0	0	230	free
Salsa, Pico de Gallo, Hot (2 Tbsp)	5	2	0	0	260	free
Salsa, Pico de Gallo, Medium (2 Tbsp)	5	2	0	0	260	free
Salsa Verde, Medium (2 Tbsp)	10	2	0	0	95	free
Taco Sauce, Extra Chunky, Medium (1 Tbsp)	5	1	0	0	80	free
Taco Sauce, Extra Chunky, Mild (1 Tbsp)	5	1	0	0	80	free
Taco Sauce, Hot (1 Tbsp)	5	1	0	0	90	free

SAUCES, CONDIMENTS, AND GRAVIES

Products	Cal.	Carb. (g)	Fat (g)	Sat. Fat (g)	Sodium (mg)	Exchanges
Taco Sauce, Medium (1 Tbsp)	5	1	0	0	70	free
Taco Sauce, Mild (1 Tbsp)	5	1	0	0	85	free
OPEN PIT						
BBQ Sauce, Hickory Flavor (2 Tbsp)	50	11	0	0	380	1 carb.
BBQ Sauce, Hot (2 Tbsp)	50	11	0	0	380	1 carb.
BBQ Sauce, Mesquite (2 Tbsp)	50	11	<1	0	440	1 carb.
BBQ Sauce, Onion Flavor (2 Tbsp)	50	11	0	0	480	1 carb.
BBQ Sauce, Original Flavor (2 Tbsp)	50	11	0	0	450	1 carb.
BBQ Sauce, Sweet & Sour (2 Tbsp)	45	10	0	0	420	1/2 carb.
BBQ Sauce, Sweet Flavor (2 Tbsp)	50	12	0	0	300	1 carb.
BBQ Sauce, Thick Tangy Onion (2 Tbsp)	50	12	0	0	380	1 carb.
BBQ Sauce, Thick Tangy Hickory (2 Tbsp)	50	12	0	0	390	1 carb.
BBQ Sauce, Thick Tangy Honey Spice (2 Tbsp)	45	11	0	0	340	1 carb.

ORTEGA

Enchilada Sauce (1/2 cup)	60	12	0	0	1040	1 carb.
Green Chiles, Strips (2)	10	3	0	0	25	free
Picante Sauce, Medium (2 Tbsp)	10	2	0	0	210	free
Picante Sauce, Mild (2 Tbsp)	10	2	0	0	210	free
Puree, Red Jalapeño (1/4 cup)	15	3	0	0	0	free
Taco Sauce, Thick & Smooth, Hot (1 Tbsp)	10	2	0	0	120	free
Taco Sauce, Thick & Smooth, Medium (1 Tbsp)	10	2	0	0	125	free
Taco Sauce, Thick & Smooth, Mild (1 Tbsp)	10	2	0	NA	125	free
Salsa, Dipping, Medium (2 Tbsp)	10	2	0	0	320	free
Salsa, Green Chile, Mild (2 Tbsp)	10	2	0	0	210	free
Sauce, Nacho Cheese (1/4 cup)	80	4	6	3	360	1 med-fat meat
Sauce/Puree, Green Chile (1/4 cup)	15	3	0	0	0	free
Sauce/Puree, Jalapeño (1/4 cup)	15	3	0	0	0	free
Sauce/Puree, Red Chile (1/4 cup)	15	3	0	0	0	free

SAUCES, CONDIMENTS, AND GRAVIES

Products	Cal.	Carb. (g)	Fat (g)	Sat. Fat (g)	Sodium (mg)	Exchanges
ORVAL KENT						
Pimento Spread (2 Tbsp)	130	3	12	2	280	2 fat
Salsa w/Green Chili, Spicy (2 Tbsp)	10	2	0	0	180	free
OSCAR MAYER						
Bacon Bits (1 Tbsp)	24	<1	1	<1	224	free
PANCHO VILLA						
Taco Sauce, Mild (2 Tbsp)	15	3	0	0	170	free
PILLSBURY						
Syrup, Pancake, Lite (1 Tbsp)	28	7	0	0	52	1/2 carb.
Syrup, Pancake, Regular (1 Tbsp)	52	13	0	0	23	1 carb.
PREGO						
Pizza Sauce, Traditional (1/4 cup)	40	6	2	0	230	1/2 carb.
Pizza Sauce w/Pepperoni Chunks (1/4 cup)	70	7	3	1	330	1/2 carb., 1 fat
Sauce, Marinara (1/2 cup)	110	12	6	2	670	1 carb., 1 fat

Spaghetti Sauce, Onion & Garlic (1/2 cup)	120	18	5	1	500	1 carb., 1 fat
Spaghetti Sauce, Three-Cheese (1/2 cup)	100	20	2	<1	480	1 carb.
Spaghetti Sauce, Tomato & Basil (1/2 cup)	110	19	3	<1	420	1 carb., 1 fat
Spaghetti Sauce, Traditional (1/2 cup)	150	22	6	2	640	1/2 carb., 1 fat
Spaghetti Sauce, Xtra Chunky, Garden Combination (1/2 cup)	90	16	1	<1	480	1 carb.
Spaghetti Sauce, Xtra Chunky, Garlic Cheese (1/2 cup)	130	22	4	1	610	1-1/2 carb., 1 fat
Spaghetti Sauce, Xtra Chunky, Mushroom Green Pepper (1/2 cup)	100	16	4	1	430	1 carb., 1 fat
Spaghetti Sauce, Xtra Chunky, Mushroom Onion (1/2 cup)	120	16	6	2	570	1 carb., 1 fat
Spaghetti Sauce, Xtra Chunky, Mushroom Spice (1/2 cup)	120	19	4	0	510	1 carb., 1 fat
Spaghetti Sauce, Xtra Chunky, Mushroom Supreme (1/2 cup)	130	21	5	<1	490	1-1/2 carb., 1 fat

SAUCES, CONDIMENTS, AND GRAVIES

Products	Cal.	Carb. (g)	Fat (g)	Sat. Fat (g)	Sodium (mg)	Exchanges
Spaghetti Sauce, Xtra Chunky, Mushroom Tomato (1/2 cup)	110	19	4	1	510	1 carb., 1 fat
Spaghetti Sauce, Xtra Chunky, Sausage Peppercorn (1/2 cup)	180	22	9	3	570	1-1/2 carb., 2 fat
Spaghetti Sauce, Xtra Chunky, Tomato Onion Garlic (1/2 cup)	120	17	6	2	550	1 carb., 1 fat
Spaghetti Sauce, Xtra Chunky, Zesty Basil (1/2 cup)	130	22	4	2	580	1-1/2 carb., 1 fat
Spaghetti Sauce, Xtra Chunky, Zesty Oregano (1/2 cup)	140	25	3	1	580	1-1/2 carb., 1 fat
Spaghetti Sauce Flavored w/Meat (1/2 cup)	160	23	6	2	700	1-1/2 carb., 1 fat
Spaghetti Sauce w/Mushrooms (1/2 cup)	150	20	5	2	500	1 carb., 1 fat
PROGRESSO						
Olives, Oil-Cured (6)	80	3	6	<1	330	1 fat
Pasta Sauce, Meat-Flavored (1/2 cup)	100	12	5	1	610	1 carb., 1 fat

Pizza Sauce (1/4 cup)	35	5	1	0	140	1/2 carb.
Salsa, Italian, Mild/Medium/Hot (2 Tbsp)	10	2	0	0	170	free
Sauce, Authentic Alfredo (1/2 cup)	310	5	27	15	670	1 med-fat meat, 4 fat
Sauce, Authentic Marinara (1/2 cup)	100	9	5	2	440	1/2 carb., 1 fat
Sauce, Authentic White Clam (1/2 cup)	90	2	7	2	470	1 med-fat meat
Sauce, Creamy Clam (1/2 cup)	100	8	6	2	560	1/2 carb., 1 fat
Sauce, Marinara (1/2 cup)	90	8	5	<1	480	1/2 carb., 1 fat
Sauce, Red Clam (1/2 cup)	80	8	3	<1	620	1/2 carb., 1 med-fat meat
Sauce, Rock Lobster (1/2 cup)	100	6	7	1	430	1/2 carb., 1 fat
Sauce, White Clam (1/2 cup)	120	1	9	2	310	1 med-fat meat, 1 fat
Spaghetti Sauce (1/2 cup)	100	12	5	1	620	1 carb., 1 fat
Spaghetti Sauce, Mushroom (1/2 cup)	100	12	5	1	580	1 carb., 1 fat

QUE BUENO

Enchilada Sauce (1/2 cup)	60	8	2	0	320	1/2 carb.
Salsa, Chunky (1 Tbsp)	5	<1	0	0	70	free
Salsa w/Green Chiles (1 Tbsp)	5	<1	0	0	80	free

SAUCES, CONDIMENTS, AND GRAVIES

Products	Cal.	Carb. (g)	Fat (g)	Sat. Fat (g)	Sodium (mg)	Exchanges
Sauce, Jalapeño Cheese (2 Tbsp)	33	3	2	<1	248	1/2 fat
Sauce, Nacho Cheese (1/2 cup)	72	10	3	2	496	1/2 carb., 1 fat
Sauce, Picante (1 Tbsp)	5	1	0	0	130	free
Taco Sauce (2 Tbsp)	15	3	0	0	130	free
REGINA						
Cooking Wine, Burgundy (2 Tbsp)	20	3	0	0	360	free
Cooking Wine, Sherry (2 Tbsp)	35	5	0	0	360	1/2 carb.
Vinegar, Red Wine, 50-grain (1 Tbsp)	0	1	0	0	0	free
Vinegar, Red Wine, 100-grain (1 Tbsp)	5	2	0	0	0	free
Vinegar, White Wine, 100-grain (1 Tbsp)	5	1	0	0		free
ROSARITA						
Enchilada Sauce, Mild (1/2 cup)	46	6	2	<1	818	1/2 carb.
Green Chilies, Diced (2 Tbsp)	6	1	<1	0	85	free
Jalapeños, Diced (2 Tbsp)	5	<1	<1	0	121	free

Jalapeños, Nacho Sliced (2 Tbsp)	4	1	0	0	448	free
Salsa, Extra Chunky, Medium (2 Tbsp)	7	1	<1	0	229	free
Salsa, Green Tomatillo, Medium (2 Tbsp)	9	2	0	0	188	free
Salsa, Roasted, Mild (2 Tbsp)	10	2	<1	0	233	free
Salsa, Traditional, Medium (2 Tbsp)	7	2	<1	0	234	free
Sauce, Zesty Jalapeño Picante, Medium (2 Tbsp)	9	2	<1	0	254	free
SIMMER CHEF						
Sauce, Creamy Mushroom Herb (1/2 cup)	90	9	5	2	670	1/2 carb., 1 fat
Sauce, Family-Style Stroganoff (1/2 cup)	100	8	6	2	740	1/2 carb., 1 fat
Sauce, Golden Honey Mustard (1/2 cup)	150	30	2	0	400	2 carb.
Sauce, Hearty Onion Mushroom (1/2 cup)	50	9	1	0	670	1/2 carb.
Sauce, Old Country Cacciatore (1/2 cup)	90	13	4	<1	400	1 carb., 1 fat
Sauce, Oriental Sweet & Sour (1/2 cup)	110	25	1	0	340	1-1/2 carb.
Sauce, Zesty Tomato Mexicali (1/2 cup)	80	15	2	<1	390	1 carb.
TABASCO						
Sauce, Pepper (1 Tbsp)	2	<1	<1	<1	93	free

SAUCES, CONDIMENTS, AND GRAVIES

Products	Cal.	Carb. (g)	Fat (g)	Sat. Fat (g)	Sodium (mg)	Exchanges
TOSTITOS						
Sauce, Picante (1/2 cup)	53	10	<1	<1	640	1/2 carb.
WEIGHT WATCHERS						
Pasta Sauce w/Mushrooms (1/2 cup)	60	11	0	0	420	1 carb.

SNACK FOODS

Products	Cal.	Carb. (g)	Fat (g)	Sat. Fat (g)	Sodium (mg)	Exchanges
Chips, Bagel (5)	298	52	7	1	419	3-1/2 strch, 1 fat
Chips, Yogurt (1 oz)	146	16	8	2	13	1 strch, 2 fat
Combos, Cheddar Pretzels Snacks (10)	143	20	6	NA	335	1 strch, 1 fat
Cracker Crumbs, Graham (1/2 cup)	254	46	6	1	363	3 strch, 1 fat
Crackers, Animal (8)	89	15	3	<1	79	1 strch, 1 fat
Crackers, Graham (3)	89	16	2	<1	127	1 strch
Crackers, Matzoh, Plain (3/4 oz)	83	18	<1	<1	0	1 strch
Crackers, Matzoh, Whole-Wheat (1)	100	22	<1	<1	<1	1-1/2 strch
Crackers, Norwegian Flatbread (5)	106	24	<1	<1	77	1-1/2 strch
Crackers, Rye Crispbread (2)	59	13	<1	<1	150	1 strch
Crispbread, Rye (1)	37	8	<1	<1	26	1/2 strch
Melba Toast (2)	40	8	1	1	84	1/2 strch

SNACK FOODS

Products	Cal.	Carb. (g)	Fat (g)	Sat. Fat (g)	Sodium (mg)	Exchanges
Oriental Snack Mix (1 oz)	155	9	12	5	235	1/2 strch, 2 fat
Popcorn, Air-Popped (1 cup)	31	6	<1	<1	<1	1/2 strch
Popcorn, Carmel (1 cup)	152	28	5	1	73	1 strch, 1 fat
Popcorn, Cheese (1 cup)	58	6	4	<1	98	1/2 strch, 1 fat
Popcorn, Oil-Popped, Salted (1 cup)	55	6	3	<1	97	1/2 strch, 1 fat
Popcorn Cakes (2)	76	16	<1	<1	58	1 strch
Pretzel Twists, Hard, Unsalted	229	47.5	2.1	.45	173	3 strch
Pretzels, Whole-Wheat (1 oz)	103	23	<1	<1	58	1-1/2 strch
Pretzels, Yogurt-Covered (2)	39	6	2	1	5	1/2 strch
Rice Cakes, Brown, Plain (1)	35	7	<1	<1	29	1/2 strch
Rice Cakes, Brown, Sesame Seed (2 cakes)	71	15	<1	<1	41	1 strch
Rice Krispies Bar (1)	109	21	3	<1	141	1-1/2 strch, 1 fat
Trail Mix (1/4 cup)	173	17	11	2	86	1 strch, 2 fat

BETTY CROCKER

Dunk Aroos (1 tray)	120	21	4	1	55	1-1/2 carb., 1 fat
Fruit By The Foot (1 roll)	80	17	2	<1	45	1 carb.
Fruit By The Foot, Cherry (1 oz)	105	23	2	<1	56	1-1/2 carb.
Fruit By The Foot, Grape (1 oz)	105	23	2	<1	56	1-1/2 carb.
Fruit By The Foot, Strawberry (1 oz)	104	22	2	<1	55	1-1/2 carb.
Fruit Gushers (1 pouch)	90	20	1	0	45	1 carb.
Fruit Roll-Ups (2)	110	24	1	0	105	1-1/2 carb.
Fruit Roll-Ups, Cherry (1)	53	12	<1	<1	40	1 carb.
Fruit Roll-Ups, Crazy Colors (1)	52	12	<1	<1	51	1 carb.
Fruit Roll-Ups, Grape (1)	53	12	<1	<1	58	1 carb.
Fruit Roll-Ups, Hot Colors (1)	53	12	<1	<1	51	1 carb.
Fruit Roll-Ups, Strawberry (1)	52	12	<1	<1	49	1 carb.
Fruit String Ling (1 pouch)	80	17	1	0	45	1 carb.

CARNATION

Breakfast Bar, Chewy Chocolate Chip (1)	150	24	6	2	80	1-1/2 carb. 1 fat

SNACK FOODS

Products	Cal.	Carb. (g)	Fat (g)	Sat. Fat (g)	Sodium (mg)	Exchanges
Breakfast Bar, Chewy Peanut Butter Chocolate Chip (1)	150	22	5	2	85	1-1/2 carb., 1 fat
Breakfast Bar, Chocolate Chunk Granola (1)	130	26	3	1	40	2 carb., 1 fat
Breakfast Bar, Honey & Oats Granola (1)	130	26	3	<1	45	2 carb., 1 fat
CRACKER JACKS						
Cracker Jacks (2/3 cup)	113	23	2	<1	84	1-1/2 carb.
Fat-Free Butter Toffee (1 cup)	110	26	0	0	95	2 carb.
Fat-Free Original (1 cup)	110	26	0	0	85	2 carb.
Original (2/3 cup)	110	23	2	0	90	1-1/2 carb.
DEL MONTE						
Trail Mix, Sierra (1/4 cup)	150	20	8	3	65	1 strch, 1 high-fat meat
Yogurt Raisins, Strawberry (0.9-oz bag)	110	20	3	3	25	1 carb., 1 fat
Yogurt Raisins, Vanilla (0.9-oz bag)	110	20	3	3	25	1 carb., 1 fat
ESTEE						
Crackers, Unsalted (5 pieces)	70	11	2	<1	20	1 strch

Fruit & Nut Mix (1/4 cup)	210	19	12	7	45	1 fruit, 1 high-fat meat, 1 fat
Pretzel Nuggets, Original (30)	120	24	2	0	180	1-1/2 strch
Pretzel Nuggets, Ranch (23)	130	24	2	<1	240	1-1/2 strch
Pretzels, Unsalted Dutch (2)	130	26	1	0	40	2 strch
Pretzels, Unsalted (23)	120	25	1	0	30	1-1/2 strch
Raisins, Chocolate-Coated (1/4 cup)	180	27	6	5	45	2 carb., 1 fat
Snack Crisps, Apple Cinnamon (1 bag)	90	16	2	0	70	1 strch
Snack Crisps, Chocolate (1 bag)	90	15	2	0	70	1 strch
Snack Crisps, Lemon (1 bag)	90	16	2	0	70	1 strch
Snack Crisps, Ranch (1 bag)	90	15	2	0	135	1 strch
FEATHERWEIGHT						
Granola Bar, High-Fiber Yogurt-Coated (1)	96	19	3	<1	6	1 carb., 1 fat
FRANKLIN						
Crunch 'N Munch (2/3 cup)	140	24	4	1	160	1-1/2 carb., 1 fat
Crunch 'N Munch, Fat-Free (3/4 cup)	110	26	0	0	190	2 carb.

SNACK FOODS

Products	Cal.	Carb. (g)	Fat (g)	Sat. Fat (g)	Sodium (mg)	Exchanges
FRITO-LAY						
Cereal Bar, Grandma's Fat-Free, Apple (1)	160	38	0	0	135	2-1/2 carb.
Cereal Bar, Grandma's Fat-Free, Strawberry (1)	160	39	0	0	140	2-1/2 carb.
Cheetos, Cheesy Checkers (1 oz)	150	15	10	3	350	1 strch, 2 fat
Cheetos, Crunchy (1 oz)	150	16	9	2	300	1 strch, 2 fat
Cheetos, Curls (1 oz)	150	16	9	3	280	1 strch, 2 fat
Cheetos, Flamin' Hot (1 oz)	160	16	9	2	240	1 strch, 2 fat
Cheetos, Puffed Balls (1 oz)	160	13	10	3	370	1 strch, 2 fat
Cheetos, Puffs (1 oz)	160	15	10	3	370	1 strch, 2 fat
Chips, Santitas 100% White Corn (1 oz)	140	19	6	1	75	1 strch, 1 fat
Chips, Santitas Restaurant-Style Tortilla (1 oz)	140	19	6	1	75	1 strch, 1 fat
Cracker Snacks, Cheddars (1 pkg)	220	27	10	3	530	2 strch, 2 fat
Crackers, Cheese Peanut Butter (1 pkg)	200	22	10	2	400	1-1/2 strch, 2 fat
Crackers, Jalapeño Cheddar (1 pkg)	200	24	10	3	470	1-1/2 strch, 2 fat

Food	Cal.	Carb.	Fat		Sod.	Exchanges
Crackers, Toast Peanut Butter (1 pkg)	190	23	9	2	380	1-1/2 strch, 2 fat
Crackers, Wheat Cheese (1 pkg)	200	24	9	2	430	1-1/2 strch, 2 fat
Doritos, Chester's Cheese (1 oz)	140	18	7	2	160	1 strch, 1 fat
Doritos, Cooler Ranch (1 oz)	140	18	7	1	160	1 strch, 1 fat
Doritos, Dunker's (1 oz)	140	19	6	1	80	1 strch, 1 fat
Doritos, Flamin Hot (1 oz)	140	17	8	1	270	1 strch, 2 fat
Doritos, Pizza Cravers (1 oz)	140	18	7	2	170	1 strch, 1 fat
Doritos, Reduced-Fat Cooler Ranch (1 oz).	130	18	5	1	200	1 strch, 1 fat
Doritos, Reduced-Fat Nacho Cheesier (1 oz)	130	19	5	1	210	1 strch, 1 fat
Doritos, Taco Bell Taco Supreme (1 oz)	140	18	7	2	200	1 strch, 1 fat
Doritos, Toasted Corn (1 oz)	140	19	6	1	65	1 strch, 1 fat
Fritos, BBQ (1 oz)	150	16	9	2	310	1 strch, 2 fat
Fritos, Chili Cheese (1 oz)	160	15	10	2	260	1 strch, 2 fat
Fritos, King Size (1 oz)	160	15	10	2	150	1 strch, 2 fat
Fritos, Original (1 oz)	160	15	10	2	170	1 strch, 2 fat
Fritos, Scoops (1 oz)	150	16	9	2	135	1 strch, 2 fat

SNACK FOODS

Products	Cal.	Carb. (g)	Fat (g)	Sat. Fat (g)	Sodium (mg)	Exchanges
Fritos, Wild N' Mild (1 oz)	160	15	10	2	170	1 strch, 2 fat
Funyuns (1 oz)	140	18	7	2	250	1 strch, 1 fat
Munchos (1 oz)	150	18	10	3	270	1 strch, 2 fat
Munchos, BBQ (1 oz)	160	15	10	2	250	1 strch, 2 fat
Popcorn, Chester's Butter (3 cups)	160	15	12	2	330	1 strch, 2 fat
Popcorn, Chester's Carmel Craze (3/4 cup)	130	27	2	0	220	2 strch
Popcorn, Chester's Cheddar Cheese (3 cups)	190	17	13	3	300	1 strch, 3 fat
Popcorn, Chester's Microwave Butter (5 cups)	200	22	12	2	300	1-1/2 strch, 2 fat
Popcorn, Chester's Triple Mix (1-1/2 cup)	140	19	6	1	240	1 strch, 1 fat
Popcorn, Smartfood Butter (3 cup)	150	15	9	2	240	1 strch, 2 fat
Popcorn, Smartfood Butter, Reduced-Fat (3-1/3 cups)	130	21	4	<1	410	1-1/2 strch, 1 fat
Popcorn, Smartfood Toffee Crunch, Low-Fat (3/4 cup)	130	28	1	0	250	2 strch
Popcorn, Smartfood White Cheddar Cheese (2 cups)	190	17	12	3	310	1 strch, 2 fat

Food	Cal.					Exchanges
Popcorn, Smartfood White Cheddar Cheese, Reduced-Fat (3 cups)	140	19	6	2	280	1 strch, 1 fat
Pork Rind, Baken-ets Fried, Hot N' Spicy (7)	70	<1	5	2	440	1 med-fat meat
Pork Rind, Baken-ets Fried, Hot V' Spicy Cracklins (8)	80	<1	5	2	370	1 med-fat meat
Pork Rind, Baken-ets Fried, Regular (9)	80	<1	5	2	330	1 med-fat meat
Pork Rind, Baken-ets Fried, Regular Cracklins (8)	50	<1	6	2	550	1 med-fat meat
Potato Chips, Lay's Baked BBQ (1 oz)	110	23	2	0	220	1-1/2 strch
Potato Chips, Lay's Baked Original (1 oz)	110	23	2	0	150	1-1/2 strch
Potato Chips, Lay's Baked Sour Cream & Onion (1 oz)	110	23	2	0	170	1-1/2 strch
Potato Chips, Lay's Flamin' Hot (1 oz)	150	15	10	3	180	1 strch, 2 fat
Potato Chips, Lay's Hickory BBQ (1 oz)	150	15	10	2	220	1 strch, 2 fat
Potato Chips, Lay's K.C. Masterpiece B.B.Q (1 oz)	150	15	9	3	270	1 strch, 2 fat
Potato Chips, Lay's Onion & Garlic (1 oz)	150	16	9	3	200	1 strch, 2 fat
Potato Chips, Lay's Original (1 oz)	150	15	10	3	120	1 strch, 2 fat
Potato Chips, Lay's Salsa & Cheese (1 oz)	160	19	9	3	180	1 strch, 2 fat
Potato Chips, Lay's Salt & Vinegar (1 oz)	160	15	10	3	340	1 strch, 2 fat

SNACK FOODS

Products	Cal.	Carb. (g)	Fat (g)	Sat. Fat (g)	Sodium (mg)	Exchanges
Potato Chips, Lay's Sour Cream & Onion (1 oz)	160	15	9	9	180	1 strch, 2 fat
Potato Chips, Lay's Wavy Hidden Valley Ranch (1 oz)	160	14	11	3	150	1 strch, 2 fat
Potato Chips, Lay's Wavy Original (1 oz)	160	15	10	3	120	1 strch, 2 fat
Potato Chips, Ruffles Cheddar & Sour Cream (1 oz)	160	15	10	3	230	1 strch, 2 fat
Potato Chips, Ruffles French Onion (1 oz)	150	15	10	3	180	1 strch, 2 fat
Potato Chips, Ruffles Golden Dijon (1 oz)	150	16	9	3	190	1 strch, 2 fat
Potato Chips, Ruffles K.C. Masterpiece Mesquite BBQ (1 oz)	150	15	9	3	120	1 strch, 2 fat
Potato Chips, Ruffles Original (1 oz)	150	14	10	3	125	1 strch, 2 fat
Potato Chips, Ruffles Ranch (1 oz)	150	15	9	3	280	1 strch, 2 fat
Potato Chips, Ruffles Reduced-Fat Regular (1 oz)	140	18	7	1	130	1 strch, 1 fat
Potato Chips, Ruffles Reduced-Fat Sour Cream & Onion (1 oz)	130	18	6	1	200	1 strch, 1 fat
Pretzels, Rold Gold Bavarian (1 oz)	110	21	2	<1	440	1-1/2 strch

Food	Cal.	Carb. (g)	Fat (g)	Sat. Fat (g)	Chol. (mg)	Sod. (mg)	Exchanges/Choices
Pretzels, Rold Gold Fat-Free Sticks (1 oz)	110	23	0	0		530	1-1/2 strch
Pretzels, Rold Gold Thins (1 oz)	110	23	0	0		520	1-1/2 strch
Pretzels, Rold Gold Tiny Twists (1 oz)	100	23	0	0		420	1-1/2 strch
Pretzels, Rold Gold Rods (1 oz)	110	22	2	2		370	1-1/2 strch
Snack Bars, Grandma's, Fudge Chocolate Chip (1)	190	29	7	3	<1	160	2 carb, 1 fat
Snack Bars, Grandma's, Oatmeal Apple Spice (1)	210	24	10	3		150	1-1/2 carb., 2 fat
Sunchips, French Onion (1 oz)	140	18	7	1		115	1 strch, 1 fat
Sunchips, Harvest Cheddar (1 oz)	140	18	7	1		180	1 strch, 1 fat
Sunchips, Original (1 oz)	140	18	7	1		160	1 strch, 1 fat
Tostitos, Baked Cool Ranch (1 oz)	120	21	3	0		170	1-1/2 strch, 1 fat
Tostitos, Baked Original (1 oz)	110	24	1	1		200	1-1/2 strch
Tostitos, Baked Unsalted (1 oz)	110	24	1	0		0	1-1/2 strch
Tostitos, Bite Size (1 oz)	140	17	8	1		110	1 strch, 2 fat
Tostitos, Crispy Rounds (1 oz)	150	17	8	1		85	1 strch, 2 fat
Tostitos, Lime N' Chili (1 oz)	150	17	7	1		180	1 strch, 1 fat
Tostitos, Restaurant-Style (1 oz)	130	19	6	1		80	1 strch, 1 fat

SNACK FOODS

Products	Cal.	Carb. (g)	Fat (g)	Sat. Fat (g)	Sodium (mg)	Exchanges
Tostitos, Sante Fe Gold (1 oz)	140	19	6	1	80	1 strch, 1 fat
Tostitos, Unsalted Restaurant-Style (1 oz)	140	18	8	1	10	1 strch, 2 fat
GARDETTO'S						
Pretzel Mix (1/2 cup)	120	23	2	0	170	1-1/2 strch
Snack Mix, Chips & Twists, Sour Cream & Chive (1/2 cup)	170	18	10	2	300	1 strch, 2 fat
Snack Mix, Snak-ens, Original (1/2 cup)	180	18	10	2	380	1 strch, 2 fat
GENERAL MILLS						
Bugles (1 oz)	145	18	8	7	290	1 strch, 2 fat
Bugles, Nacho Cheese (1 oz)	152	16	9	8	270	1 strch, 2 fat
HEALTH VALLEY						
Caramel Corn Puffs, Fat-Free (1 oz)	104	23	0	0	57	1-1/2 carb.
Caramel Corn Puffs, Fat-Free Apple Cinnamon (1 cup)	110	24	0	0	60	1-1/2 carb.

Caramel Corn Puffs, Fat-Free Original (1 cup)	110	24	0	0	60	1-1/2 carb.
Cheese Flavor Puffs, Fat-Free Original (1 cup)	73	15	0	0	173	1 strch
Cheese Puffs, Fat-Free (1 oz)	104	22	0	0	246	1-1/2 strch
Cheese Puffs, Fat-Free Original (1-1/2 cup)	110	23	0	0	260	1-1/2 strch
Cheese Puffs, Fat-Free Zesty Chili (1 oz)	104	22	0	0	246	1-1/2 strch
Crackers, Fat-Free Amaranth Graham (8)	100	23	0	0	30	1-1/2 strch
Crackers, Fat-Free Fire, Hot 3-Chili Cheese (6)	50	11	0	0	80	1 strch
Crackers, Fat-Free Fire, Medium Jalapeño Cheese (6)	50	11	0	0	80	1 strch
Crackers, Fat-Free Fire, Mild Chili Cheese (6)	50	11	0	0	80	1 strch
Crackers, Fat-Free Healthy Pizza, Cheese (6)	50	11	0	0	140	1 strch
Crackers, Fat-Free Healthy Pizza, Garlic (6)	50	11	0	0	140	1 strch
Crackers, Fat-Free Oat Bran Graham (8)	100	23	0	0	30	1-1/2 strch
Crackers, Fat-Free Whole-Wheat (5)	50	11	0	0	80	1 strch
Crackers, Fat-Free Whole-Wheat, Cheese (5)	50	11	0	0	80	1 strch
Crackers, Fat-Free Whole-Wheat, Herb (5)	50	11	0	0	80	1 strch
Crisp Rice Bar, Fat-Free Apple Raisin (1)	110	26	0	0	5	1-1/2 carb.

SNACK FOODS

Products	Cal.	Carb. (g)	Fat (g)	Sat. Fat (g)	Sodium (mg)	Exchanges
Crisp Rice Bar, Fat-Free Orange Date (1)	110	26	0	0	5	2 carb.
Crisp Rice Bar, Fat-Free Tropical Fruit (1)	110	26	0	0	5	2 carb.
Granola Bar, Fat-Free Blueberry (1)	140	35	0	0	5	2 carb.
Granola Bar, Fat-Free Date Almond (1)	140	35	0	0	5	2 carb.
Granola Bar, Fat-Free Raisin (1)	140	35	0	0	5	2 carb.
KEEBLER						
Cracker Sandwiches, Cheese & Peanut Butter (1 pkg)	190	22	9	2	420	1-1/2 strch, 2 fat
Cracker Sandwiches, Club & Cheddar (1 pkg)	190	20	11	3	320	1 strch, 2 fat
Cracker Sandwiches, Toast & Peanut Butter (1 pkg)	190	23	9	2	300	1-1/2 strch, 2 fat
Cracker Sandwiches, Town House & Cheddar (1 pkg)	200	19	13	3	300	1 strch, 3 fat
Crackers, Club, 33% Reduced-Fat (5)	70	12	2	0	200	1 strch
Crackers, Club Partners, 50% Reduced-Sodium (4)	70	9	3	1	80	1/2 strch, 1 fat
Crackers, Club Partners, Original (4)	70	9	3	1	160	1/2 strch, 1 fat
Crackers, Toasteds Complements, Buttercrisp (9)	140	19	7	2	280	1 strch, 1 fat

	Cal	Carb	Fat	Sat Fat	Sodium	Exchanges
Crackers, Toasteds Complements, Onion (9)	140	19	6	1	310	1 strch, 1 fat
Crackers, Toasteds Complements, Sesame (9)	140	19	6	1	320	1 strch, 1 fat
Crackers, Toasteds Complements, Wheat (9)	140	19	6	2	270	1 strch, 1 fat
Crackers, Town House (5)	80	9	5	1	150	1/2 strch, 1 fat
Crackers, Town House, 50% Reduced-Sodium (5)	80	10	5	1	75	1/2 strch, 1 fat
Crackers, Town House, Reduced-Fat (6)	70	11	2	<1	180	1 strch
Crackers, Town House, Wheat (5)	80	10	4	1	140	1/2 strch, 1 fat
Crackers, Zesta Saltines, 50% Reduced-Sodium (5)	60	11	2	<1	95	1 strch
Crackers, Zesta Saltines, Fat-Free (5)	50	11	0	0	90	1 strch
Crackers, Zesta Saltines, Original (5)	60	10	2	<1	190	1 strch
Crackers, Zesta Saltines, Unsalted Tops (5)	70	10	2	<1	90	1 strch
Crackers, Zesta Soup & Oyster (42)	70	10	3	1	160	1/2 strch, 1 fat
Crisp, Low-Fat Cinnamon (8)	110	24	2	<1	190	1-1/2 strch
Graham Selects, Original (8)	130	23	3	1	135	1-1/2 strch, 1 fat
Graham Selects, Honey (8)	150	21	6	2	140	1-1/2 strch, 1 fat
Graham Selects, Low-Fat French Vanilla (8)	110	24	2	<1	90	1-1/2 strch

SNACK FOODS

Products	Cal.	Carb. (g)	Fat (g)	Sat. Fat (g)	Sodium (mg)	Exchanges
Munch'ems, 33% Reduced-Fat, Chili Cheese (28)	130	23	4	2	470	1-1/2 strch, 1 fat
Munch'ems, 33% Reduced-Fat, Salsa (28)	130	23	4	1	290	1-1/2 strch, 1 fat
Munch'ems, 55% Reduced-Fat, Cheddar (30)	130	21	4	1	330	1-1/2 strch, 1 fat
Munch'ems, 55% Reduced-Fat, Original (35)	130	21	4	<1	450	1-1/2 strch, 1 fat
Munch'ems, 55% Reduced-Fat, Ranch (33)	130	21	4	<1	310	1-1/2 strch, 1 fat
Munch'ems, 55% Reduced-Fat, Sour Cream & Onion (33)	130	22	4	<1	390	1-1/2 strch, 1 fat
Munch'ems, Seasoned Original (30)	130	20	5	1	350	1 strch, 1 fat
Toasteds, Reduced-Fat Sesame (10)	120	21	3	<1	310	1-1/2 strch, 1 fat
Toasteds, Reduced-Fat Wheat (10)	120	22	3	1	300	1-1/2 strch, 1 fat
Wheatables, 30% Reduced-Fat, French Onion (27)	130	21	4	1	320	1-1/2 strch, 1 fat
Wheatables, 30% Reduced-Fat, Ranch (29)	130	21	4	1	340	1-1/2 strch, 1 fat
Wheatables, 30% Reduced-Fat, White Cheddar (27)	130	21	4	1	330	1-1/2 strch, 1 fat
Wheatables, 50% Reduced-Fat (29)	130	21	4	1	320	1-1/2 strch, 1 fat

Food	Cal.	Carb.	Fat	Sat. Fat	Sod.	Exchanges
Wheatables, Original (26)	150	18	7	2	320	1 strch, 1 fat
KELLOGG'S						
Nutri-Grain Bar, Apple (1)	150	25	5	1	65	1-1/2 carb., 1 fat
Nutri-Grain Bar, Blueberry (1)	150	25	5	1	65	1-1/2 carb., 1 fat
Nutri-Grain Bar, Raspberry (1)	150	25	5	1	65	1-1/2 carb., 1 fat
Nutri-Grain Bar, Strawberry (1)	150	25	5	1	65	1-1/2 carb., 1 fat
KRAFT						
Handi-Snacks, Cheez 'n Breadsticks (1 pkg)	130	11	7	4	340	1 strch, 1 fat
Handi-Snacks, Cheez 'n Crackers (1 pkg)	130	10	8	5	340	1/2 strch, 2 fat
Handi-Snacks, Cheez 'n Pretzels (1 pkg)	110	11	6	4	420	1 strch, 1 fat
Handi-Snacks, Mozzarella String Cheese (1 pkg)	80	<1	6	4	240	1 med-fat meat
Handi-Snacks, Peanut Butter'n Cracker (1)	180	12	12	3	150	1 strch, 2 fat
Handi-Snacks Peanut Butter'n Graham (1 pkg)	170	14	10	3	130	1 strch, 2 fat
M&M MARS						
Granola Bars, Kudos Chocolate Chip (1)	120	20	5	3	70	1 carb., 1 fat
Granola Bars, Kudos Peanut Butter (1)	130	19	5	2	80	1 carb., 1 fat

SNACK FOODS

Products	Cal.	Carb. (g)	Fat (g)	Sat. Fat (g)	Sodium (mg)	Exchanges
MEDICAL FOODS						
Nite Bite, Chocolate Fudge (1)	100	15	4	1	40	1 carb., 1/2 fat
Nite Bite, Peanut Butter (1)	100	15	4	1	80	1 carb., 1/2 fat
NABISCO						
Air Crisps, Ritz (24)	140	22	5	1	250	1-1/2 strch, 1 fat
Air Crisps, Wheat Thins (24)	130	21	5	1	290	1-1/2 strch, 1 fat
Arrowroot Biscuits, National (6)	120	18	3	<1	60	1 strch, 1 fat
Better Cheddars (22)	150	17	8	2	290	1 strch, 2 fat
Better Cheddars, Reduced-Fat (24)	140	19	6	2	350	1 strch, 1 fat
Cereal Bar, Snackwell's Blueberry (1)	120	29	0	0	110	2 carb.
Cereal Bar, Snackwell's Strawberry (1)	120	29	0	0	105	2 carb.
Cheese Nips (29)	150	18	6	2	310	1 strch, 1 fat
Cheese Nips, Reduced-Fat (31)	130	21	4	1	310	1 strch, 1 fat
Chicken-In-A-Biskit (14)	160	17	9	2	270	1 strch, 2 fat

Food	Cal.	Carb.	Fat		Sodium	Exchanges
Crackers, Barnum's Animal (10)	120	22	4	<1	140	1-1/2 strch, 1 fat
Crackers, American Classic (4)	70	9	3	<1	160	1/2 strch, 1 fat
Crackers, Honey Maid Cinnamon Graham (8)	120	24	2	<1	170	1-1/2 strch
Crackers, Honey Maid Graham (2)	60	11	2	0	110	1 strch
Crackers, Honey Maid Honey Graham (8)	120	22	2	<1	180	1-1/2 carb.
Crackers, Honey Maid Plain Graham (8)	120	22	2	<1	180	1-1/2 carb.
Crackers, Premium Saltine (4)	50	8	2	<1	200	1/2 strch
Crackers, Premium Saltine, Unsalted Tops (4)	50	8	1	0	100	1/2 strch
Crackers, Ritz (10)	151	18	8	2	254	1 strch, 2 fat
Crackers, Ritz Bits (24)	80	9	5	<1	130	1/2 strch, 1 fat
Crackers, Ritz Bits Cheese (24)	80	9	4	<1	140	1/2 strch, 1 fat
Crackers, Snackwell's Classic Golden (6)	60	11	1	0	140	1 strch
Crackers, Snackwell's Fat-Free Cracked Pepper (7)	60	13	0	0	150	1 strch
Crackers, Snackwell's Fat-Free Wheat (7)	60	12	<1	<1	169	1 strch
Crackers, Snackwell's French Onion (32)	120	24	2	0	290	1-1/2 strch
Crackers, Snackwell's Salsa Cheddar (32)	120	23	2	0	340	1-1/2 strch

SNACK FOODS

Products	Cal.	Carb. (g)	Fat (g)	Sat. Fat (g)	Sodium (mg)	Exchanges
Crackers, Snackwell's Wheat (5)	60	12	0	0	170	1 strch
Crackers, Snackwell's Zesty Cheese (32)	120	23	2	<1	330	1-1/2 strch
Crackers, Swiss Cheese (15)	140	18	7	2	350	1 strch, 1 fat
Crackers, Triscuits (7)	150	21	6	1	160	1-1/2 strch, 1 fat
Crackers, Triscuits, Wheat 'n Bran (3)	48	8	2	<1	65	1/2 strch
Crackers, Wheat Thins, Original (16)	140	19	6	1	170	1 strch, 1 fat
Crackers, Wheat Thins, Reduced-Fat (18)	120	21	4	<1	220	1-1/2 strch, 1 fat
Granola Bar, Snackwell's Carmel (1)	110	22	3	3	40	1-1/2 carb., 1 fat
Granola Bar, Snackwell's Original (1)	110	22	3	3	40	1-1/2 carb., 1 fat
Harvest Crisps, 5-Grain (13)	130	23	4	<1	340	1-1/2 strch, 1 fat
Pretzel Twists, Mister Salty (7)	120	23	2	0	810	1-1/2 strch
Sandwiches w/Cheese, Ritz Bitz (14)	170	16	10	3	300	1 strch, 2 fat
Sandwiches w/Peanut Butter, Ritz Bitz (14)	150	18	8	2	200	1 strch, 2 fat
Snack Mix, Doo Dads (1/2 cup)	130	19	6	1	361	1 strch, 1 fat

Sociables (7)	80	9	4	<1	150	1/2 strch, 1 fat
NATURE VALLEY						
Granola Bars, Crunchy, Oats N' Honey (2)	200	35	6	1	170	2 carb, 1 fat
Granola Bars, Low-Fat Chewy (1)	110	21	2	0	65	1-1/2 strch
Granola Clusters (1)	140	24	5	2	48	1-1/2 strch, 1 fat
NESTLE						
Snack Bar, Sweet Success Chocolate Brownie (1)	120	23	4	2	45	1-1/2 carb, 1 fat
Snack Bar, Sweet Success Chocolate Chip (1)	120	23	4	2	40	1-1/2 carb., 1 fat
Snack Bar, Sweet Success Chocolate Peanut Butter (1)	120	23	4	2	35	1-1/2 carb., 1 fat
OLD EL PASO						
Tortilla Chips, Nachips (1 oz = 9 chips)	150	17	8	2	85	1 strch, 2 fat
Tortilla Chips, White Corn (1 oz = 11 chips)	140	16	8	1	60	1 strch, 2 fat
ORVILLE REDENBACHER'S						
Mini Popcorn Cake, Apple Cinnamon (11)	97	26	<1	<1	42	2 carb.
Mini Popcorn Cake, Butter (13)	99	23	2	<1	170	1-1/2 carb.

SNACK FOODS

Products	Cal.	Carb. (g)	Fat (g)	Sat. Fat (g)	Sodium (mg)	Exchanges
Mini Popcorn Cake, Carmel (11)	97	26	<1	<1	34	2 carb.
Mini Popcorn Cake, Honey Nut (11)	97	26	<1	<1	30	2 carb.
Mini Popcorn Cake, White Cheddar Cheese (13)	98	23	2	<1	98	1-1/2 carb.
Popcorn Cake, Butter (3)	113	26	2	<1	192	2 carb.
Popcorn Cake, Carmel (2)	84	23	<1	<1	29	1-1/2 carb.
Popcorn Cake, White Cheddar Cheese (3)	111	26	2	<1	111	2 carb.
PEPPERIDGE FARM						
Chips, Onion Multi-Grain Bagel (1 oz)	120	19	4	0	200	1 strch, 1 fat
Crackers, Butter-Flavored Thins (4)	71	10	3	1	97	1/2 strch, 1 fat
Crackers, Cracked Wheat (3)	108	14	4	2	230	1 strch, 1 fat
Crackers, Distinctive Assortment, Three (3)	60	9	3	0	90	1/2 strch, 1 fat
Crackers, English Wafer Biscuit (4)	72	13	2	0	97	1 strch
Crackers, Goldfish, Cheddar, LoSalt (1/2 cup)	71	9	3	<1	66	1/2 strch, 1 fat
Crackers, Goldfish, Cheddar Cheese (1/2 cup)	66	9	3	<1	95	1/2 strch, 1 fat

	Cal.	Carb.	Fat	Sat. Fat	Sod.	Exchanges/Choices
Crackers, Goldfish, Original (1/2 cup)	66	9	3	<1	109	1/2 strch, 1 fat
Crackers, Goldfish, Parmesan Cheese (1/2 cup)	66	9	2	<1	142	1/2 strch
Crackers, Goldfish, Pizza Flavor (1/2 cup)	66	9	3	<1	76	1/2 strch, 1 fat
Crackers, Goldfish, Pretzel Flavor (1/2 cup)	57	10	1	<1	204	1/2 strch
Crackers, Hearty Wheat (4)	104	13	5	0	130	1 strch, 1 fat
Crackers, Pretzel Distinctive (9)	130	23	3	0	440	1-1/2 strch, 1 fat
Crackers, Sesame (4)	95	12	3	0	128	1 strch, 1 fat
Crisps, Garlic Butter Crunch Baked Bread (1 oz)	140	16	8	2	230	1 strch, 2 fat
Crisps, Original Tortilla (1 oz)	130	18	6	1	290	1 strch, 1 fat
Crisps, Salsa Tortilla (1 oz)	130	18	7	1	350	1 strch, 1 fat
Crisps, Tortilla, Chili Cheese (1 oz)	130	18	7	1	340	1 strch, 1 fat
Snack Mix, Extra Nutty (1/2 cup)	180	20	9	2	330	1 strch, 2 fat
Snack Mix, Goldfish, Original (1/2 cup)	170	21	8	2	360	1-1/2 strch, 2 fat
Snack Mix, Goldfish, Zesty Cheddar (1/2 cup)	180	19	10	2	390	1 strch, 2 fat
Snack Mix, Honey Mustard & Onion (1/2 cup)	180	19	10	2	390	1 strch, 2 fat
Snack Mix, Lightly Seasoned (1/2 cup)	170	22	8	1	400	1-1/2 strch, 2 fat

SNACK FOODS

Products	Cal.	Carb. (g)	Fat (g)	Sat. Fat (g)	Sodium (mg)	Exchanges
Snack Sticks, Pumpernickel (9)	150	20	6	<1	340	1 strch, 1 fat
Snack Sticks, Sesame (9)	150	20	6	<1	340	1 strch, 1 fat
Snack Sticks, Three-Cheese (9)	140	20	5	2	410	1 strch, 1 fat
PLANTERS						
Fiddle Faddle (3/4 cup)	150	21	7	4	160	1-1/2 carb., 1 fat
Fiddle Faddle, Fat-Free (1 cup)	110	28	0	0	210	2 carb.
Fiddle Faddle, Reduced-Fat (1/2 cup)	110	24	1	0	200	1-1/2 carb.
QUAKER						
Granola Bars, Chewy, All Flavors, Low-Fat (1)	110	22	2	<1	100	1-1/2 carb.
Granola Bars, Chewy, Chocolate Chip (1)	120	21	4	2	70	1-1/2 carb., 1 fat
Granola Bars, Chewy, Peanut Butter & Chocolate Chip (1)	120	19	5	2	85	1 carb., 1 fat
Mini Popcorn Cakes, Butter Flavor (6)	50	11	<1	0	140	1 carb.
Mini Popcorn Cakes, Carmel (5)	50	12	<1	0	70	1 carb.

Mini Popcorn Cakes, Cheddar Cheese (6)	50	11	<1	0	200	1 carb.
Mini Popcorn Cakes, Lightly Salted (7)	50	11	<1	0	110	1 carb.
Mini Rice Cakes, Apple Cinnamon (5)	50	12	0	0	0	1 carb.
Mini Rice Cakes, Banana Nut (5)	50	12	0	0	25	1 carb.
Mini Rice Cakes, Carmel Corn (5)	50	12	0	0	25	1 carb.
Mini Rice Cakes, Honey Nut (5)	50	12	0	0	25	1 carb.
Mini Rice Cakes, Mini Chocolate Crunch (5)	50	12	0	0	10	1 carb.
Mini Rice Cakes, White Cheddar (6)	50	11	0	0	120	1 carb.
Rice Cakes, Apple Cinnamon (1)	50	11	0	0	0	1/2 carb.
Rice Cakes, Banana Nut (1)	50	11	0	0	45	1 carb.
Rice Cakes, Blueberry Crunch (1)	50	12	0	0	0	1 carb.
Rice Cakes, Butter Popped Corn (1)	35	7	0	0	45	1/2 carb.
Rice Cakes, Carmel Corn (1)	50	12	0	0	30	1 carb.
Rice Cakes, Chocolate Crunch (1)	50	11	0	0	10	1 carb.
Rice Cakes, Cinnamon Crunch (1)	50	11	0	0	25	1 carb.
Rice Cakes, Monterey Jack Corn (1)	40	8	0	0	80	1/2 carb.

SNACK FOODS

Products	Cal.	Carb. (g)	Fat (g)	Sat. Fat (g)	Sodium (mg)	Exchanges
Rice Cakes, Salt Free (1)	35	7	0	0	0	1 carb.
Rice Cakes, Salted (1)	35	7	0	0	15	1/2 carb.
Rice Cakes, Strawberry Crunch (1)	50	12	0	0	0	1 carb.
Rice Cakes, White Cheddar Corn (1)	40	8	0	0	90	1/2 carb.
RALSTON						
Party Mix, Chex, Homemade (2/3 cup)	120	19	5	<1	288	1 strch, 1 fat
Snack Mix, Chex, Bold & Zesty (1/2 cup)	160	17	7	2	390	1 strch, 1 fat
Snack Mix, Chex, Golden Cheddar Cheese (2/3 cup)	140	24	5	1	250	1-1/2 strch, 1 fat
Snack Mix, Chex, Traditional (2/3 cup)	130	22	4	1	280	1-1/2 strch, 1 fat
RY KRISP						
Crackers, Seasoned Rye (2)	60	10	2	0	90	1/2 strch
Crackers, Sesame Rye (2)	60	10	1.5	0	80	1/2 strch
SUNSHINE						
Cheez-its (10)	50	6	3	<1	100	1/2 strch, 1 fat

Crackers, Hi-Ho (4)	70	8	4	1	130	1/2 strch, 1 fat

WEIGHT WATCHERS

Sweet Success Chocolate Raspberry Bar (1)	120	23	4	2	35	1-1/2 carb., 1 fat
Sweet Success Oatmeal Raisin Bar (1)	120	23	4	2	30	1-1/2 carb., 1 fat

ZBAR

Chocolate Crunch (1)	110	22	3	0	95	1 strch, 1 fat

SOUPS AND STEWS

SOUPS AND STEWS

BANQUET

Products	Cal.	Carb. (g)	Fat (g)	Sat. Fat (g)	Sodium (mg)	Exchanges
Beef Stew (1 cup)	160	16	4	2	1110	1 strch, 1 med-fat meat
CAMPBELL'S, READY-TO-SERVE						
Chunky Beef Pasta (1 cup)	150	18	3	1	970	1 strch, 1 lean meat
Chunky Beef w/Country Vegetable (1 cup)	160	18	4	1	900	1 strch, 1 med-fat meat
Chunky Chicken Broccoli Cheese (1 cup)	250	17	15	6	1399	1 strch, 1 med-fat meat, 2 fat
Chunky Chicken Corn Chowder (1 cup)	250	18	15	7	870	1 strch, 1 med-fat meat, 2 fat
Chunky Chicken Mushroom Chowder (1 cup)	210	15	12	4	970	1 strch, 1 med-fat meat, 1 fat
Chunky Chicken Noodle w/Mushroom (1 cup)	140	15	5	2	830	1 strch, 1 med-fat meat
Chunky Chicken Nuggets w/Vegetable (1 cup)	150	19	5	2	830	1 strch, 1 med-fat meat
Chunky Chicken Rice (1 cup)	130	15	4	2	940	1 strch, 1 med-fat meat
Chunky Chicken Vegetable (1 cup)	90	11	2	<1	800	1 strch, 1 lean meat
Chunky Chili Beef w/Beans (1 cup)	230	30	6	2	850	2 strch, 1 med-fat meat

Item	Cal	Carb	Fat	Sat Fat	Sodium	Exchanges
Chunky Creamy Chicken w/Mushroom (1 cup)	210	12	17	8	1020	1 strch, 1 med-fat meat, 2 fat
Chunky Creole-Style Bean & Rice (1 cup)	210	27	8	3	720	2 strch, 1 med-fat meat, 1 fat
Chunky Manhattan Clam Chowder (1 cup)	130	20	4	1	900	1 strch, 1 fat
Chunky Mediterranean Vegetable (1 cup)	140	21	5	2	850	1-1/2 strch, 1 fat
Chunky Minestrone (1 cup)	140	22	5	2	800	1-1/2 strch, 1 fat
Chunky New England Clam Chowder (1 cup)	250	21	15	6	1079	1-1/2 strch, 1 med-fat meat, 2 fat
Chunky Old-Fashioned Chicken (1 cup)	130	12	3	2	950	1 strch, 1 lean meat
Chunky Old-Fashioned Vegetable (1 cup)	150	17	5	2	870	1 strch, 1 med-fat meat
Chunky Pepper Steak (1 cup)	140	18	3	1	830	1 strch, 1 lean meat
Chunky Potato Ham Chowder (1 cup)	220	16	14	8	840	1 strch, 3 fat
Chunky Sirloin Burger w/Vegetables (1 cup)	190	20	9	4	930	1 strch, 1 med-fat meat, 1 fat
Chunky Split Pea n'Ham (1 cup)	190	27	3	1	1119	2 strch, 1 lean meat
Chunky Steak Potato (1 cup)	160	20	4	1	890	1 strch, 1 med-fat meat
Chunky Vegetable (1 cup)	130	22	3	1	870	1-1/2 strch, 1 fat
Old-Fashioned Bean & Ham (1 cup)	190	29	2	<1	880	2 strch, 1 lean meat

SOUPS AND STEWS

CAMPBELL'S CONDENSED (PREPARED W/WATER)

Products	Cal.	Carb. (g)	Fat (g)	Sat. Fat (g)	Sodium (mg)	Exchanges
Beef Consomme (1 cup)	25	2	0	0	820	1 very lean meat
Black Bean (1 cup)	120	19	2	<1	1030	1 strch
Broccoli Cheese (1 cup)	110	9	7	3	860	1/2 strch, 1 fat
Cheddar Cheese (1 cup)	150	10	10	5	1119	1/2 strch, 2 fat
Chicken & Stars (1 cup)	70	9	2	<1	1010	1/2 strch
Chicken Alphabet w/Vegetable (1 cup)	80	11	2	<1	880	1 strch
Chicken Dumpling (1 cup)	80	10	3	<1	1049	1/2 strch, 1 fat
Chicken Gumbo (1 cup)	60	9	2	<1	990	1/2 strch
Chicken Noodle (1 cup)	80	10	3	<1	980	1/2 strch, 1 fat
Chicken Vegetable (1 cup)	80	12	2	<1	940	1 strch
Chicken w/Rice (1 cup)	70	9	3	<1	830	1/2 strch, 1 fat
Chicken w/Wild Rice (1 cup)	70	9	2	<1	900	1 strch
Chicken Won Ton (1 cup)	45	5	<1	0	940	1 very lean meat

Food (1 cup)	Cal	Carb	Fat		Sodium	Exchanges
Chili Beef w/Bean (1 cup)	170	24	5	3	910	1-1/2 strch, 1 fat
Cream of Asparagus (1 cup)	110	9	7	2	910	1/2 strch, 1 fat
Cream of Broccoli (1 cup)	100	9	6	3	770	1/2 strch, 1 fat
Cream of Celery (1 cup)	110	9	7	3	900	1/2 strch, 1 fat
Cream of Chicken (1 cup)	130	11	8	3	890	1 strch, 2 fat
Cream of Chicken Broccoli (1 cup)	120	9	8	3	860	1/2 strch, 2 fat
Cream of Chicken Mushroom (1 cup)	130	9	9	3	1000	1/2 strch, 2 fat
Cream of Chicken Noodle (1 cup)	130	12	7	2	880	1 strch, 1 fat
Cream of Mexican Pepper (1 cup)	110	10	7	2	860	1/2 strch, 1 fat
Cream of Mushroom (1 cup)	110	9	7	3	870	1/2 strch, 1 fat
Cream of Potato (1 cup)	100	16	3	2	890	1 strch, 1 fat
Cream of Shrimp (1 cup)	100	8	7	2	890	1/2 strch, 1 fat
Creamy Onion (1 cup)	110	13	6	2	910	1 strch, 1 fat
Curly Noodle & Chicken Broth (1 cup)	80	12	3	<1	840	1 strch, 1 fat
Double Noodle & Chicken Broth (1 cup)	100	15	3	<1	810	1 strch, 1 fat
Fiesta Tomato (1 cup)	60	13	0	0	720	1 strch

SOUPS AND STEWS

Products	Cal.	Carb. (g)	Fat (g)	Sat. Fat (g)	Sodium (mg)	Exchanges
French Onion w/Beef Stock (1 cup)	70	10	3	0	980	1/2 strch, 1 fat
Golden Corn (1 cup)	120	20	4	1	730	1 strch, 1 fat
Golden Mushroom (1 cup)	80	10	3	1	930	1/2 strch, 1 fat
Green Pea (1 cup)	180	29	3	<1	890	2 strch, 1 fat
Hearty Vegetable w/Pasta (1 cup)	90	18	<1	0	830	1 strch
Homestyle Chicken Noodle (1 cup)	70	9	3	2	970	1/2 strch, 1 fat
Homestyle Cream Tomato (1 cup)	110	21	3	1	860	1-1/2 strch, 1 fat
Homestyle Vegetable (1 cup)	70	10	2	<1	970	1/2 strch
Italian Tomato Basil/Oregano (1 cup)	100	23	<1	0	820	1-1/2 strch
Manhattan Clam Chowder (1 cup)	70	12	2	<1	910	1 strch
Minestrone (1 cup)	100	16	2	<1	960	1 strch
Nacho Cheese Soup/Dip (1 cup)	140	11	8	4	810	1 strch, 2 fat
New England Clam Chowder (1 cup)	90	13	3	<1	970	1 strch, 1 fat
Noodles & Ground Beef (1 cup)	100	11	4	2	900	1 strch, 1 fat

Old-Fashioned Tomato Rice (1 cup)	120	23	2	<1	790	1 /12 strch
Old-Fashioned Vegetable (1 cup)	70	10	3	<1	950	1/2 strch, 1 fat
Oyster Stew (1 cup)	90	6	6	4	940	1/2 strch, 1 fat
Scotch Broth (1 cup)	80	9	3	2	870	1/2 strch, 1 fat
Split Pea, Ham, & Bacon (1 cup)	180	28	4	2	860	2 strch, 1 fat
Teddy Bear (1 cup)	80	12	2	<1	840	1 strch
Tomato (1 cup)	100	18	2	0	730	1 strch
Tomato Bisque (1 cup)	130	24	3	2	900	1-1/2 strch, 1 fat
Turkey Noodle (1 cup)	80	10	3	<1	970	1/2 strch, 1 fat
Turkey Vegetable (1 cup)	80	11	3	<1	840	1 strch, 1 fat
Vegetable (1 cup)	90	17	<1	0	750	1 strch
Vegetable Beef (1 cup)	80	10	2	<1	810	1/2 strch
Vegetarian Vegetable (1 cup)	70	14	<1	0	770	1 strch

CAMPBELL'S HEALTHY REQUEST

Bean w/Bacon (1 cup)	180	25	5	2	480	1-1/2 strch, 1 med-fat meat
Chicken Broth (1 cup)	20	1	0	0	480	free

SOUPS AND STEWS

Products	Cal.	Carb. (g)	Fat (g)	Sat. Fat (g)	Sodium (mg)	Exchanges
Chicken Corn Chowder (1 cup)	140	22	3	1	480	1-1/2 strch, 1 fat
Chicken Noodle (1 cup)	70	8	3	<1	480	1/2 strch, 1 fat
Chicken Vegetable (1 cup)	80	12	2	<1	480	1 strch
Chicken w/Rice (1 cup)	70	9	3	<1	480	1/2 strch, 1 fat
Cream of Broccoli (1 cup)	70	9	2	1	480	1/2 strch
Cream of Celery (1 cup)	70	11	2	<1	480	1 strch
Cream of Chicken (1 cup)	80	11	3	1	480	1 strch, 1 fat
Cream of Mushroom (1 cup)	70	9	3	1	480	1/2 strch, 1 fat
Hearty Chicken Noodle (1 cup)	110	11	3	1	480	1 strch, 1 lean meat
Hearty Chicken Rice (1 cup)	120	17	3	1	480	1 strch, 1 fat
Hearty Chicken Vegetable (1 cup)	120	17	3	1	480	1 strch, 1 lean meat
Hearty Minestrone (1 cup)	120	24	2	<1	480	1-1/2 strch
Hearty Vegetable (1 cup)	100	20	1	0	470	1 strch
Hearty Vegetable Beef (1 cup)	140	20	3	1	480	1 strch, 1 lean meat

Minestrone (1 cup)	90	17	<1		480	1 strch
New England Clam Chowder (1 cup)	110	15	4	1	480	1 strch, 1 fat
Southwest-Style Vegetable (1 cup)	150	28	2	<1	480	2 strch
Split Pea w/Ham (1 cup)	170	27	3	1	480	2 strch, 1 fat
Tomato (1 cup)	90	18	2	<1	460	1 strch
Tomato Vegetable (1 cup)	120	22	2	<1	480	1-1/2 strch
Turkey Vegetable Rice (1 cup)	120	17	3	1	480	1 strch, 1 lean meat
Vegetable (1 cup)	90	15	2	<1	480	1 strch
Vegetable Beef (1 cup)	80	11	2	<1	480	1 strch
CAMPBELL'S HOME COOKIN'						
Chicken Noodle (1 cup)	100	11	4	1	980	1 strch, 1 med-fat meat
Cream of Mushroom (1 cup)	170	9	13	4	970	1/2 strch, 3 fat
Hearty Lentil (1 cup)	150	26	2	<1	860	2 strch
Italian Vegetable (1 cup)	100	14	4	2	860	1 strch, 1 fat
Minestrone (1 cup)	120	19	2	1	990	1 strch
Southwest Vegetable (1 cup)	130	24	3	<1	750	1-1/2 strch, 1 fat

SOUPS AND STEWS

Products	Cal.	Carb. (g)	Fat (g)	Sat. Fat (g)	Sodium (mg)	Exchanges
Tuscany Minestrone (1 cup)	160	21	7	2	880	1-1/2 strch, 1 fat
Vegetable Beef (1 cup)	120	18	2	1	1009	1 strch, 1 lean meat
CHEF MATE						
Beef Stew (1 cup)	203	20	7	4	959	1 strch, 2 med-fat meat
Chili w/Beans (1 cup)	383	29	25	11	1179	2 strch, 2 med-fat meat, 3 fat
Chili w/Beans, Chicken (1 cup)	210	29	5	2	1100	2 strch, 2 lean meat
Chili w/o Beans (1 cup)	439	18	33	14	1621	1 strch, 2 med-fat meat, 5 fat
Spice Chili (1/2 cup)	203	16	12	6	739	1 strch, 1 med-fat meat, 1 fat
HEALTH VALLEY						
14-Garden Vegetable (7-1/2 oz)	71	15	0	0	221	1 strch
5-Bean Vegetable (7-1/2 oz)	124	28	0	0	221	2 strch
Black Bean & Carrot (7-1/2 oz)	97	21	0	0	248	1-1/2 strch, 1 very lean meat
Chicken Broth (7-1/2 oz)	27	0	0	0	151	1 very lean meat
Country Corn & Vegetable (7-1/2 oz)	71	15	0	0	213	1 strch

Fat-Free 14-Garden Vegetable (1 cup)	80	17	0	0	250	1 strch
Fat-Free Beef Broth (1 cup)	18	0	0	0	74	free
Fat-Free Beef Broth Soup (1 cup)	30	2	0	0	160	1 very lean meat
Fat-Free Black Bean & Vegetable (1 cup)	110	24	0	0	280	1-1/2 strch, 1 very lean meat
Fat-Free Carotene Soup w/Vegetable Powder (1 cup)	70	17	0	0	240	1 strch
Fat-Free Chicken Broth (1 cup)	30	0	0	0	170	free
Fat-Free Country Corn & Vegetable (1 cup)	80	17	0	0	240	1 strch
Fat-Free Five Bean Vegetable (1 cup)	140	32	0	0	250	2 strch, 1 very lean meat
Fat-Free Hearty Lentil w/Vegetables (5 oz)	80	12	0	0	140	1 strch, 1 very lean meat
Fat-Free Italian Minestrone (1 cup)	80	21	0	0	210	1-1/2 strch, 1 very lean meat
Fat-Free Lentil & Carrot (1 cup)	90	25	0	0	220	1-1/2 strch, 1 very lean meat
Fat-Free Pasta Cacciatore (1 cup)	90	19	0	0	210	1 strch
Fat-Free Pasta Fagioli (1 cup)	80	17	0	0	250	1 strch
Fat-Free Pasta Primavera (1 cup)	80	21	0	0	210	1-1/2 strch, 1 very lean meat
Fat-Free Pasta Romano (1 cup)	140	32	0	0	250	2 strch, 1 very lean meat
Fat-Free Rotini Vegetable Pasta (1 cup)	100	20	0	0	290	1 strch

SOUPS AND STEWS

Products	Cal.	Carb. (g)	Fat (g)	Sat. Fat (g)	Sodium (mg)	Exchanges
Fat-Free Split Pea & Carrot (1 cup)	110	17	0	0	230	1 strch, 1 very lean meat
Fat-Free Tomato Vegetable (1 cup)	80	17	0	0	240	1 strch
Fat-Free Vegetable Barley (1 cup)	90	19	0	0	210	1 strch
Hearty Lentil w/Garden Vegetable (5 oz)	80	12	0	0	140	1 strch, 1 very lean meat
Lentil & Carrot (7-1/2 oz)	80	22	0	0	195	1-1/2 strch
Real Italian Minestrone (7-1/2 oz)	71	19	0	0	186	1 strch, 1 very lean meat
Split Pea & Carrot (7-1/2 oz)	97	15	0	0	204	1 strch, 1 very lean meat
Tomato Vegetable (7-1/2 oz)	71	15	0	0	213	1 strch
Vegetable Barley (7-1/2 oz)	80	17	0	0	186	1 strch
HEALTHY CHOICE						
Bean & Ham (1 cup)	184	34	3	1	465	2 strch, 1 lean meat
Beef & Potato (1 cup)	119	18	2	<1	635	1 strch, 1 lean meat
Chicken Corn Chowder (1 cup)	176	30	3	1	466	2 strch, 1 fat
Chicken Pasta (1 cup)	118	18	3	1	493	1 strch, 1 lean meat

Food					Exchanges
Chicken w/Rice (1 cup)	108	15	3	1	426	1 strch, 1 lean meat
Chili Beef (1 cup)	166	30	1	<1	384	2 strch, 1 very lean meat
Clam Chowder (1 cup)	123	23	1	<1	481	1-1/2 strch
Country Vegetable (1 cup)	104	23	<1	<1	431	1-1/2 strch
Cream of Chicken w/Mushroom (1 cup)	127	20	2	<1	421	1 strch, 1 lean meat
Cream of Chicken w/Vegetable (1 cup)	127	21	2	<1	384	1-1/2 strch
Cream of Mushroom (1 cup)	77	14	<1	<1	450	1 strch
Garden Vegetable (1 cup)	118	26	<1	<1	405	2 strch
Hearty Chicken (1 cup)	132	20	3	<1	461	1 strch, 1 lean meat
Lentil (1 cup)	146	28	<1	<1	419	2 strch
Minestrone (1 cup)	112	23	1	<1	392	1-1/2 strch
Old-Fashioned Chicken Noodle (1 cup)	137	19	3	1	402	1 strch, 1 lean meat
Split Pea & Ham (1 cup)	155	26	2	1	399	2 strch, 1 lean meat
Tomato Garden (1 cup)	106	21	2	<1	424	1-1/2 strch
Turkey w/Wild Rice (1 cup)	92	13	2	<1	355	1 strch
Vegetable Beef (1 cup)	130	22	<1	<1	422	1-1/2 strch, 1 very lean meat

SOUPS AND STEWS

Products	Cal.	Carb. (g)	Fat (g)	Sat. Fat (g)	Sodium (mg)	Exchanges
LIBBY'S						
Beef Stew (1 cup)	279	18	19	4	819	1 strch, 1 med-fat meat, 3 fat
Chili, No Beans (1 cup)	481	16	38	18	1581	1 strch, 3 med-fat meat, 5 fat
Chili & Beans (1 cup)	421	29	28	13	1211	2 strch, 1 med-fat meat, 5 fat
LIPTON CUP-A-SOUP						
Chicken Broth (6 oz)	20	3	1	0	580	free
Chicken Noodle (6 oz)	60	10	1	<1	540	1/2 strch
Chicken Vegetable (6 oz)	50	10	1	<1	520	1/2 strch
Cream of Chicken (6 oz)	70	11	3	<1	650	1 strch, 1 fat
Cream of Mushroom (6 oz)	60	10	2	0	590	1/2 strch
Creamy Broccoli & Cheese (6 oz)	70	8	3	2	550	1/2 strch, 1 fat
Creamy Chicken-Flavored Vegetable (6 oz)	90	10	4	2	590	1/2 strch, 1 fat
Green Pea (6 oz)	110	17	4	1	620	1 strch, 1 fat
Harvest Vegetable (6 oz)	90	17	2	<1	450	1 strch

Hearty Chicken Supreme (6 oz)	90	13	4	2	650	1 strch, 1 fat
Ring Noodle (6 oz)	50	9	1	<1	560	1/2 strch
Spring Vegetable (6 oz)	50	9	1	0	500	1/2 strch
Tomato (6 oz)	90	19	2	1	490	1 strch
Virginia Pea (6 oz)	130	19	5	2	630	1 strch, 1 fat
OLD EL PASO						
Black Bean w/Bacon (1 cup)	160	26	2	<1	960	1-1/2 strch, 1 lean meat
Chicken Vegetable (1 cup)	110	13	3	<1	620	1 strch, 1 lean meat
Chicken w/Rice (1 cup)	90	10	3	<1	680	1/2 strch, 1 lean meat
Chili w/Beans (1 cup)	200	15	7	2	420	1 strch, 2 lean meat
Garden Vegetable (1 cup)	110	17	3	<1	710	1 strch, 1 fat
Hearty Beef (1 cup)	120	14	3	2	690	1 strch, 1 lean meat
Hearty Chicken Noodle (1 cup)	110	10	3	1	NA	1/2 strch, 1 lean meat
PROGRESSO						
Bean & Ham (1 cup)	160	25	2	<1	870	1-1/2 strch, 1 lean meat
Beef Barley (1 cup)	130	13	4	2	780	1 strch, 1 med-fat meat

SOUPS AND STEWS

Products	Cal.	Carb. (g)	Fat (g)	Sat. Fat (g)	Sodium (mg)	Exchanges
Beef Minestrone (1 cup)	140	14	4	2	850	1 strch, 1 med-fat meat
Beef Noodle (1 cup)	140	15	4	2	950	1 strch, 1 med-fat meat
Beef Vegetable & Rotini (1 cup)	120	10	4	2	830	1/2 strch, 1 med-fat meat
Broccoli & Shells (1 cup)	70	14	1	0	720	1 strch
Chickarina (1 cup)	120	10	5	2	710	1/2 strch, 1 med-fat meat
Chicken & Wild Rice (1 cup)	130	15	2	<1	820	1 strch
Chicken Barley (1 cup)	110	14	3	<1	720	1 strch, 1 lean meat
Chicken Broth (1 cup)	20	1	<1	NA	860	free
Chicken Minestrone (1 cup)	120	12	4	1	790	1 strch, 1 med-fat meat
Chicken Noodle (1 cup)	80	8	2	<1	730	1/2 strch, 1 lean meat
Chicken Rice & Vegetables (1 cup)	110	12	3	1	750	1 strch, 1 lean meat
Chicken Vegetable & Penne (1 cup)	100	11	3	<1	780	1 strch, 1 lean meat
Clam & Rotini Chowder (1 cup)	200	21	9	2	800	1-1/2 strch, 2 fat
Corn Chowder (1 cup)	180	20	10	4	780	1 strch, 2 fat

Cream of Chicken (1 cup)	170	11	10	4	880	1 strch, 2 fat
Cream of Mushroom (1 cup)	140	12	8	4	920	1 strch, 2 fat
Creamy Tortellini (1 cup)	210	15	15	8	830	1 strch, 3 fat
Escarole in Chicken Broth (1 cup)	25	2	1	0	980	free
Green Split Pea (1 cup)	170	25	3	1	870	1-1/2 strch, 1 fat
Healthy Classics Beef Barley (1 cup)	140	20	2	1	490	1 strch, 1 lean meat
Healthy Classics Beef Vegetable (1 cup)	150	25	2	<1	410	1-1/2 strch, 1 lean meat
Healthy Classics Chicken Noodle (1 cup)	80	10	2	<1	480	1/2 strch, 1 lean meat
Healthy Classics Chicken Rice w/Vegetables (1 cup)	90	12	2	0	450	1 strch, 1 lean meat
Healthy Classics Cream of Broccoli (1 cup)	90	13	3	<1	580	1 strch, 1 fat
Healthy Classics Garlic & Pasta (1 cup)	100	18	2	0	450	1 strch
Healthy Classics Lentil (1 cup)	130	20	2	0	440	1 strch, 1 lean meat
Healthy Classics Minestrone (1 cup)	120	20	3	0	510	1 strch, 1 fat
Healthy Classics New England Clam Chowder (1 cup)	120	20	2	<1	530	1 strch
Healthy Classics Split Pea (1 cup)	180	30	3	1	420	2 strch, 1 lean meat
Healthy Classics Tomato Garden Vegetable (1 cup)	100	19	1	0	480	1 strch

SOUPS AND STEWS

Products	Cal.	Carb. (g)	Fat (g)	Sat. Fat (g)	Sodium (mg)	Exchanges
Healthy Classics Vegetable (1 cup)	80	13	2	0	470	1 strch
Hearty Black Bean (1 cup)	170	30	2	0	730	2 strch
Hearty Chicken (10.5 oz can)	120	10	3	<1	1070	1/2 strch, 2 very lean meat
Hearty Minestrone/Shells (1 cup)	120	20	2	0	700	1 strch
Hearty Penne/Chicken Broth (1 cup)	70	12	1	0	930	1 strch
Hearty Tomato & Rotini (1 cup)	90	16	1	0	820	1 strch
Hearty Vegetable/Rotini (1 cup)	110	20	1	0	720	1 strch
Homestyle Chicken & Vegetable (1 cup)	100	10	3	<1	680	1/2 strch, 1 lean meat
Lentil (1 cup)	140	22	2	0	750	1-1/2 strch, 1 lean meat
Lentil & Shells (1 cup)	130	22	2	0	840	1-1/2 strch, 1 lean meat
Lentil w/Sausage (1 cup)	170	19	7	2	780	1 strch, 1 med-fat meat
Macaroni & Bean (1 cup)	160	23	4	1	800	1-1/2 strch, 1 fat
Manhatten Clam Chowder (1 cup)	110	11	2	0	710	1 strch, 1 lean meat
Meatballs & Pasta Pearls (1 cup)	140	13	7	3	700	1 strch, 1 med-fat meat

Minestrone (1 cup)	130	22	3	<1	960	1-1/2 strch, 1 fat
New England Clam Chowder (1 cup)	180	17	10	4	1050	1 strch, 1 med-fat meat, 1 fat
Spicy Chicken & Penne (1 cup)	120	13	4	1	680	1 strch, 1 med-fat meat
Split Pea w/Ham (1 cup)	160	20	4	2	830	1 strch, 1 med-fat meat
Tomato Beef & Rotini (1 cup)	140	15	5	2	750	1 strch, 1 med-fat meat
Tomato Soup (1 cup)	90	15	2	0	990	1 strch
Tomato Tortellini (1 cup)	120	13	5	2	910	1 strch, 1 fat
Tortellini/Chicken Broth (1 cup)	80	10	2	<1	750	1/2 strch
Vegetable (1 cup)	90	15	2	<1	850	1 strch
Zesty Minestrone (1 cup)	150	17	6	3	790	1 strch, 1 fat
UNCLE BEN'S						
Club Black Bean & Rice Soup (1 cup)	150	28	2	0	430	2 strch
WEIGHT WATCHERS						
Chicken & Rice (10-1/2 oz)	110	17	2	0	720	1 strch
Minestrone (10-1/2 oz can)	130	23	2	4.5	760	1-1/2 strch
Vegetable (10-1/2 oz can)	130	27	1	0	680	2 strch

VEGETABLES AND VEGETABLE JUICES

VEGETABLES AND VEGETABLE JUICES

Products	Cal.	Carb. (g)	Fat (g)	Sat. Fat (g)	Sodium (mg)	Exchanges
Alfalfa Sprouts (1 cup)	10	1	<1	<1	2	free
Artichoke Hearts (1/2 cup)	36	7	<1	0	42	1 vegetable
Artichokes, Cooked (1/2)	30	7	<1	0	57	1 vegetable
Asparagus, Frozen (1/2 cup)	23	4	<1	<1	3	1 vegetable
Asparagus, Spears, Canned (1/2 cup)	23	3	<1	<1	472	1 vegetable
Bamboo Shoots, Canned (1 cup)	25	4	<1	<1	9	1 vegetable
Bamboo Shoots, Sliced, Cooked (1 cup)	14	2	<1	<1	5	free
Bamboo Shoots, Sliced, Raw (1 cup)	41	8	<1	<1	6	1 vegetable
Bean Sprouts (1 cup)	31	6	<1	<1	6	1 vegetable
Beans, Green or Wax, Canned (1/2 cup)	14	3	<1	0	171	1 vegetable
Beans, Green, Frozen (1/2 cup)	18	4	<1	0	9	1 vegetable
Beets, Canned (1/2 cup)	26	6	<1	0	233	1 vegetable
Beets, Harvard, Diced (1/2 cup)	136	25	4	<1	287	1 carb., 1 vegetable, 1 fat

Beets, Pickled (1/2 cup)	74	19	<1	<1	301	1 carb., 1 vegetable
Broccoli, Cooked w/Cheese Sauce (1/2 cup)	110	6	7	4	365	1 vegetable, 1 fat
Broccoli, Cooked w/Cream Sauce (1/2 cup)	93	8	6	2	346	1 vegetable, 1 fat
Broccoli, Raw, Chopped (1 cup)	25	5	<1	<1	24	1 vegetable
Broccoli, Spears, Frozen (1/2 cup)	26	5	<1	0	22	1 vegetable
Brussel Sprouts, Frozen, Cooked (1/2 cup)	33	7	<1	<1	18	1 vegetable
Cabbage, Bok Choy, Cooked (1 cup)	20	3	<1	<1	58	1 vegetable
Cabbage, Chinese, Raw (1 cup)	12	3	<1	0	7	1 vegetable
Cabbage, Fresh, Cooked (1/2 cup)	16	3	<1	0	6	1 vegetable
Cabbage, Raw, Green (1 cup)	18	4	<1	0	13	1 vegetable
Cabbage, Red, Cooked (1/2 cup)	16	4	<1	<1	6	1 vegetable
Carrot Juice, Canned (1/2 cup)	49	11	<1	<1	36	2 vegetable
Carrots, Canned (1/2 cup)	17	4	<1	0	176	1 vegetable
Carrots, Fresh, Cooked (1/2 cup)	35	8	<1	0	52	1 vegetable
Carrots, Raw (1 cup)	47	11	<1	0	38	2 vegetable
Cauliflower, Frozen, Cooked (1/2 cup)	17	3	<1	0	16	1 vegetable

VEGETABLES AND VEGETABLE JUICES

Products	Cal.	Carb. (g)	Fat (g)	Sat. Fat (g)	Sodium (mg)	Exchanges
Cauliflower, Raw (1 cup)	25	5	<1	0	30	1 vegetable
Celery, Fresh, Cooked (1/2 cup)	14	3	<1	0	68	1 vegetable
Celery, Raw (1 cup)	19	4	<1	0	104	1 vegetable
Coleslaw Salad (1/2 cup)	89	8	7	1	162	1 vegetable, 1 fat
Collard Greens, Fresh, Cooked (1/2 cup)	17	4	<1	0	10	1 vegetable
Corn, Canned (1/2 cup)	83	20	<1	<1	286	1 strch
Corn, Cream-Style, Canned (1/2 cup)	92	23	<1	<1	365	1-1/2 strch
Corn, Frozen, Cooked (1/2 cup)	66	17	<1	0	4	1 strch
Corn on the Cob, Cooked, (1 medium)	83	19	1	<1	13	1 strch
Corn on the Cob, Frozen (1, 3-inch)	70	14	<1	NA	5	1 strch
Cucumber, Raw (1 cup)	14	3	<1	0	2	1 vegetable
Cucumber Salad, Marinated in Vinegar (1 cup)	48	13	<1	<1	350	1/2 carb., 1 vegetable
Eggplant, Fresh, Cooked (1/2 cup)	13	3	<1	0	1	1 vegetable
Endive/Escarole, Raw (1 cup)	9	2	<1	0	11	1 vegetable

Escarole/Curly Endive, Chopped (1 cup)	9	2	<1	<1	11	free
French Fries, Frozen, Oven-Heated (10)	163	19	9	4	307	1 strch, 2 fat
Hominy, Yellow, Canned (1/2 cup)	58	12	<1	<1	168	1 strch
Jicama (1 cup)	46	11	<1	<1	5	2 vegetable
Kale, Fresh, Cooked (1/2 cup)	21	4	<1	0	15	1 vegetable
Kohlrabi, Cooked (1/2 cup)	24	6	<1	0	17	1 vegetable
Leeks, Cooked (1/2 cup)	16	4	<1	0	6	1 vegetable
Lettuce, Iceburg, Raw (1 cup)	7	1	<1	0	5	1 vegetable
Lettuce, Romaine, Chopped (1 cup)	9	1	<1	<1	5	free
Lettuce, Romaine, Raw (1 cup)	9	1	<1	0	5	1 vegetable
Lima Beans, Frozen, Cooked (1/2 cup)	95	18	<1	<1	26	1 strch
Mixed Vegetables, No Corn, Peas, or Pasta (1/2 cup)	20	3	0	0	15	1 vegetable
Mixed Vegetables w/Corn (1 cup)	80	18	0	0	80	1 strch
Mixed Vegetables w/Pasta (1 cup)	80	15	0	0	85	1 strch
Mushrooms, Canned (1/2 cup)	19	4	<1	0	331	1 vegetable
Mushrooms, Fresh, Cooked (1/2 cup)	21	4	<1	<1	2	1 vegetable

VEGETABLES AND VEGETABLE JUICES

Products	Cal.	Carb. (g)	Fat (g)	Sat. Fat (g)	Sodium (mg)	Exchanges
Mushrooms, Raw (1 cup)	18	3	<1	0	3	1 vegetable
Mustard Greens, Fresh, Cooked (1/2 cup)	10	2	<1	0	11	1 vegetable
Okra, Batter-Fried (1/2 cup)	88	6	7	1	67	1 vegetable, 1 fat
Okra, Frozen, Cooked (1/2 cup)	34	8	<1	<1	3	1 vegetable
Onions, Creamed (1/2 cup)	100	11	6	2	334	2 vegetable, 1 fat
Onions, Fresh, Cooked (1/2 cup)	46	11	<1	0	3	2 vegetable
Onions, Green, Raw (1 cup)	32	7	<1	0	16	1 vegetable
Onions, Raw (1 cup)	61	14	<1	0	5	2 vegetable
Palm Hearts, Cooked (1/2 cup)	75	20	<1	<1	10	1 strch
Parsnips, Raw Slices (1/2 cup)	50	12	<1	<1	7	2 vegetable
Pea Pods, Fresh, Cooked (1/2 cup)	34	6	<1	0	3	1 vegetable
Pea Pods, Raw (1 cup)	61	11	<1	<1	6	2 vegetable
Peas, Green, Canned (1/2 cup)	59	11	<1	<1	186	1 strch
Peas, Green, Fresh, Cooked (1/2 cup)	67	13	<1	0	2	1 strch

Food						Exchanges
Peas, Green, Frozen, Cooked (1/2 cup)	62	11	<1	0	70	1 strch
Peppers, Green, Fresh, Cooked (1/2 cup)	19	5	<1	0	1	1 vegetable
Peppers, Green, Raw (1 cup)	27	6	<1	0	2	1 vegetable
Peppers, Hot Green Chili, Raw (1 cup)	60	14	<1	0	10	2 vegetable
Peppers, Jalapeño, Canned (1/2 cup)	16	3	<1	<1	995	1 vegetable
Peppers, Sweet, Red, Cooked (1/2 cup)	19	5	<1	<1	1	1 vegetable
Plantain, Cooked (1/2 cup)	89	24	<1	0	4	1 strch
Potatoes, Baked w/Skin (3 oz)	93	22	<1	0	7	1-1/2 strch
Potatoes, Cooked, Peeled (3 oz)	73	17	<1	0	4	1 strch
Potatoes, Hash Brown, Frozen, Cooked (1/2 cup)	170	22	9	4	27	1-1/2 strch, 2 fat
Potatoes, Mashed, Flakes, Milk/Fat Added (1/2 cup)	119	16	6	4	349	1 strch, 1 fat
Potatoes, Scalloped (1 cup)	211	27	9	3	821	2 strch, 2 fat
Potatoes, Sweet, Canned (1/2 cup)	92	22	<1	0	53	1-1/2 strch
Potatoes Au Gratin, Homemade w/Margarine (1 cup)	323	28	19	10	1060	2 strch, 4 fat
Radishes (1 cup)	20	4	<1	0	28	1 vegetable
Sauerkraut, Canned (1/2 cup)	22	5	<1	0	780	1 vegetable

VEGETABLES AND VEGETABLE JUICES

Products	Cal.	Carb. (g)	Fat (g)	Sat. Fat (g)	Sodium (mg)	Exchanges
Spinach, Canned (1/2 cup)	25	4	<1	<1	29	1 vegetable
Spinach, Frozen, Cooked (1/2 cup)	27	5	<1	0	82	1 vegetable
Spinach, Raw (1 cup)	12	2	<1	0	44	1 vegetable
Spinach Salad, No Dressing (1 cup)	89	10	4	<1	157	2 vegetable, 1 fat
Squash, Spaghetti, Cooked (1/2 cup)	23	5	<1	<1	14	1 vegetable
Squash, Summer, Fresh, Cooked (1/2 cup)	18	4	<1	<1	1	1 vegetable
Squash, Summer, Raw (1 cup)	26	6	<1	<1	3	1 vegetable
Squash, Winter (1 cup)	83	22	<1	0	8	1-1/2 strch
Succotash, Canned (1/2 cup)	81	18	<1	<1	282	1 strch
Succotash, Cooked (1/2 cup)	111	24	<1	<1	16	1-1/2 strch
Tater Tots, Frozen, Oven-Heated (10)	155	21	8	4	522	1-1/2 strch, 2 fat
Tomato Juice (1/2 cup)	21	5	<1	0	440	1 vegetable
Tomato Paste, Canned (1/2 cup)	110	25	1	<1	1034	1 strch, 1 vegetable
Tomato Sauce (1/2 cup)	37	9	<1	0	738	1 vegetable

Tomatoes, Canned (1/2 cup)	24	5	<1	0	196	1 vegetable
Tomatoes, Raw (1 cup)	38	8	<1	<1	16	1 vegetable
Tossed Green Salad (3/4 cup)	19	4	<1	<1	11	1 vegetable
Turnip Greens, Fresh, Cooked (1/2 cup)	14	3	<1	0	21	1 vegetable
Turnips, Fresh, Cooked (1/2 cup)	14	4	<1	0	39	1 vegetable
Vegetable Juice (1/2 cup)	23	6	<1	0	442	1 vegetable
Vegetable Juice Cocktail (1/2 cup)	23	6	<1	<1	442	1 vegetable
Water Chestnuts (1/2 cup)	35	9	0	0	6	1 vegetable
Watercress, Raw (1 cup)	4	<1	0	0	14	1 vegetable
Yam, Plain (1/2 cup)	79	19	<1	0	6	1 strch
Zucchini Squash, Fresh, Cooked (1/2 cup)	14	4	0	0	3	1 vegetable
Zucchini, Raw (1 cup)	18	4	<1	0	4	1 vegetable
BIRD'S EYE						
Artichoke Hearts, Deluxe (1/2 cup)	38	8	<1	<1	47	1 vegetable
Japanese-Style Vegetables (1/2 cup)	78	8	5	2	320	1 vegetable, 1 fat
Spinach, Creamed (1/2 cup)	111	7	8	5	565	1 vegetable, 2 fat

VEGETABLES AND VEGETABLE JUICES

Products	Cal.	Carb. (g)	Fat (g)	Sat. Fat (g)	Sodium (mg)	Exchanges
Stir-Fry, Sugar Snap (3/4 cup)	35	5	0	0	20	1 vegetable
Stir-Fry Vegetables, Broccoli (1 cup)	51	9	<1	0	53	2 vegetable
Stir-Fry Vegetables, Chinese (1/2 cup)	44	9	<1	<1	302	2 vegetable
Stir-Fry Vegetables, Japanese (1/2 cup)	35	7	<1	<1	439	1 vegetable
Stir-Fry Vegetables, Pepper (1 cup)	29	6	<1	0	18	1 vegetable
CAMPBELL'S						
Tomato Juice (1 cup)	44	9	0	0	859	2 vegetable
V8 100% Vegetable Juice (1 cup)	56	11	0	0	687	2 vegetable
V8 Light Tangy 100% Vegetable Juice (1 cup)	58	12	0	0	349	2 vegetable
V8 Picante Vegetable Juice (1 cup)	51	10	0	0	684	2 vegetable
V8 Spicy Hot 100% Vegetable Juice (1 cup)	51	10	0	0	786	2 vegetable
CONTADINA						
Tomato Paste (2 Tbsp)	30	6	0	0	20	1/2 strch
Tomato Paste, Italian (2 Tbsp)	40	7	1	0	330	1/2 strch

VEGETABLES AND VEGETABLE JUICES 395

Tomato Puree (1/2 cup)	38	8	0	0	29	1 vegetable
Tomato Sauce (1/2 cup)	40	8	0	0	560	1 vegetable
Tomato Sauce, Italian (1/2 cup)	31	8	0	0	651	1 vegetable
Tomato Sauce, Thick & Zesty (1/2 cup)	40	6	0	0	680	1 vegetable
Tomato Tidbits (1/4 cup)	20	4	0	0	10	1 vegetable
Tomatoes, Crushed, in Puree (1/2 cup)	40	8	0	0	295	1 vegetable
Tomatoes, Italian (Pear) (1/2 cup)	25	4	0	0	218	1 vegetable
Tomatoes, Italian Stewed (1/2 cup)	40	8	0	0	262	1 vegetable
Tomatoes, Mexican Stewed (1/2 cup)	42	10	0	0	230	2 vegetable
Tomatoes, Pasta-Ready (1/2 cup)	42	5	3	0	650	1 vegetable, 1 fat
Tomatoes, Recipe-Ready (1/2 cup)	32	5	0	0	220	1 vegetable
Tomatoes, Stewed (1/2 cup)	43	9	0	0	252	2 vegetable
Tomatoes, Whole Peeled (1/2 cup)	25	4	0	0	218	1 vegetable
GREEN GIANT						
Beets, Harvard, Canned (1/3 cup)	64	15	<1	0	266	1/2 carb, 1 vegetable
Broccoli Spears in Butter Sauce (1/2 cup)	50	7	2	1	330	1 vegetable

VEGETABLES AND VEGETABLE JUICES

Products	Cal.	Carb. (g)	Fat (g)	Sat. Fat (g)	Sodium (mg)	Exchanges
Broccoli, Cauliflower, Carrots in Butter Sauce (3/4 cup)	54	8	2	1	303	1 vegetable
Broccoli, Pasta, Sweet Peas in Butter Sauce (3/4 cup)	70	11	2	1	283	1/2 strch, 1 vegetable
Corn, Shoepeg White, in Sauce (3/4 cup)	120	21	3	1	316	1-1/2 strch, 1 fat
Corn Niblets in Butter Sauce (2/3 cup)	129	23	3	1	347	1-1/2 strch, 1 fat
Baby Peas & Butter Sauce, LeSueur (3/4 cup)	100	16	2	1	370	1 strch
Baby Peas & Mushrooms, LeSueur (3/4 cup)	56	10	<1	0	107	2 vegetable
Mixed Vegetables in Butter Sauce (3/4 cup)	65	11	2	1	235	2 vegetable
Pasta Accents, Alfredo (2 cups)	130	16	5	2	297	3 vegetable, 1 fat
Pasta Accents, Creamy Cheddar (2-1/3 cup)	250	36	8	3	700	2 strch, 1 vegetable, 1 fat
Pasta Accents, Florentine (2 cup)	336	44	9	3	908	2 strch, 2 vegetable, 2 fat
Pasta Accents, Garlic (2 cups)	254	36	10	5	641	2-1/2 strch, 2 fat
Pasta Accents, Primavera (2-1/4 cup)	320	40	12	5	500	2 strch, 2 vegetable, 2 fat
Pasta Accents, White Cheddar (1-3/4 cup)	310	38	12	4	568	2 strch, 1 vegetable, 2 fat

Peas, Sweet, in Butter Sauce (3/4 cup)	97	16	2	2	397	1 strch
Rice, Oriental (1 cup)	190	37	<1	0	981	2 strch, 1 vegetable
Stir-Fry, Asian (2-1/4 cup)	230	45	2	0	2160	1-1/2 strch, 4 vegetable
Stir-Fry, Broccoli (2-1/3 cup)	117	16	3	<1	1099	3 vegetables, 1 fat
Stir-Fry, Vegetable Almond (1-3/4 cup)	150	22	5	0	1110	1 strch, 1 vegetable, 1 fat
Stir-Fry Vegetables, Lo Mein (2 1/3 cup)	176	32	<1	0	1067	1 strch, 3 vegetable
Stir-Fry Vegetables, Sweet & Sour (1-3/4 cup)	128	29	<1	0	394	1 strch, 3 vegetable
Stir-Fry Vegetables, Szechuan (1-3/4 cup)	154	21	5	<1	1222	1/2 strch, 2 vegetable, 1 fat
Stir-Fry Vegetables, Teriyaki (1-3/4 cup)	101	19	<1	0	872	4 vegetable
Three-Bean Salad, Canned (1/2 cup)	68	16	<1	0	466	1 strch
Vegetables, English Cheddar (1/2 cup)	115	15	5	2	391	1 strch, 1 fat
Vegetables, Japanese Teriyaki (1/2 cup)	50	9	<1	0	400	2 vegetable
Vegetables, Normandy Mushroom (1/2 cup)	77	11	3	2	270	1 strch, 1 fat

LIBBY'S

Pumpkin, Solid Pack, Canned (1/2 cup)	41	9	0	0	5	2 vegetable

VEGETABLES AND VEGETABLE JUICES

Products	Cal.	Carb. (g)	Fat (g)	Sat. Fat (g)	Sodium (mg)	Exchanges
MRS. PAUL'S						
Onion Rings, Old-Fashioned (7 rings)	230	29	12	3	450	2 strch, 2 fat
Sweet Potatoes, Candied (1/2 cup)	276	67	1	<1	109	1 strch, 3-1/2 carb.
ORE IDA						
Baked Potato, Topped, Broccoli & Cheese (1/2)	150	25	4	2	410	1-1/2 strch, 1 fat
Baked Potato, Twice, Cheddar Cheese (1)	190	26	8	2	450	2 strch, 2 fat
Cheddar Browns (1 patty)	80	14	2	1	370	1 strch
Cottage Fries (3 oz or 13 fries)	130	21	4	1	25	1-1/2 strch, 1 fat
Country Fries (3 oz or 15 fries)	120	19	4	<1	280	1 strch, 1 fat
Crispers (3 oz or 15 fries)	220	24	13	3	460	2 strch, 3 fat
Crispy Crowns (3 oz or 12 pieces)	190	20	11	2	410	1 strch, 2 fat
Crispy Crunchies (3 oz or 12 fries)	160	20	8	2	310	1 strch, 2 fat
Deep Fries Crinkle Cuts (3 oz or 18 fries)	160	23	6	1	25	1-1/2 strch, 1 fat
Deep Fries French Fries (3 oz or 22 fries)	160	22	7	2	20	1-1/2 strch, 1 fat

Fast Fries (3 oz or 23 fries)	150	20	6	1	330	1 strch, 1 fat
Golden Crinkles (3 oz or 14 fries)	140	23	4	1	20	1-1/2 strch, 1 fat
Golden Fries (3 oz or 15 fries)	120	20	4	<1	20	1 strch, 1 fat
Golden Patties (1 patty)	160	17	9	2	180	1 strch, 2 fat
Golden Twirls (3 oz or 10 fries)	150	23	6	2	270	1-1/2 strch, 1 fat
Hash Browns, Country-Style (1 cup)	60	14	0	0	20	1 strch
Hash Browns, Microwave (1 pkg)	220	26	12	4	290	2 strch, 2 fat
Hash Browns, Shredded (1 patty)	70	15	0	0	25	1 strch
Hash Browns, Southern-Style (3/4 cup)	80	17	0	0	30	1 strch
Hash Browns, Toaster (2 patties)	190	25	11	2	470	1-1/2 strch, 2 fat
Hot Tots (3 oz or 9 pieces)	160	20	7	2	370	1 strch, 1 fat
Onion Ringers (6 rings)	230	26	13	3	300	2 strch, 3 fat
Pixie Crinkles (3 oz or 32 fries)	130	21	5	1	25	1-1/2 strch, 1 fat
Potato Wedges w/skin, Homestyle (3 oz or 7 fries)	110	19	3	<1	15	1 strch, 1 fat
Potatoes, Mashed (2/3 cup)	90	16	3	0	150	1 strch, 1 fat
Potatoes O'Brien (3/4 cup)	60	15	0	0	20	1 strch

VEGETABLES AND VEGETABLE JUICES

Products	Cal.	Carb. (g)	Fat (g)	Sat. Fat (g)	Sodium (mg)	Exchanges
Shoestrings (3 oz or 39 fries)	150	22	6	1	20	1-1/2 strch, 1 fat
Snackin' Fries (1 pkg)	340	36	20	4	590	2-1/2 strch, 4 fat
Steak Fries (3 oz or 7 fries)	110	19	3	<1	20	1 strch, 1 fat
Stew Vegetables (2/3 cup)	50	11	0	0	45	1 strch
Sweet Potatoes w/Candied Sauce Pkt (5 pieces w/sauce)	170	40	0	0	75	2 carb, 2 vegetable
Tater Tots (3 oz or 9 pieces)	160	21	8	2	300	1-1/2 strch, 2 fat
Tater Tots, Microwave (1 pkg)	180	27	8	2	280	2 strch, 2 fat
Tater Tots, Onion (3 oz or 9 pieces)	150	21	7	2	400	1-1/2 strch, 1 fat
Texas Crispers (3 oz or 7 pieces)	170	20	9	3	280	1 strch, 2 fat
Waffle Fries (3 oz or 9 fries)	150	21	7	1	250	1-1/2 strch, 1 fat
Zesties (3 oz or 12 fries)	160	20	8	2	390	1 strch, 2 fat
PROGRESSO						
Artichoke Hearts (2 pieces)	35	6	0	0	240	1 vegetable

Zucchini, Italian-Style (1/2 cup)	40	7	2	0	400	1 vegetable
STOUFFER'S						
Green Bean Mushroom Casserole, Side Dish (1)	130	13	8.2	2	530	1/2 strch, 1 vegetable, 2 fat
Spinach, Cream, Side Dish (1)	150	8	12	4	380	1 vegetable, 2 fat

VEGETARIAN FOODS

VEGETARIAN FOODS

Products	Cal.	Carb. (g)	Fat (g)	Sat. Fat (g)	Sodium (mg)	Exchanges
Miso (1/2 cup)	284	39	8	1	5032	2-1/2 strch, 1 med-fat meat, 1 fat
Miso Sauce (1 cup)	383	72	7	<1	4015	5 strch, 1 fat
Tempeh (1 cup)	330	28	13	2	10	2 strch, 4 lean meat
Tofu, Firm, Raw (1/2 cup)	181	5	11	2	18	3 lean meat
Tofu (Regular) (1/2 cup)	94	2	6	<1	9	1 med-fat meat
Tofu Yogurt (1 cup)	254	43	5	<1	92	3 strch, 1 fat
Vegetarian Bacon Strips (3 strips)	75	2	7	1	352	1/2 med-fat meat, 1 fat
Vegetarian Breakfast Links (1 link)	64	3	5	<1	222	1 med-fat meat
Vegetarian Breakfast Patties (1)	97	4	7	1	337	1 med-fat meat
Vegetarian Chicken Slices (2)	132	4	8	1	474	1 med-fat meat, 1 fat
Vegetarian Chicken, Breaded, Fried (1 slice)	97	3	7	1	228	1 med-fat meat
Vegetarian Chili (2/3 cup)	186	20	3	<1	694	1 strch, 3 very lean meat

Vegetarian Fillets (1)	136	4	9	1	230	2 med-fat meat
Vegetarian Fish Sticks (2)	165	5	10	2	279	2 med-fat meat
Vegetarian Frankfurter (1)	102	4	5	<1	219	1 med-fat meat
Vegetarian Luncheon Meat (1/2-inch slice)	188	6	11	2	576	1/2 strch, 2 med-fat meat
Vegetarian Meat Patties (1)	142	6	6	1	391	1/2 strch, 2 lean meat
Vegetarian Meatballs (7)	140	6	6	<1	385	1/2 strch, 2 lean meat
Vegetarian Pot Pie (1)	524	41	34	10	538	3 strch, 1 med-fat meat, 6 fat
Vegetarian Sandwich Spread (3 Tbsp)	72	4	4	<1	302	1 med-fat meat
Vegetarian Scallops, Breaded & Fried (1/2 cup)	257	8	16	3	434	1/2 strch, 3 med-fat meat
Vegetarian Soyburger (1)	142	6	6	1	391	1/2 strch, 2 lean meat
GREEN GIANT						
Breakfast Links (3)	110	5	5	<1	340	2 lean meat
Breakfast Patties (2)	100	5	4	<1	280	1 med-fat meat
Harvest Burger, Italian (1)	140	8	5	2	370	1/2 strch, 2 lean meat
Harvest Burger, Original (1)	140	8	4	2	380	1/2 strch, 2 lean meat
Harvest Burger, Southwestern-Style (1)	140	9	4	2	370	1/2 strch, 2 lean meat

VEGETARIAN FOODS

Products	Cal.	Carb. (g)	Fat (g)	Sat. Fat (g)	Sodium (mg)	Exchanges
HEALTH VALLEY						
Soy Moo Milk, Fat-Free (1 cup)	110	22	0	0	60	1-1/2 strch
LIFE LITE						
Soft Serve Tofutti, Chocolate (1/2 cup)	90	20	<1	NA	80	1 carb.
Soft Serve Tofutti, Vanilla (1/2 cup)	90	20	<1	NA	80	1 carb.
Tofutti, All Flavors (1/2 cup)	200	21	11	2	90	1-1/2 carb., 2 fat
Tofutti, Better Than Cheese Cake (1 slice)	180	16	10	4	110	1 carb., 2 fat
Tofutti, Better Than Cream Cheese (2 Tbsp)	80	1	8	3	200	2 fat
Tofutti, Egg Watchers (1/4 cup)	50	2	2	<1	100	1 lean meat
LOMA LINDA						
Big Franks (1)	110	2	7	1	240	1 med-fat meat
Chicken Supreme (1/3 cup dry)	90	6	1	0	720	1/2 strch, 2 very lean meat
Chik Nuggets (5)	240	13	16	3	710	1 strch, 1 med-fat meat, 2 fat
Corn Dogs (1)	200	18	9	2	240	1 strch, 1 med-fat meat, 1 fat

Food						Exchanges
Dinner Cuts (1 slice)	80	3	2	<1	350	2 very lean meat
Fried Chik'n (1 piece)	180	<1	15	2	500	2 med-fat meat, 1 fat
Fried Chik'n/Gravy (2 pieces)	390	6	31	5	810	1/2 strch, 3 med-fat meat, 3 fat
Griddle Steaks (1)	130	4	7	1	410	2 lean meat
Linketts (1)	70	1	5	<1	160	1 med-fat meat
Little Links (2)	90	2	6	1	230	1 med-fat meat
Nuteena (3/8-inch slice)	160	6	13	5	120	1/2 strch, 1 med-fat meat, 2 fat
Ocean Platter (1/3 cup)	90	8	1	0	450	1/2 strch, 2 very lean meat
Patty Mix (1/3 cup)	90	7	1	0	480	1/2 strch, 2 very lean meat
Redi-Burger (5/9-inch slice)	170	5	10	2	460	2 med-fat meat
Sandwich Spread (1/4 cup)	80	7	5	1	260	1/2 strch, 1 fat
Sizzle Burger (1)	200	10	12	2	540	1/2 strch, 2 med-fat meat
Swiss Stake (1)	120	8	6	1	430	1/2 strch, 1 med-fat meat
Tender Bits (6)	110	7	5	<1	440	1/2 strch, 1 med-fat meat

VEGETARIAN FOODS

Products	Cal.	Carb. (g)	Fat (g)	Sat. Fat (g)	Sodium (mg)	Exchanges
Tender Rounds (8)	120	5	5	1	330	2 lean meat
Vege-Burger (1/4 cup)	70	2	2	<1	115	1 lean meat
Vita-Burger Chunks (1/4 cup)	70	6	1	0	350	1/2 strch, 1 very lean meat
Vita-Burger Granules (3 Tbsp)	70	6	1	0	350	1/2 strch, 1 very lean meat
MORNING STAR FARMS						
Better'n Burgers (1)	70	6	0	0	360	1/2 strch, 1 very lean meat
Better'n Eggs (1/4 cup)	20	0	0	0	90	1 very lean meat
Breakfast Links (2)	60	2	3	<1	340	1 lean meat
Breakfast Patties (1)	70	2	3	<1	270	1 lean meat
Breakfast Strips (2)	60	2	5	<1	220	1 fat
Chik Patties (1)	170	13	10	2	570	1 strch, 1 med-fat meat, 1 fat
Deli Franks (1)	110	3	7	1	520	1 med-fat meat
Garden Grain Pattie (1)	120	18	3	1	280	1 strch, 1 fat
Garden Vege Pattie (1)	100	9	3	<1	350	1/2 strch, 1 lean meat

Food						Exchanges
Grillers (1)	140	5	7	2	260	2 lean meat
Homestyle Noodles (1/2 cup)	160	33	0	0	10	2 strch
Prime Patties (1)	130	4	5	2	240	2 lean meat
Scramblers (1/4 cup)	35	2	0	0	95	1 very lean meat
Spicy Black Bean Burger (1)	100	16	1	0	470	1 strch, 1 very lean meat

NATURAL TOUCH

Food						Exchanges
Dinner Entree (1)	220	2	15	3	380	3 med-fat meat
Garden Vege Pattie (1)	110	8	4	1	280	1/2 strch, 1 med-fat meat
Lentil Rice Loaf (1-inch slice)	170	14	9	3	370	1 strch, 1 med-fat meat, 1 fat
Nine Bean Loaf (1-inch slice)	160	13	8	2	350	1 strch, 1 med-fat meat, 1 fat
Okara Patty (1)	110	4	5	1	360	2 lean meat
Vegan Burger (1)	70	6	0	0	370	1/2 strch, 1 very lean meat
Vege Burger (1)	140	4	6	1	320	2 lean meat
Vege Frank (1)	100	2	6	1	470	1 med-fat meat
Vegetarian Chili (1 cup)	270	21	12	2	1330	1-1/2 srch, 2 med-fat meat

VEGETARIAN FOODS

Products	Cal.	Carb. (g)	Fat (g)	Sat. Fat (g)	Sodium (mg)	Exchanges
WORTHINGTON						
Beef Slices, Smoked (6)	120	6	6	1	730	1/2 strch, 1 med-fat meat
Beef-Style Meatless (3/8-inch slice)	110	4	7	1	620	1 med-fat meat
Bolono (3 slices)	80	2	4	1	720	1 med-fat meat
Chic-ketts (2-3/8-inch slices)	120	2	7	1	390	2 lean meat
Chicken, Sliced (2)	80	1	5	1	370	1 med-fat meat
Chik, Diced (1/4 cup)	60	1	4	<1	240	1 med-fat meat
Chik, Diced, Meatless (1/4 cup)	80	1	5	1	360	1 med-fat meat
Chik, Sliced (3)	90	1	6	1	390	1 med-fat meat
ChikStiks (1)	110	3	7	1	360	1 med-fat meat
Chili (1 cup)	290	21	15	3	1130	1-1/2 strch, 2 med-fat meat, 1 fat
Choplets (2)	90	3	2	1	500	2 very lean meat
Corned Beef, Sliced (4)	140	5	9	2	520	1 med-fat meat, 1 fat

Food						Exchanges
Country Stew (1 cup)	210	20	9	2	830	1 strch, 1 med-fat meat, 1 fat
CrispyChik Patties (1)	170	15	9	2	600	1 strch, 1 med-fat meat, 1 fat
Cutlets (1)	70	3	1	0	340	2 very lean meat
Dinner Roast (3/4-inch slice)	180	5	12	2	580	2 med-fat meat
Fillets (2)	180	8	10	2	750	1/2 strch, 2 med-fat meat
FriChik (2)	120	1	8	1	430	1 med-fat meat, 1 fat
FriPats (1)	130	4	6	1	320	2 lean meat
Golden Croquettes (4)	210	14	10	2	600	1 strch, 2 med-fat meat
Granburger (3 Tbsp)	60	3	<1	0	410	1 very lean meat
Leanies (1)	110	2	8	2	430	1 med-fat meat, 1 fat
Multi-Grain Cutlet (2)	100	5	2	<1	390	2 very lean meat
Numete (3/8-inch slice)	130	5	10	3	270	1 med-fat meat, 1 fat
Prime Stakes (1)	140	4	9	2	440	1 med-fat meat, 1 fat
Prosage Links (2)	60	2	3	2	340	1 lean meat
Prosage Patties (1)	100	1	7	2	370	1 med-fat meat
Prosage Roll (5/8-inch slice)	140	2	10	2	390	1 med-fat meat, 1 fat

VEGETARIAN FOODS

Products	Cal.	Carb. (g)	Fat (g)	Sat. Fat (g)	Sodium (mg)	Exchanges
Protose (3/8-inch slice)	130	5	7	1	280	2 lean meat
Salami, Meatless (3)	130	2	8	1	930	2 med-fat meat
Saucettes (1)	90	1	6	1	200	1 med-fat meat
Savory Slices (3)	150	6	9	4	540	1/2 strch, 1 med-fat meat, 1 fat
Stakelets (1)	140	6	8	2	480	1/2 strch, 2 med-fat meat
Stripples (2)	60	2	5	<1	220	1 fat
Super-Links (1)	110	2	8	1	350	1 med-fat meat, 1 fat
Tuno, drained (1/2 cup)	80	2	6	1	290	1 med-fat meat
Turkee Slices (3 slices)	190	3	14	3	580	2 med-fat meat, 1 fat
Turkey Slices, Smoked (3)	140	3	10	2	620	1 med-fat meat, 1 fat
Veelets (1 pattie)	180	10	9	2	390	1/2 strch, 2 med-fat meat
Vegetable Scallops (1/2 cup)	90	3	2	<1	410	2 very lean meat
Vegetable Steaks (2)	80	3	2	<1	300	2 very lean meat

Vegetarian Beef Pie (1)	410	40	24	4	1340	2-1/2 strch, 5 fat
Vegetarian Burger (1/4 cup)	60	2	2	0	270	1 lean meat
Vegetarian Chicken Pie (1)	450	44	27	6	1080	3 strch, 5 fat
Vegetarian Egg Rolls (1)	180	20	8	2	380	1 strch, 2 fat
Vegetarian Beef, Ground Meatless (1/2 cup)	80	3	3	<1	270	2 very lean meat
Vegetarian Sausage, Ground Meatless (1/2 cup)	110	3	6	2	330	2 lean meat
Veja-Links (1)	50	1	3	<1	190	1 lean meat
Wham (2 slices)	80	1	5	1	430	1 med-fat meat

Resources

Self-Care Titles

NEW!
*Type 2 Diabetes: Your Healthy Living
Guide, 2nd Edition*   #CTIIHG
Nonmember: $16.95/ADA Member: $14.95

NEW!
*The Ten Keys to Helping Your Child
Grow Up With Diabetes*   #CSMTK
Nonmember: $14.95/ADA Member: $13.95

NEW!
Women & Diabetes   #CSMWD
Nonmember: $14.95/ADA Member: $13.95

ADA Complete Guide to Diabetes   #CSMCGD
Nonmember: $29.95/ADA Member: $25.95

*101 Tips for Staying Healthy with
Diabetes*   #CSMFSH
Nonmember: $12.50/ADA Member: $10.50

How to Get Great Diabetes Care   #CSMHGGDC
Nonmember: $11.95/ADA Member: $9.95

413

Sweet Kids #CSMSK
Nonmember: $14.95/ADA Member: $11.95

Reflections on Diabetes #CSMROD
Nonmember: $9.95/ADA Member: $8.95

*101 Tips for Improving Your
Blood Sugar* #CSMTBBGC
Nonmember: $12.50/ADA Member: $10.50

Diabetes A to Z #CGFDAZ
Nonmember: $9.95/ADA Member: $8.95

Managing Diabetes on a Budget #CSMMDOAB
Nonmember: $7.95/ADA Member: $6.95

*The Fitness Book: For People with
Diabetes* #CSMFB
Nonmember: $18.95/ADA Member: $16.95

Raising a Child with Diabetes #CSMRACWD
Nonmember: $14.95/ADA Member: $12.95

The Dinosaur Tamer #CSMDTAOS
Nonmember: $9.95/ADA Member: $8.95

*Grilled Cheese at Four O'Clock in
the Morning* #CCHGC
Nonmember: $6.95/ ADA Member: $5.95

The Take-Charge Guide to Type I Diabetes #CSMT1
Nonmember: $16.95/ADA Member: $13.50

Diabetes & Pregnancy: What to Expect #CPREDP
Nonmember: $9.95/ADA Member: $8.95

Gestational Diabetes: What to Expect #CPREGD
Nonmember: $9.95/ADA Member: $8.95

Necessary Toughness #CGFNT
Nonmember: $7.95/ADA Member: $6.95

Diabetes: A Positive Approach—Video #CVIDPOS
Nonmember: $19.95/ADA Member: $17.95

1997 Buyer's Guide #CMISBUY97
Nonmember: $4.95/ADA Member: $3.95

Cookbooks & Meal Planners

NEW!
Brand-Name Diabetic Meals #CCBBNDM
Nonmember: $12.95/ADA Member: $10.95

NEW!
How to Cook for People with Diabetes #CCBCFPD
Nonmember: $11.95/ADA Member: $9.95

NEW!
World-Class Diabetic Cooking #CCBWCC
Nonmember: $12.95/ADA Member: $10.95

NEW!
Southern-Style Diabetic Cooking #CCBSSDC
Nonmember: $11.95/ADA Member: $9.95

Flavorful Seasons Cookbook   #CCBFS
Nonmember: $16.95/ADA Member: $14.95

Diabetic Meals In 30 Minutes—
Or Less!   #CCBDM
Nonmember: $11.95/ADA Member: $9.95

Diabetes Meal Planning Made Easy   #CCBMP
Nonmember: $14.95/ADA Member: $12.95

Month of Meals   #CMPMOM
Nonmember: $12.50/ADA Member: $10.50

Month of Meals 2   #CMPMOM2
Nonmember: $12.50/ADA Member: $10.50

Month of Meals 3   #CMPMOM3
Nonmember: $12.50/ADA Member: $10.50

Month of Meals 4   #CMPMOM4
Nonmember: $12.50/ADA Member: $10.50

Month of Meals 5   #CMPMOM5
Nonmember: $12.50/ADA Member: $10.50

Great Starts & Fine Finishes   #CCBGSFF
Nonmember: $8.95/ADA Member: $7.15

Easy & Elegant Entrees   #CCBEEE
Nonmember: $8.95/ADA Member: $7.15

Savory Soups & Salads #CCBSSS
Nonmember: $8.95/ADA Member: $7.15

Quick & Hearty Main Dishes #CCBQHMD
Nonmember: $8.95/ADA Member: $7.15

Simple & Tasty Side Dishes #CCBSTSD
Nonmember: $8.95/ADA Member: $7.15

To order call: 1-800-232-6733

To join ADA call: 1-800-806-7801

About The American Dietetic Association

The American Dietetic Association is the world's largest organization of food and nutrition professionals. Founded in 1917, The American Dietetic Association promotes optimal nutrition to improve public health and well-being. The Association has nearly 70,000 members, of whom approximately 75 percent are registered dietitians (RD). The membership also includes dietetic technicians (DTR) and others holding advanced degrees in nutrition and dietetics. As the public education center of the Association, the National Center for Nutrition and Dietetics provides programs and services to inform and educate the public about food and nutrition issues. The Center and The American Dietetic Association are located at 216 W. Jackson Boulevard, Chicago, IL 60606.

Registered dietitians offer preventive and therapeutic nutrition services in a variety of settings, including health care, business, research, and educational organizations, as well as private practice. Registered dietitians working in the health care field serve as vital members of medical teams providing medical nutrition therapy to treat illnesses, injuries, and chronic conditions such as diabetes.

The credentials "RD" signify that a practitioner has completed a rigorous program of education and training. The registered dietitian must have at least a baccalaureate degree in an approved program of dietetics or related field from an accredited U.S. college or university. In addition, he or she must complete an internship or similar experience and pass a national credentialing exam. To retain RD status, dietitians must fulfill continuing education requirements to update and enhance their knowledge and skills.

To find a registered dietitian, the expert in diet, health, and nutrition, ask your physician or call your local hospital. You can also access The American Dietetic Association's toll-free dietitian referral service by calling 800/366-1655 or visiting the web site at www.eatright.org.

About the American Diabetes Association

The American Diabetes Association is the nation's leading voluntary health organization supporting diabetes research, information, and advocacy. Founded in 1940, the Association provides services in communities across the country. Its mission is to prevent and cure diabetes and to improve the lives of all people affected by diabetes.

For more than 50 years, the American Diabetes Association has been the leading publisher of comprehensive diabetes information for people with diabetes and the health care professionals who treat them. Its huge library of practical and authoritative books for people with diabetes covers every aspect of self care—cooking and nutrition, fitness, weight control, medications, complications, emotional issues, and general self care. The Association also publishes books and medical treatment guides for physicians and other health care professionals.

Membership in the Association is available to health professionals and people with diabetes and includes subscriptions to one or more of the association's periodicals. People with diabetes receive

Diabetes Forecast, the nation's leading lifestyle magazine for people with diabetes. Health care professionals receive one or more of the Association's five scientific and medical journals.

For More Information

Please call toll-free

**Questions about
diabetes:**   1-800-DIABETES

**Membership,
people with diabetes:**   1-800-806-7801

**Membership,
health professionals:**   1-800-232-3472

**Free catalog of
ADA books:**   1-800-232-6733